W9-CNK-155

Clinical Pediatric Optometry

Leonard J. Press, O.D., F.A.A.O.
Associate Professor of Optometry
State University of New York, State College of Optometry
New York, New York

Bruce D. Moore, O.D., F.A.A.O.
Adjunct Associate Professor of Optometry
New England College of Optometry
Director, Contact Lens Service and Staff Optometrist
Children's Hospital
Boston, Massachusetts

With Four Contributing Authors

Butterworth–Heinemann
Boston   London   Oxford   Singapore   Sydney   Toronto   Wellington

Every effort has been made to ensure that the drug dosage schedules within this text are accurate and
conform to standards accepted at time of publication. However, as treatment recommendations vary in
the light of continuing research and clinical experience, the reader is advised to verify drug dosage
schedules herein with information found on product information sheets. This is especially true in cases
of new or infrequently used drugs.

Recognizing the importance of preserving what has been written, it is the policy of Butterworth–
Heinemann to have the books it publishes printed on acid-free paper, and we exert our best efforts to
that end.

Library of Congress Cataloging-in-Publication Data

Press, Leonard J.
    Clinical pediatric optometry / Leonard J. Press, Bruce D. Moore ; with 4 contributing
authors.
        p.   cm.
    Includes bibliographical references and index.
    ISBN 0-7506-9080-1 (alk. paper)
    1. Pediatric optometry I. Moore, Bruce D. II. Title.
    [DNLM: 1. Eye Diseases—in infancy & childhood. 2. Vision Disorders—in infancy &
childhood. WW 600 P935c]
    RE952.5.C45P74   1993
    618.92'09775—dc20
    DNLM/DLC
    for Library of Congress   92-13562
                                                                                         CIP

British Library Cataloguing-in-Publication Data

Press, Leonard J.
    Pediatric Optometry: Clinical Guide
    I. Title II. Moore, Bruce D.
    618.92

    ISBN 0-7506-9080-1

Butterworth–Heinemann
313 Washington Street
Newton, MA 02158

10 9 8 7 6 5 4 3 2

Printed in the United States of America

To Sarina, Adena, Elli, and Daniel for hours stolen from your development to develop this book, and to Miriam for love and nurturing too strong to be served justice by words on a printed page.

To Rachel, Eric, and Kate for the hours away from you and to Marcia for her love and understanding during this long endeavor.

Contributors

Brian Altman, M.D.
Director of Pediatric Ophthalmology
Eastern State School and Hospital, Trevose, Pennsylvania
and the Woodhauen Center, Philadelphia, Pennsylvania

Paul B. Freeman, O.D., F.A.A.O.
Chief of Low Vision Services
Allegheny General Hospital
Pittsburgh, Pennsylvania

John Griffin, O.D.
Professor of Optometry
Southern California College of Optometry
Fullerton, California

Bruce D. Moore, O.D., F.A.A.O.
Clinical Assistant in Ophthalmology
Harvard Medical School
Associate Professor
New England College of Optometry
Boston, Massachusetts

Rudolph S. Wagner, M.D.
Assistant Professor of Ophthalmology
University of Medicine and Dentistry of New Jersey—New Jersey Medical School
Newark, New Jersey

Contents

Preface

Advances in neuroscience during the past three decades have focused attention on the significance of normal and abnormal visual development. The opportunity to influence vision development at an early age has heightened interest in pediatric optometry as a specialty area. Residency programs in pediatric optometry have been established at many of the colleges of optometry, facilitating the application of basic science to clinical practice.

Rather than dictating standards for optometric practice, discoveries in vision science must be tempered by the clinical observations of practitioners experienced in children's vision care. As an example, claims for critical periods of visual development as derived from laboratory experiments are valid for extreme conditions of deprivation under controlled conditions. The majority of clinical cases, however, present with subtle degrees of deprivation and with inadequate documentation of age of onset. The management of individual patients therefore calls upon the professional judgements of the clinician, who must stay abreast of developments in contemporary vision science.

The information gathering process during visual examination of the infant or child is similar to the process during visual examination of the adult. The ability to obtain this information, however, is as much an art as it is a science. With the advent of equipment and procedures to examine young children, it is now less acceptable to indicate on one's examination record that the child was uncooperative or unresponsive. Our intent is to assist the reader in gathering clinical findings and obtaining more insight into the pediatric patient. This, in turn, will enhance the reader's ability to design, implement, and monitor effective treatment regimens.

Until recently, the area of pediatric eye disease was one with which optometrists had relatively little clinical contact. The typical referral pattern for children with eye disease was for pediatricians to channel patients to ophthalmologists. With the recent expansion of the scope and practice of optometry into the realm of diagnosis and treatment of eye diseases along with the inclusion of optometry into multidisciplinary environments such as clinics, HMOs (health maintenance organizations), and hospitals, however, optometrists are now coming into contact with these patients. The reader will therefore notice a significant allocation of space in this text to the discussion of pediatric eye disease in the context of optometric care, emphasizing the clinical characteristics, differential diagnosis, and treatment of these disorders in a manner consistent with the practice of optometry. No attempt has been made to be encyclopedic as there are pediatric ophthalmology texts that address the rare conditions likely to be seen in tertiary care settings by subspecialists. Rather the material included on eye disease is reflective of the experience of an optometrist in a multidisciplinary environment.

There is no longer discussion about optometric entry into ocular disease management, rather, the discussion centers in the melding of behavioralism with structuralism. Paradoxically medicine is expanding in the direction of behavioralism and the need to treat the patient rather than the disease, while optometry, which evolved from this approach, is burgeoning in the direction of structuralism. The challenge to optometrists is not to lose the art of behavioral optometry in the face of time constraints in practice or under the economic pressures of third-party dictates.

The goal of this text is to present a comprehensive guide for optometric care of the infant and child. We have tried to emphasize the "how to" aspect of pediatric care rather than surveying the literature as an academic venture. The style invites the reader to a chairside chat and is geared toward a middle ground between the novice seeking introduction and integration and the experienced clinician seeking refinement and reference. In this context, we have endeavored to be timely, relevant, and futuristic. Welcome to our journey.

Leonard J. Press, O.D.
Bruce Moore, O.D.

Acknowledgments

The impetus for this text came from Dr. D. Leonard Werner, who suggested to Dr. Leonard Press seven years ago that he undertake this task. Dr. Israel Press merits recognition for his sage counsel to pursue pediatric optometry as a professional niche. We wish to express our gratitude to the professionals and support staff at our respective institutions. We are blessed with illustrious colleagues who lent their constant support and encouragement, in particular, Drs. Barry Tannen, Stuart Rothman, Robert Duckman, Irwin Suchoff, Harold Solan, Harold Friedman, Martin Birnbaum, and Marie Marrone, and Ms. Margaret Lewis, Claudia Perry, and Diane Schiumo and Mr. Wayne Grofik at the SUNY College of Optometry; Drs. Richard Robb (Department of Ophthalmology Chair), Robert Petersen, Anne Fulton, Lois Smith, Luisa Mayer, and Ron Hansen and Ms. Dorothy Rodier, Carol Zimmer, Regina Harvey, and Elizabeth Burns at The Children's Hospital, Boston. We also acknowledge the use of the extensive slide collection of the Ophthalmology Department at The Children's Hospital, Boston.

1

Case History

Leonard J. Press

The case history of a pediatric patient differs from that of an adult in that the questions are predominantly addressed to the parent or caretaker rather than to the child. There are numerous ways to gather information prior to the child's examination. Most common is the process of completing a preexamination questionnaire. The form used for all new patients in our office is reproduced as Figure 1.1. Some offices have the practice of mailing an extensive preexamination questionnaire to the parents of all new pediatric patients. Figure 1.2 is an example of this form.

Having gathered all preexamination information including any pertinent reports from other professionals, the flow of the case history is dictated by three primary factors.

1. The purpose of the examination
2. The age of the child
3. Whether the child is a new or established patient

PURPOSE OF THE EXAMINATION

The motivation for having a child's eyes examined stems largely from observations or concerns of a parent or from the advice of a professional.

Observations

The most common observations or concerns of parents are related to the outward appearance of the eyes. The examiner should pinpoint what is being observed, when it was first noticed, whether the observation varies, and how long it has persisted. As an example, consider the parental concern of strabismus.

Parental observation: Eyes crossed or floating.
Questions to be asked: When did you first notice this?
                     How often does it occur?
                     Does it happen any special time of the day?
                     Does anyone else in the family have this?
                     Has there been any prior intervention?

FAMILY EYECARE ASSOCIATES
—welcome to our office—

DATE: _____

NAME: _____ DATE OF BIRTH: _____

ADDRESS: _____ PHONE: (___) _____

No. & Street　　　　City　　　　Zip code

PEDIATRIC PATIENT: _____

Name of parent(s)　　　　Name of school　　　Grade

_____

Pediatrician's name　　　　Date of last eye exam

ADULT PATIENT: _____

Name of your spouse　　　　Your occupation

_____

Business phone　　　Your physician's name　　　Date of last eye exam

WHO MAY WE THANK FOR REFERRING YOU TO US? _____

Please check if you have had any of the following conditions:
___ Allergies (to _____)
___ Arthritis
___ Diabetes
___ Heart disease
___ High blood pressure

___ Eye disease (circle: lazy eye, eye turn, cataract, glaucoma)
___ Eye surgery (for _____)
___ Eye or head injury
___ Eye discomfort or headaches

Has anyone in your family had:
___ Diabetes
___ Heart disease

___ Eye disease (circle: lazy eye, eye turn, cataract, glaucoma)

Current or recent medications: _____

Have contact lenses ever been prescribed for you? _____

Do you wear glasses for distance vision? ___ For near vision? ___
Is your vision clear at all distances? ___
Are your eyes comfortable at work? ___ Do you use a VDT screen? ___
(Note: parents should add appropriate observations of children)

INSURANCE INFORMATION:

Name of insurance company _____

Policy holder _____ Identification # _____

Medicare # _____ Medicaid # _____

Patient's social security # _____

METHOD OF PAYMENT TODAY: ___ BY CASH ___ BY CHECK
___ BY VISA/MASTERCARD

Figure 1.1　New patient history form

The significance of the answers to these questions is apparent in the discussion on strabismus in Chapter 13. This example is being used to illustrate the maxim in clinical care that states that case history is an ongoing process as well as the concept that taking a history involves a series of branching questions. Consider the simplest case in which the parent's observation is that the eye turn seems constant and is not specific to the time of day. In addition, there has been no prior intervention nor is there a family history of strabismus. If you determine that there is no strabismus present, the parent should be asked to demonstrate the observation. Have an assistant hold the baby and look over the parent's shoulder so that you can agree on the nature of what that parent is observing. If you determine that the cause of the apparent esotropia is wide epicanthal skin folds, no further questions are necessary. Rather reassurance is in order by demonstrating to the parent the significance of symmetrical corneal light reflexes in relation to pseudostrabismus.

Conversely if the child proves to have accommodative esotropia or intermittent exotropia, additional and specific lines of questioning should be pursued. In accommodative esotropia, the eye turn should be more pronounced when the child is making eye contact. In intermittent exotropia at distance, the deviation should be most noticeable when the child is tired, feverish, or daydreaming. The child is also usually observed to close one eye in sunlight. If the parents confirm these observations, further insight is gained into the duration of the condition, and this serves to establish the caretakers as reliable observers. In addition, improvement in the condition with treatment or the passage of time can be gauged in part by any change in these observations. Parents should be advised that an optometrist can make certain observations of the child during examination but is not with the child as often and does not know the child as well as the parents do. When the optometrist can establish an adult as a reliable observer, through the case history, that adult becomes an important partner in the clinical care of the child. It is then advisable to have the same adult return with the child for future care.

Physical Signs

Most transient physical signs are reported accurately by parents. The more common signs include red eyes, sties, eyelids stuck together in the morning, eyelids twitching, eyes tearing, and rubbing of the eyes. Checklist pamphlets available from the Optometric Extension Program (OEP) and the American Optometric Association (AOA) (see Appendix A) serve as a convenient guide to these observations, which can be capsulized into the *ABCs* (Appearance, Behavior, Complaints) of vision difficulties (Kavner, 1985) (see Table 1.1). In addition to questions about onset and duration, the examiner will need to know if the parent has instituted any treatment prior to the examination that has lessened the signs or symptoms.

Performance Problems

The parent may express concern over some aspect of the child's development that is delayed. This may include the extent to which the child is using vision.

Name _____

Address _____

Telephone _____

Date of Birth _____

Date of Exam _____

Age _____

1. My child is here today because:
   ___ eye turns in   ___ eye turns out
   ___ squints a lot   ___ rubs eyes a lot
   ___ eyes don't seem to focus   ___ no problems—general checkup
   ___ recheck examination   ___ check because of visual problems in
   ___ initial visit—2nd opinion   other family members
                                       ___ other _____

   _____
   _____

2. My child is: ___ natural ___ adopted ___ foster ___ other

3. Mother's age when child was born:
   ___ under 25 ___ 26–30 ___ 31–35 ___ over 35

4. Are there any known genetic or familial disorders? ___ No ___ Yes
   Please explain: _____
   _____

5. How long was pregnancy? ___ less than 7 months ___ between 7 and 8 months
                           ___ between 8 and 9 months ___ over 9 months

6. During the pregnancy of this child, which, if any, of the following occurred?
   ___ excessive nausea   ___ use of alcohol
   ___ staining   ___ use of drugs
   ___ toxemia   ___ use of megadose vitamins
   ___ injury by falling   ___ regular obstetrical care
   ___ severe illness   ___ little medical care
   ___ trauma   ___ poor nutrition
   ___ smoking   ___ poor hygiene
   ___ prescribed medication   ___ other
   Please explain: _____
   _____
   _____

7. Labor, during delivery, lasted _____ hours.

8. Labor (___ was ___ was not) induced.

9. Type of delivery: ___ natural ___ Caesarian ___ forceps or instruments
                     ___ anesthesia ___ other _____

Figure 1.2   Parent questionnaire for infant exam

10. Were there any problems during delivery? ___ Yes ___ No
   If yes, please explain: _____
   _____
   _____

11. This child's birth weight was _____ lbs and ozs.
12. APGAR scores (if known) were: _____ at one min., _____ at five mins.

13. Immediately after birth this child was:
   ___ doing well   ___ having sucking problems
   ___ in need of medical attention   ___ having breathing difficulty
   ___ placed in an incubator   ___ having swallowing difficulty
   ___ placed in an isolette   ___ having colic problems
   ___ having Rh problems   ___ feverish
   ___ allergic   ___ other
   If other, please explain _____
   _____
   _____

14. This child was: ___ breast fed ___ bottle fed ___ both

15. Was any medication prescribed during the first year of life? ___ Yes ___ No

16. Is the child's development normal in:
   Sitting: ___ Yes ___ No   Crawling: ___ Yes ___ No   Creeping: ___ Yes ___ No
   Walking: ___ Yes ___ No   Speech: ___ Yes ___ No   Emotional: ___ Yes ___ No

17. Family History (Check all appropriate spaces):

	Nearsighted	Farsighted	Astigmatism	Amblyopia (lazy eye)	Strabismus (eye turn)	Poor color vision	Other (please specify)
Father	____	____	____	____	____	____	____
Mother	____	____	____	____	____	____	____
Brother or sister	____	____	____	____	____	____	____
Uncle or aunt	____	____	____	____	____	____	____
Grand-parent	____	____	____	____	____	____	____

18. List all previous evaluations done on your child (if necessary use other side of page):

Doctor or institution   Date   Type of evaluation   Results

_____   _____   _____   _____

Table 1.1   Common signs/symptoms of vision disorders and their probable significance

APPEARANCE

Closing one eye/one eye turning inward or outward
  Probe binocular problems
Excessive blinking
  Probe tic due to emotional considerations such as pressure at home or in school
  Probe anterior segment irritation
  Probe accommodative—vergence flexibility
Excessive tearing
  Probe asthenopia
  Probe anterior segment irritation
Red eyes or lids/crust on eyelids/frequent sties or swollen lids
  Probe anterior segment disorders
Squinting in normal sunlight or under fluorescents
  Probe photophobia
  Probe binocular problems
  Probe refractive status

BEHAVIOR (AND PERFORMANCE)

Difficulty staying on task or concentrating
  Probe history of attention deficit disorder (ADD)
  Probe cognitive style (see Chapter 9)
  Probe history of medications (e.g., Ritalin)
  Probe accommodative/binocular problems
  Probe auditory-visual integration
Loss of place when reading, skipping or re-reading lines, omitting or transposing letters
  Probe ocular-motor disorder
  Probe visual-perceptual skills
  Probe lateral and vertical binocular imbalance
Excessive tongue/body movement during gross or fine-motor tasks
  Probe perceptual-motor skills
  Probe binocular problems

Occasionally parents will be concerned about a young child who is clumsy or bumps into things repeatedly. The parent who has older children with whom the patient can be compared has a different frame of reference than does the first-time parent. New parents tend to be anxious about innocuous conditions whereas experienced parents are more likely to pinpoint conditions requiring intervention. The practitioner must be knowledgeable about general developmental timetables (Table 1.2) to know the significance of observations about development.

Preventive Care

If your practice is efficient in educating parents about potential problems through newsletters, in-office literature, or otherwise, the motivation for the

Table 1.1   *(continued)*

Inaccuracy/lack or relying on vision when engaged in visual tasks
  Probe motivation
  Probe relative modality preference in broad perceptual evaluation
Poor eye-hand coordination (large-motor such as sports, vs. fine-motor such as sewing, pencil-paper, or visually guiding the use of small tools)
  Probe developmental level
Organizational errors (poor spacing, columnar orientation)
  Probe spatial-perception and form perception
Inaccuracy in copying from the blackboard
  Probe all of the above
Decoding errors (difficulty deciphering printed instructions or reading maps)
  Probe all of the above

COMPLAINTS
  Headaches, eye fatigue, or discomfort after prolonged viewing
    Probe accommodative-vergence complex
    Probe general health, sinuses, allergies
    Probe motivation
  Instability of print at near
    Probe accommodative-vergence-ocular-motor complex
    Probe ergonomics
    Probe general health
  Blurred vision
    Probe refractive profile
    Probe accommodative-vergence facility
    Probe trauma-related possibilities
    Probe general health and medications
  Inexplicable rubbing or itching of eyes
    Probe seasonal or environmental allergies
    Probe anterior segment
    Probe refractive profile

examination may be preventive care. The impetus for the examination may have come from at-risk conditions identified when you previously examined the parent or a sibling, or it may stem from a history of visual or ocular problems outside the immediate family (Rosner & Rosner, 1990).

Referral

Despite all attempts to educate the public about preventive care, parents usually bring children for their initial examination when they are required to do so by the school or when they have been referred by another practitioner. Public schools tend to have periodic school screenings that the child may have failed, whereas private schools tend to have periodic requisite examinations. If another professional has

Table 1.2 Developmental timetable

Motor	No. of mos.	Language	No. of mos.
Sits unsupported	8	Syllable	6
Creeps	9	Double syllable (ma-ma)	9
Walks, supported	12	Two words	12
Climbs stairs	15	5–10 word set	15–18
Stands/walks unsupported	15–18	Three word sentence	24
Walks up/down stairs	24	Refers to self by name	24
Alternates feet on stairs	36	Gives full name	30
Rides tricycle	36	Knows a few rhymes	36
		Counts to 10	60
		Knows colors	60
		Knows alphabet	60–72

Adapted from RW Lowry, Handbook of diagnostic tests for the developmental optometrist (Worthington, Minn.: RW Lowry, 1970).

evaluated the child, a copy of that report should be brought to the initial examination. If the parents are seeking a second opinion on the management plan of another practitioner, such as the need for bifocals, vision therapy, or surgery, they may intentionally conceal some of the history until after you have rendered an opinion. Occasionally one encounters a parent who states: "Well, we saw Dr. Jones who said that Susan needs to take these eyedrops. We didn't tell you this before because we wanted to see what you had to say without being biased." Finding the reason why that parent was dissatisfied with the management plan of a previous practitioner can be useful in implementing one's own management plan.

AGE OF THE CHILD

The age of the child at the time of the first examination determines the extent to which the optometrist must delve into prenatal, perinatal, and postnatal history. When the child is 12 years old and presents with a chief complaint of recent onset distance blur, questions about pregnancy, delivery, and early development are irrelevant and not time-efficient. Conversely when the patient is a 6-month-old infant with no apparent visual responses, questions about maternal health during pregnancy, APGAR scores (see Chapter 18), and neonatal care provide potentially important diagnostic clues.

Questioning the Child

When the pediatric patient is of school age, it is appropriate to direct as many questions to the child as possible. This isn't always productive with younger children who have little frame of reference for reporting visual abnormalities and who assume that others see things the same way that they do. Rarely will children be overheard in Kiddie City saying: "Gee Jimmy, I used to be able to read toy box labels from across the store, but lately it's been all downhill." Conversely there are children who complain of subjective visual disturbance that seems exaggerated for the extent of the clinical findings. In this instance, you will want to inquire of the parent whether the child is generally a complainer.

Children who are in middle and upper grades can be questioned about visual efficiency: losing place when reading, skipping or re-reading lines, running together of words when reading or copying, blurring when looking at the blackboard at the end of the school day, or doubling of the pencil tip when writing or copying. Having the parent in the examination room while taking a history from the child can be a mixed blessing. If the child responds positively to one of the preceding questions, the parent may say, "You never told me that happens," to which the child may respond, "I did, but you never listen."

If the examiner detects an extreme reaction on the part of the child to the presence of the parent during the taking of the case history, in the direction of either anxiety or overdependence, the parent should be tactfully excused from the examination room. In some instances, the parent tends to speak for the child, and the child would do better with the opportunity to give an independent history.

NEW OR ESTABLISHED PATIENT

The child who has been to the office previously can be administered a more streamlined history than can the child who is new to the office. Questions center on new developments since the last examination or compliance with the treatment regimen previously instituted. As an example, if patching or glasses were prescribed, were they used as directed? If visual development techniques were given to the parents, were they implemented at home? If the child was asked to do home therapy procedures, was there an argument about getting them done?

When school-aged children return for progress evaluation visits, the history usually centers on change in school performance. By virtue of optometric intervention, the parent or teacher may notice an improvement in school achievement. Change may be related to functions being performed more efficiently or to tasks that once required much effort now being performed automatically. This should be well documented in the record for future reference.

REFERENCES

Kavner RS. Your child's vision. New York: Simon and Schuster, 1985:102–105.
Lowry RW. Handbook of diagnostic tests for the developmental optometrist. Worthington, Minn., 1970.
Rosner J, Rosner J. Pediatric optometry. Boston: Butterworth–Heinemann, 1990:22.

2

Common Genetic Problems in Pediatric Optometry

John R. Griffin

Genetic traits are often found at birth and in early childhood, but not always. Huntington disease, for example, may not appear until adulthood and sometimes relatively late in life. The terms *congenital* and *genetic* are therefore not synonymous. Genetic traits discussed and listed in this chapter are mainly pediatric. The mode of transmission may be Mendelian, multifactorial, or chromosomal. The Suggested Reading section at the end of this chapter provides information sources to augment this brief overview of ocular genetics.

MENDELIAN TRAITS

Mendelian traits lend themselves to pedigree analysis. The modes of transmission include autosomal dominant (AD), autosomal recessive (AR), X-linked recessive (XR), and X-linked dominant (XD). These are all single-gene traits.

Autosomal Dominant (AD) Transmission

Only one deleterious gene of a pairing is required for an individual to have an AD disease. A pedigree example is shown in Figure 2.1. A square indicates a male, a circle a female. A darkened symbol indicates an individual affected with the trait. If one parent is affected, the theoretical risk to offspring is 50 percent. It does not matter whether the affected parent is male or female; the risk to offspring is the same. Moreover male and female offspring are equally at risk. There are exceptions, for example, baldness in males, and Fuchs endothelial-epithelial dystrophy in females. Generally, however, there is no sex-influence in most AD traits.

Pedigree analysis is usually easy in AD traits since they follow a vertical pattern of transmission as shown in Figure 2.1 with an affected phenotype in each generation. Occasionally there is *skipping of a generation* due either to reduced penetrance (abnormal genotype not clinically evident) or low expressivity (trait almost subclinical and undetectable). Caution in genetic counseling must always be used because of these possibilities.

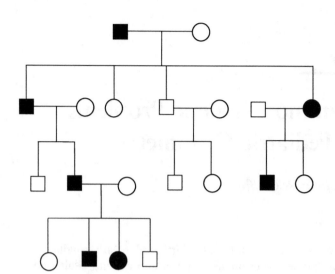

Figure 2.1 Typical pedigree in AD transmission.

Ocular traits that may be AD include Adie syndrome, albinism, aniridia, Best disease, cataract (several types), coloboma, cornea plana, corneal dystrophy (many types), Duane retraction syndrome, dyslexia (dyseidetic type), hypertelorism (ocular), Marfan syndrome, myopia (high), night blindness (congenital stationary), nystagmus, optic atrophy (congenital) ptosis, retinal cone degeneration, retinitis pigmentosa, retinoblastoma, and Waardenburg syndrome.

Autosomal Recessive (AR) Transmission

The AR mode is more difficult to analyze from pedigrees. This is because the affected phenotype often appears sporadically in one generation and does not follow a vertical pattern as is the case in AD pedigrees. An example of an AR pedigree is shown in Figure 2.2 in which the trait is found only in the third generation. The double line in the second generation indicates consanguinity (blood relationship) between the mates who are first cousins. The theoretical risk to offspring is 25 percent when both parents are carriers of the trait. It takes a double dose in AR traits for the phenotype to be expressed. Isolated ethnic communities sometimes share a common gene pool, and consanguinity should be particularly looked into during genetic counseling of individuals of the same ethnic group who live in such isolated communities.

Although pedigree analysis is difficult, compared with AD traits, it is fortunate that biochemical assay for enzyme abnormalities is a possibility for many AR diseases, for example, Tay-Sachs disease. Most AR diseases are *inborn errors of metabolism* and allow for prenatal screening of parents or testing of the fetus with amniocentesis. AR traits include albinism (Types I and II), anophthalmos, Bardet-Biedl syndrome, Behr

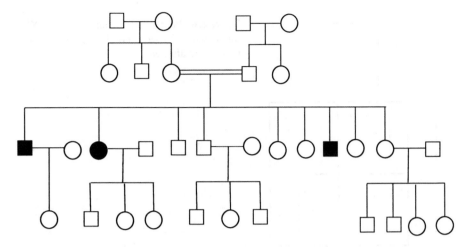

Figure 2.2 Typical pedigree in AR transmission.

syndrome, cataract (several types), choroidal sclerosis, fundus flavimacalatus, glaucoma (buphthalmos), macular degeneration (juvenile), microphthalmos, oguchi disease, retinitis pigmentosa, Tay-Sachs disease, Usher syndrome, and Wilson disease.

X-linked Recessive (XR) Transmission

The XR mode is easy to analyze from pedigrees. Affected phenotypes are usually only males and often each generation is represented. The carrier status of mothers of their affected sons can often be identified through pedigree analysis. This is shown in Figure 2.3 by a dot in the circle, representing a carrier female. Carrier status is often

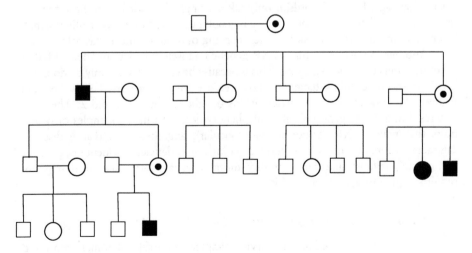

Figure 2.3 Typical pedigree in XR transmission.

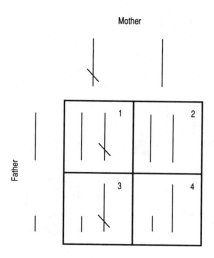

Figure 2.4 Punnett square analysis in an XR trait in which 50 percent of the sons of a carrier mother are affected.

detectable with ophthalmoscopy in ocular albinism, XR retinitis pigmentosa, and choroideremia (XR); the fundi are patchy.

Punnett square analysis is also helpful in genetic counseling. See Figure 2.4 showing a carrier mother (with, for example, ocular albinism) and a genotypically and phenotypically normal father. Each vertical line represents a chromosome and a slash indicates the deleterious gene on the chromosome. The mother is XX (represented by two long lines), and the father is XY (represented by a long line, the X, and a short line, the Y). In square 1, the daughter is a carrier but phenotypically normal. The daughter in square 2 is both genotypically and phenotypically normal. The son in square 3 is affected with the trait. This is because he is hemizygous as to the X chromosome and has no coverage. In other words, it only takes a single dose for him to have the XR trait. The son in square 4 is unaffected; he is genotypically and phenotypically normal. Therefore, the theoretical risk to male offspring of a carrier mother is 50 percent.

Another important feature in XR genetic counseling is that an affected father never transmits the trait to his sons. This is because he can have sons only by donating his Y chromosome. All his daughters, however, are obligate carriers. This is shown in Figure 2.5, showing obligate carriers in his daughters, squares 1 and 2. The sons, squares 3 and 4, are genotypically and phenotypically normal. Examples of ocular traits that may be XR include albinism (ocular), angiokeratoma (Fabry disease), cataract (congenital total), choroideremia, color vision deficiencies (deutans, protans, and possibly tritans), macular dystrophy, megalocornea, Norrie disease, nystagmus, retinitis pigmentosa, and retinoschisis.

X-linked Dominant (XD) Transmission

The XD mode is listed in this overview chapter for the sake of nomenclature and for heuristic reasons. Very few, if any, ocular traits are documented for this mode.

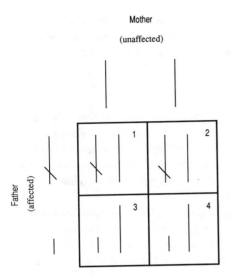

Figure 2.5 Punnett Square analysis in an XR in which all daughters of an affected father are carriers but no sons are affected.

Idiopathic congenital nystagmus may have several different modes of inheritance, one of which may be XD.

Other Considerations

Heterogeneity is a factor to be considered in genetic counseling. Many Mendelian traits can have more than one mode of transmission. Retinitis pigmentosa, for example, may be AR (the most common), XR (common but mainly in males), or AD (the least common). The *exact diagnosis* and the *exact mode of transmission* must be known before genetic counseling can be given. In other words, advice is not given without exact information.

Severity is another factor to consider. The burden (financial and emotional drain on a family) must be considered in all cases when genetic counseling is given. Dominant traits are generally less severe than are recessive traits. For example, AD retinitis pigmentosa is less severe in most cases than is AR or XR. This may be an important consideration in genetic counseling. The burden of AD retinitis pigmentosa may not be great enough to consider options (for example, therapeutic abortion) that may be decided on when the mode of transmission is, for example, XR (more severe).

Cytoplasmic (mitochondrial) inheritance is another mode to consider. It acts similarly to the XR mode in that only females transmit the trait to their offspring. The exception is that both male and female offspring may inherit the trait from their mother. An example of mitochondrial inheritance is Leber optic atrophy.

Prevalence of each Mendelian trait tends to be rare, but the rate of heterozygous individuals carrying the trait is much higher, particularly in the recessive modes. For example, the prevalence of cystic fibrosis in North American Caucasians is approximately .04 percent, but the carrier rate of this AR disease is approximately 4 percent. Fortunately screening for carriers is becoming feasible for many genetic diseases.

MULTIFACTORIAL TRAITS

Multifactorial has been referred to as polygenic inheritance. This is only partly true; environment also plays an important role in multifactorial traits. For example, height is a multifactorial trait. Several or many "tallness" genes are additive in determining an individual's height. Along with summation of genes are environmental factors. Nutrition is probably the principal factor, although exercise, climate, and other influences may have an effect on height.

Intelligence is also multifactorial. An individual may inherit ample "smartness" genes, but development of intelligence depends on environmental factors such as an enriching environment, good education, and encouragement by others to learn.

Hypertension is yet another multifactorial trait. Diet and emotional stress interact with genetic predisposition to hypertension. Although high blood pressure is thought to be mainly a problem for adults, this can occur in the pediatric population. Hypertensive retinopathy is the result of prolonged and untreated high blood pressure.

Three of the most common conditions seen by pediatric optometrists will be discussed as examples of the multifactorial mode of inheritance—strabismus, refractive errors, and dyslexia.

Strabismus

Several factors interact to cause an individual to become strabismic. Esotropia may occur if the individual has a high tonic convergence (eso tendency at far), high AC/A ratio, and sufficiently high hyperopia. Environmental stress may also play a part in an esophoria decompensating into an esotropia. An infant is at risk for esotropia if there is hyperopia over 2.00 diopters, particularly if there is esotropia in other members of the family. In multifactorial traits, the more members of a kinship having the trait puts future offspring at risk. Furthermore, the more severe the trait in the kinship, the greater is the risk to future offspring. Multifactorial inheritance, however, does not follow mathematical rules of chance as do the Mendelian traits (for example, 50 percent in AD, 25 percent in AR). Rather than theoretical chance, the *empirical* risk in multifactorial traits is determined for each trait from many other case histories with the particular trait.

Pedigree analysis, therefore, is not feasible. Generally in most multifactorial traits, for example, strabismus, the second child has approximately a 5 percent chance of having strabismus, the third child 10 percent, and the fourth child 15 percent.

Most family studies of strabismus have been on esotropia, but exotropia can also be assumed to be influenced by several factors such as low tonic convergence, low AC/A ratio, and myopic anisometropia, along with possible environmental influences, for example, eye infection necessitating patching of an eye and breaking fusion. Exotropia is probably a multifactorial trait.

Refractive Errors

Ametropia is either high (component type) or low (correlational type). High degrees of hyperopia and myopia are thought to be monogenic (Mendelian) traits. This is particularly so for progressive pathological myopia. On the other hand, low hyperopia and myopia are most likely multifactorial. Several factors cause myopia, for example, a steep cornea and long axial length. Factors such as accommodative excess and poor nutrition probably play a role in exacerbating the genetic myopic predisposition of an individual. Myopia can be both genetically and environmentally caused. The nature-nurture question is solved by adopting the multifactorial theory of myopia; this seems to hold true for correlation (low) myopia. Although most studies of ametropia have concentrated on myopia with the consensus being that myopia is a multifactorial trait, it is likely that hyperopia is also a multifactorial trait. The genetic studies of astigmatism, however, are indecisive. The probability is that astigmatism is also a multifactorial trait. Clinicians observe that indigent people with poor nutrition (that is, an environmental factor) tend to have high degrees of astigmatism.

Dyslexia

The three basic types of dyslexia are dysnemkinesia (motoric problem with letter reversals when writing), dysphonesia (poor ability to apply phonics and syllabication in coding of words), and dyseidesia (poor ability to code whole words with their sounds). Dyseidesia seems to be an AD trait. It does not respond to educational, vision, medical, or psychological therapy or to any other kind of therapy. The dyseidetic individual must work around the problem to achieve success in school, work, and play.

The other types of dyslexia are most likely multifactorial. Because environmental influences play a part in causing the problem, appropriate therapy (an environmental influence) can often ameliorate the problem. For example, dysphonesia tends to be less prevalent in adults than it is in children. (About 5 percent of children have dyseidesia, 5 percent have dysphonesia, and 5 percent have dysnemkinesia or various combinations of the three basic types of dyslexia.) By adulthood, the prevalence of dysphonesia is much less than dyseidesia, which remains at approximately 5 percent. Time may help dysphonesia lessen in severity, but educational therapy certainly speeds up this process. This is even more true in dysnemkinesia in which letter reversal problems are normally resolved by the third grade. If not, laterality and directionality perceptual therapy quickly abates these problems in about 90 percent of the cases. With the exception of dyseidesia, therefore, dyslexia is a multifactorial trait. Dyslexia is not a hopeless condition. It can be attacked directly with appropriate educational therapy. In the case of dyseidesia, the trait can be attacked indirectly with appropriate educational therapy. The role of the pediatric optometrist is to detect dyslexia as early as possible. Otherwise, secondary emotional problems result. The child may avoid school (leading to dropout), have behavioral problems (leading to delinquency), or withdraw (leading to substance abuse). A child is at risk if parents and other members of the family have a history of reading, writing, and spelling problems (indicating possible dyslexia). Dyslexia screening is possible as early as the first grade. Letter decoding and encoding studies on kindergartners show promise in predicting dyslexia. Poor visual perceptual-motor skills in toddlers may also be cause for concern and put a child predisposed to dyslexia at greater risk. The pediatric optometrist may administer or guide a program of visual perceptual-motor therapy to address this component of the problem.

Guidelines

Some characteristics of multifactorial traits in contrast to Mendelian traits are:

1. The empirical risk increases with each affected sibling. In Mendelian traits the theoretical risk is by mathematical chance with each new sibling having the same odds.
2. Multifactorial traits have a continuous variation of the condition, for example, height and intelligence. The variation can be plotted on a bell-shaped (Gaussian) curve. Mendelian traits tend to be all-or-none although many AD traits have varying expressivity.
3. Severity of the condition in the family increases the risk to future offspring. Unusually tall parents, for example, are more likely to have tall offspring than are just moderately tall parents. On the other hand, a Marfan (AD) parent may be severely affected but the child may be only slightly affected or vice versa.
4. Severity of many multifactorial traits is significantly affected by environmental influences. This is not so in most Mendelian traits.
5. Pedigree analysis is not feasible in multifactorial traits; pedigree analysis, however, is usually very useful in genetic counseling in Mendelian traits.

CHROMOSOMAL ABNORMALITIES

Chromosomal traits occur if there are numerical errors or if there are structural defects in the chromosomes. Chromosomal disorders are found in approximately 50 percent of spontaneous abortions but in only about 0.5 percent of live births.

Numerical Errors

Until the 1950s, the exact number of chromosomes in a normal human being was undetermined. The normal number (euploidy) is 46, 22 pairs of autosomes and 1 pair of sex chromosomes. Down syndrome is the most common chromosomal disorder seen by pediatric optometrists, and it has several etiologies, for example, trisomy 21 (most often the case), translocation, and, mosaicism. The most common cause is nondisjunction during the process of meiosis (gamete reduction in the female) leading to an extra chromosome in the pair numbered 21, thus trisomy 21. Down syndrome patients are short in stature; have a flat facial profile, protruding tongue, and brushfield spots (yellow or white spots on the iris); and are mentally retarded. They often have epicanthus and esotropia. Nondisjunction becomes more frequent with advanced maternal age. The chance of a woman over 40 having a Down syndrome baby is approximately 5 percent and at least 10 percent for all types of chromosomal numerical errors (aneuploidy). Genetic counseling, therefore, is recommended in advanced maternal age.

Turner syndrome, occurring in about 0.2 percent of female babies, is a chromosomal numerical error affecting the pair of sex chromosomes in females. Nondisjunction results in one of the X chromosomes missing, thus, monosomy X. These females are sterile, short in stature, and have webbed necks. They are usually normal mentally. Interestingly, Turner females have the same prevalence of color vision deficiencies as do males because they are hemizygous X as are normal males.

Some males have an XXY karyotype and therefore have the same prevalence of color vision deficiencies as females. This is the Klinefelter syndrome.

Structural Defects

Chromosomal structure may be abnormal for several reasons, such as deletions, translocations, and inversions. Two deletion abnormalities will be discussed as examples.

The 5 p- syndrome is known as the *cri du chat* (cat-cry) syndrome). Mental retardation may be severe. An infant has a mewing cry like that of a kitten. There are several ocular defects associated with this syndrome such as salt-and-pepper fundi, optic atrophy, and strabismus. Karyotype analysis shows a portion of the small arm (P) of chromosome number 5 missing. The missing genetic material is responsible for the syndrome.

Retinoblastoma may be either an AD or a chromosomal (deletion) trait. The long arm (Q) of chromosome 13 has a partial deletion causing this disease. This is life threatening and requires immediate treatment.

The fragile X syndrome was identified relatively recently and is fairly common—about 0.1 percent in males and 0.05 percent in females. Severity is generally greater in males than it is in females. The etiology is unknown but loci on the X chromosome are considered "fragile." Common problems may include strabismus, refractive errors, epicanthal folds, and visual perceptual-motor problems along with mental retardation. Physical characteristics are often prominent ears, long-narrow face, large head circumference, and hyperelastic skin. An affected father will transmit the fragile X chromosome to all daughters but to no sons since they receive the father's Y chromosome. The daughters may either have no evidence of the trait or mildly expressed severity compared with more severely affected males who have the fragile X syndrome. Nevertheless these daughters may pass the fragile X chromosome on to their sons, who are more likely to show the trait. Because pediatric optometrists see many children who have learning disabilities, the fragile X syndrome should be considered and referral for genetic counseling should be made in appropriate cases.

Guidelines

Some general guidelines for chromosomal abnormalities are:

1. There are relatively few survivors except for a few traits such as Down syndrome.
2. Mental retardation in survivors is the rule.

3. The occurrence is usually sporadic, except in translocation inheritance.
4. Down syndrome is usually due to advanced maternal age with nondisjunction rather than being genetically inherited.
5. Pedigree analysis is not feasible except in translocation inheritance.
6. Biochemical analysis is not feasible.
7. A chromosomal syndrome affects the individual in a general way, for example Down syndrome.
8. Karyotype analysis is of great importance.

GENETIC COUNSELING

Patients may need genetic counseling. For the pediatric optometrist, it is usually the parents and often prospective parents who receive counseling. There are two types of genetic counseling, *informal* and *formal*.

Informal

Informal genetic counseling can be done by the pediatric optometrist. This involves less serious genetic traits such as XR color vision deficiencies. The theoretical risks can be calculated in such Mendelian traits; true paternal parenthood, however, must be known (Figure 2.6). Lack of information on true fatherhood can result in the genetic counseling errors.

Genetic counseling is fraught with possible errors for many other reasons, such as reduced penetrance (skipping of a generation), heterogeneity, and mistaken diagnoses. This why caution must be used, even when informal genetic counseling is given.

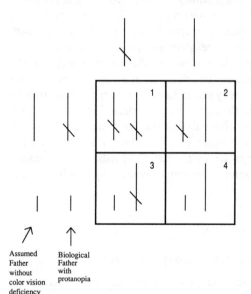

Figure 2.6 Punnett square analysis for assumed versus biological fatherhood in an XR trait.

Assumed Father without color vision deficiency

Biological Father with protanopia

When there is uncertainty and when serious conditions are involved, the optometrist should refer patients for formal genetic counseling.

Formal

Mendelian traits such as Tay-Sachs disease (AR) obviously are serious, and genetic counseling for them is recommended. A medical geneticist may recommend parental blood testing to determine carrier status of prospective parents. If neither parent is a carrier (determined by sufficient level of hexosaminidase A), no risk to the offspring is expected (see Figure 2.7a). If the mother is a carrier, no abnormal phenotype is expected (see Figure 2.7b) although two children are theoretically by chance expected to be carriers. If both the mother and father are carriers, the risk to offspring is 25 percent having Tay-Sachs disease, 50 percent expected to be carriers, and 25 percent being genotypically normal.

At this point, the genetic counselor may advise amniocentesis to determine the hexosaminidase A level of the fetus. If the fetus is shown to be either heterozygous or homozygous normal, the parents will be advised that test results indicate the probability of their having a baby who does not have Tay-Sachs disease. If the biochemical assay results from amniocentesis indicates homozygous abnormal for Tay-Sachs disease, however, the genetic specialist will present a hard question for the couple to answer. Do they wish to choose a therapeutic abortion? The genetic counselor is nondirective and must respect the wishes of the couple, whatever their decision.

Another example of referral for formal genetic counseling is in cases of ocular albinism. Suppose the pediatric optometrist is managing the case of a young boy with ocular albinism and his mother, who is pregnant, asks about the risk of having "another blind child." Since the mother can be identified as a carrier by pedigree analysis (and possibly with ophthalmoscopy because of patchy fundi—characteristic of carriers in certain XR traits), the optometrist can state that the theoretical risk for male offspring is 50 percent but probably not much risk (theoretically 0 percent but it is not wise to say *never*) for female offspring. On referral to a genetic specialist, amniocentesis may be recommended for sex determination of the fetus. If it is a female, the problem is solved. If it is a male, a difficult dilemma arises. The 50–50 chance of having

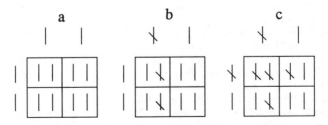

Figure 2.7 Punnett square analysis in an autosomal recessive trait: (a) no risk to offspring; (b) no phenotype risk but 50 percent chance of carrier status; (c) phenotypic risk of 25 percent and chance of carrier status of 50 percent in offspring.

a second child with ocular albinism may be too much for the parents to take. The genetic counselor will have to present the option of therapeutic abortion, but not in a directive manner. The choice belongs to the parents, not the geneticist or anyone else.

Genetic counseling takes great compassion and understanding and extensive training. It is, therefore, wise for the optometrist to say just enough of the right thing—not too little or not too much. Extensive formal genetic counseling is left to the specialist. Genetics is a specialty in medicine, probably the most elite of all specialties. On the other hand, the optometrist is negligent if too little (or if nothing) is said to advise patients, or parents of children, on genetic questions. The case of ocular albinism in this discussion is a perfect example of the need for optometrists to make exact diagnoses and referrals to genetic specialists for formal genetic counseling.

SUGGESTED READING

Bartlett JD. Congenital cone dysfunction. Am J Optom 1979;56:208–210.

Bloome MA, Garcia CA. Manual of retinal and choroidal dystrophies. New York: Appleton-Century-Crofts, 1982:3.

Boder E. Developmental dyslexia: A diagnostic approach based on three atypical reading-spelling patterns. Developmental Medicine and Child Neurology 1973; 15:663–687.

Bunin GR, Emanuel BS, Meadows AT, et al. Frequency of 13q- abnormalities among 203 patients with retinoblastoma. J Ntnl Cancer Inst 1989;81:370–374.

Catalano RA. Down syndrome. Survey of Ophthalmol 1990;34:385–398.

Cavender JC, Schwartz LG, Spivey BE. Hereditary macular dystrophies. In Duane TD, ed., Clinical Ophthalmology, vol. 3. Philadelphia: Lippincott, 1979;1–29.

Cline D, Hofstetter HW, Griffin JR. Dictionary of visual science, 4th ed. Radnor, PA: Chilton, 1989.

Cowel JK, Rutland P, Hungerford J, Jay M. Deletion of chromosome region 13q14 is transmissible and does not always predispose to retinoblastoma. Hum Gene, 1988;80:43–45.

Curtin BJ. Physiologic versus pathologic myopia: Genetics versus environment. Ophthalmology 1979;86:681–690.

Fatt HV, Griffin JR, Lyle WM. Genetics for primary eye care practitioners, 2nd ed. Boston: Butterworth–Heinemann, 1992.

Fatt HV, Grisham JD. Genetic counseling in optometry: A case study of congenital bilateral ptosis. Am J Optom and Physiol Optics 1981;58:342–346.

Gelehrter TD, Collins FS. Principles of medical genetics. Baltimore: Williams & Wilkins, 1990;73–75.

Griffin JR, Asano GW, Somers RJ, et al. Heredity in congenital esotropia. J Am Optom Assoc 1979;50:1237–1242.

Griffin JR, Walton HN. Dyslexia screener for first-graders (DSF). Culver City, Calif. Reading and Perception Therapy Center, 1990.

Griffin JR, Walton HN. Dyslexia determination test (DDT). Los Angeles: Instructional Materials and Equipment Distributors, 1987.

Griffin JR, Walton HN, Christenson GN. The dyslexia screener (TDS). Culver City, Calif.: Reading and Perception Therapy Center, 1988.

Hallgren B. Specific dyslexia ("congenital word-blindness"): A clinical and genetic study. Acta Psychiatricia et Neurologica Supplement (Scandinavia), 1950;65.

Hirsch MJ, Ditmars DL. Refraction of young myopes and their parents: A re-analysis. Am J Optom Arch Am Acad Optom 1969;46:30–32.

Jay M. On the hereditary of retinitis pigmentosa. Brit J Ophthalmol 1982;66:405–416.

Jones WL. The work-up of the diabetic patient. Rev Optom 1982;119:50–56.

Kelly TE. Clinical Genetics and Genetic Counseling, 2nd ed. Chicago: Year Book Medical Publishers, 1986:28–29.

Krupin T, Podos SM. In Heilmann KH, Richardson KT, eds. Glaucoma: Conceptions of a Disease, Stuttgart: Thieme, 1978:351.

Leary GA. The reconciliation of genetically determined myopia with environmentally induced myopia. Am J Optom Arch Am Acad Optom 1970;47:702–709.

Levitan M. Textbook of Human Genetics. Oxford, Eng.: Oxford University Press, 1988:51.

Lyle WM. Genetic risk: A reference for eye care practitioners. Waterloo, Can.: University of Waterloo Press. 1990:6–29.

McKusick VA. Mendelian inheritance in man, 9th ed. Baltimore: Johns Hopkins University Press, 1990.

McKusick VA. Maternal genes: Mitochondrial diseases. In Mori J, Paul NW, Roderick TH, Wallace DC, eds. Medical and experimental mammalian genetics: A perspective. New York: Alan R. Liss, 1987;137–190.

Maino DM, Wesson M, Schlange D, et al. Optometric findings in the Fragile X syndrome. Optom Vision Sci 1991; 68(8):634–640.

Maumenee IH. Classification of hereditary cataracts in children by linkage analysis. Ophthalmology 1979;86:1554–1558.

Mets MB, Maumenee IH. The eye and the chromosome. Survey of Ophthalmology 1983;28:21.

Muench KH. The genetic basis for human disease. New York: Elsevier, 1979;36.

Pearce WG. Congenital nystagmus: Genetic and environmental causes. Canadian J Ophthalmol. 1978;13:1–9.

Pokorny J, Smith VC, Verriest G. Congenital and acquired color vision defects. New York: Grune and Stratton, 1979;216.

Schechter RJ. Ocular findings in a newborn with *cri du chat* syndrome. Ann Ophthalmol 1978;10:339–344.

Singh G, Lott MT, Wallace DC. A mitochondrial DNA mutation as a cause of Leber's hereditary optic neuropathy. New Engl J Medicine 1989, 320:1300–1305.

Stine GJ. The new human genetics. Dubuque, Iowa: Wm. C. Brown, 1989;256.

Witkop CJ, Jr., Nance WE, Rawls RF, et al. Autosomal recessive oculocutaneous albinism in man: Evidence for genetic heterogeneity. Am J Hum Genet 1970;22: 55–74.

3

Examination of the Infant

Leonard J. Press

Clinical examination of the infant centers on the evaluation of ocular health and visual function. There are important methodological, anatomical, and perceptuocognitive considerations that are unique to infant assessment. Included in the methodological considerations are case history, the time of day at which the examination is performed, the physical surroundings, and the materials or procedures used. First an overview of these considerations and then a systematic approach to examination comprise the body of Chapter 3.

METHODOLOGICAL CONSIDERATIONS
Case History

In contrast with the adult, the infant offers no symptoms, few reliable signs, and therefore only an indirect case history. The issues involved in taking a case history from the infant's caretakers were explored in Chapter 1.

Time of Examination

The ideal time to examine an infant is when she is awake and attentive, which is usually in the morning. It is advisable that the infant not be fed just prior to the examination because infants tend to become very drowsy after feeding. Procedures such as visual acuity and ocular motility assessment are predicated on an alert and attentive state. In contrast, it is better to conduct direct ophthalmoscopy when the infant is drowsy. An alert infant tends to foveate the center of the light, giving the examiner an exquisite view of the macula but little else. Parents should therefore be reminded to bring a bottle to the office, and ophthalmoscopy should be done while the infant is being fed. When sucking, the infant's eyelids remain open, gaze is stable, and calmness is exhibited (Saint-Anne Dargassies, 1986).

Physical Surroundings

The environment in which the infant is examined should be non-threatening. The examiner must gain the infant's trust and cooperation. Many examiners elect not to wear a white doctor's jacket because children associate this with potentially uncomfortable experiences. The room should be bright and decorated with pleasant animal or cartoon characters. This should not be overdone, however, as it may detract attention from the stimuli presented by the examiner. A caretaker must accompany the infant to serve as an assistant in holding the child as well as providing a familiar and comforting face.

Materials and Procedures

The equipment necessary to examine an infant should be readily available in the examining area. These include acuity cards or apparatus, eye patch, occluder, finger puppets, penlight, lens racks, loose prisms, optokinetic nystagmus (OKN) drum, Styrofoam balls, retinoscope, ophthalmoscope, and diagnostic pharmaceutical agents. Given the limited attention span of infants, one cannot afford to expend time looking for equipment or alternate procedures.

Perceptuocognitive Factors: Habituation

The concept of habituation plays a central role in every phase of infant vision testing. Experimental psychologists have demonstrated that infants will not maintain interest in objects that are presented repeatedly (Vurpillot, 1976). The examiner must therefore be ready to intersperse a variety of targets. For example, one might find that a particular finger puppet captures the infant's interest for pursuit testing. When the same target is used to test convergence, however, the infant tunes out the target and stares at the examiner's face. The introduction of a different finger puppet or facial contour picture after the first is withdrawn will momentarily recapture the infant's attention.

Systems Analysis

Woodruff (1973) described the use of a systems examination of the infant's visual function. He recommended an order of examination that proceeded from bony skeleton to the soft tissues, the glandular and lymphatic systems, the vascular system, the neuromuscular system and binocular relationships, and the eyes as optical systems. Gesell and colleagues (1949) recommended the systematic visual behavior examination of infants that followed the ontogenetic sequence of eye-hand coordination, postural orientation, fixation, retinal reflex, and spatial projection. Mohindra (1979) presented a developmental inventory for infants that mirrored the Denver Developmental Test and included gross-motor, fine-motor adaptive, language, personal social, and visual areas.

A systems approach has been adopted that is a blend of the procedures already discussed. Any systems approach should allow one to document the integrity of basic functions as well as to investigate the integration of systems. The evaluation of infants will be approached with emphasis on external observations (bony skeleton and soft tissue structure as well as motor response), pupillary responses and ocular motility (the neuromuscular system), ocular alignment (binocular relationships), visual acuity and refractive state (the eyes as optical components of a behavioral system), and internal ocular health.

SYSTEM I: EXTERNAL STRUCTURES

Physical Size

The examiner should obtain a general impression of whether the child appears to be within the expected range of weight, height, and head circumference. Useful formulae for these variables have been developed (Behrman & Vaughan, 1983) and are listed in Table 3.1. In addition, the top of the head may be palpated to gain an impression of the fontanels. The posterior fontanel is generally closed by 4 months and the anterior fontanel by 9–18 months. Persistence of excessively large fontanels have been associated with specific disorders (Table 3.2) that can influence visual or ocular development.

Table 3.1 Formulas for approximate average height and weight

Weight	Kilograms	Pounds
At birth	3.25	7
3–12 months	Age (mo) + 9/2	Age (mo) + 11
1–6 years	Age (yr) × 2 + 8	Age (yr) × 5 + 17
Height	Centimeters	Inches
At birth	50	20
At 1 year	75	30
2–6 years	Age (yr) × 6 + 77	Age (yr) × 2.5 + 30

After RE Behrman and VC Vaughan, Nelson textbook of pediatrics, 12th ed. (Philadelphia: WB Saunders, 1983).

Table 3.2 Disorders associated with persistently large anterior fontanel

Achondroplasia	Osteogenesis imperfecta
Apert's syndrome	Prematurity
Athyrototic hypothyroidism	Rubella syndrome
Hydrocephaly	Trisomies 13, 18, 21
Intrauterine growth retardation	Vitamin D deficiency rickets

After RE Behrman and VC Vaughan, Nelson textbook of pediatrics, 12th ed. (Philadelphia: WB Saunders, 1983).

Orbit and Facial Symmetry

The general appearance of the face should be inspected with regard to features such as epicanthal folds, spacing of the eyes, and relative placement of the ears. Abnormalities in or asymmetries of these features may be associated with isolated congenital ocular anomalies or with congenital syndromes. The average newborn interpupillary distance is 49 mm. Vertical asymmetry of the eyes within the orbit may result in the head being tilted toward the side of the eye with the higher placement. The vertical palpebral apertures may be of different sizes. Although this is usually a benign physiological variant, it must be differentiated from microphthalmia and documented accordingly in the record.

Head Posture

Adaptive or compensatory head turns are usually first observed when the child is older than one year but may be noted in infancy. The most common causes of head tilt or turn are related to nystagmus or noncomitant strabismus. If the examiner observes abnormal head posture, she should place her hand on the infant's head to restrain movement. She should then conduct an ocular motility investigation as is discussed in Section III. If the infant strongly objects to having her head restrained when she is looking in one direction but does not object to restraint when she is looking in the opposite direction, a purposeful head turn can be assumed.

Eyelids

Minor and usually transient damage to the lids, orbit, or eye is common during difficult labor or forceps delivery. Swelling or redness of the lids or orbital area is therefore not uncommon following birth. Damage to the lids, orbit skull and central nervous system has been estimated to occur in up to 25 percent of normal deliveries and as high as 50 percent in births where the labor was difficult or where forceps were used.

The most common lid abnormality observed in infants is ptosis. Ecchymosis and swelling of the upper eyelid may produce a secondary ptosis or obscure a true ptosis. A variable degree of lid retraction is a normal finding in the neonatal period.

Sclera

The sclera has a translucent bluish cast at birth that becomes more opaque and whitens during the first year. Abnormal coloration may signify collagen abnormality, and localized thinning may be associated with inflammation or trauma. Melanosis and nevi are common in the sclera of darkly pigmented infants.

Conjunctiva

Conjunctivitis is common in the newborn period and may extend to hyperemia, mucopurulent discharge, lid edema, and photophobia. The neonate is particularly susceptible to infectious conjunctivitis because of the microbial environment to which she has been exposed. In addition, the newborn loses the protection of maternal antibodies before fully generating her own immune components and has poor resistance due to the absence of lymphoid tissue. One percent silver nitrate, used as prophylaxis against gonococcal ophthalmia neonatorum, frequently causes chemical conjunctivitis. A Burton ultraviolet lamp or head-borne loupe are helpful in obtaining a good view.

Cornea

Clarity and size are the principal features to be noted during routine examination of the anterior segment. Corneal diameter may be approximated with a millimeter rule. The newborn's cornea measures approximately 10 mm in horizontal diameter, reaching the adult dimension of 12 mm by two years of age. Clarity of the cornea should be judged with a transilluminator, magnifying loupe, or hand-held slit lamp. Corneal insult should be judged with ultraviolet light and fluorescein. The Burton lamp is well-suited for this purpose, providing a wide field of light to capture the infant's attention as well as a wide field of view for the examiner.

Iris

Coloration of the iris should be noted. Heterochromia, a difference in color between the two irides, may be partial or complete. Congenital heterochromia, usually an autosomal dominant trait, should be photodocumented. Noninherited congenital heterochromia may occur in congenital Horner's syndrome, wherein birth injury is responsible for lighter iris pigmentation on the sympathetically denervated side.

Pupils

Infants tend to have small pupil sizes until about 12 months of age (Riordan-Eva, 1989). Infants with darkly pigmented irides tend to have smaller pupillary diameters than do infants with lighter irides (Martin, 1989). This makes it more difficult to elicit direct and consensual pupillary reflexes in infants with dark irides. Pupil size in infancy can vary widely. The state of alertness and attentiveness influences pupil size (Banks, 1980).

Lacrimal Apparatus

The lacrimal gland is not usually developed until after birth, but the examiner should observe reflex tear secretion beginning two weeks after birth. Psychic tearing (due to crying) is not usually observed until after two months. The most probable cause of excessive lacrimation is obstruction of the nasolacrimal duct. This is usually due to incomplete canalization, as the thin membrane that closes the end of the duct fails to disappear following birth. Occurring in 1–4 percent of newborns, most congenital nasolacrimal obstruction clears spontaneously by 3 months of age.

SYSTEM II: PRIMITIVE REFLEXES

Primitive reflexes of the neonate are essential to progressive development of central nervous system (CNS) control. In normal maturation, primitive spinal and brain stem reflexes present from birth gradually diminish so that midbrain and cortical patterns of righting and equilibrium can predominate. Neurologic dysfunction resulting from CNS disease is manifest in uncoordinated sensorimotor activity. CNS lesions release primitive reflexes from the inhibition normally exerted by higher centers. This results in phylogenetically immature movement, which is dramatized in cerebral palsied children. A listing of infant visual reflexes and their normal time course is given in Table 3.3.

SYSTEM III: OCULAR MOTILITY
Position Maintenance

Steady, accurate fixation is subject in part to development of the fovea and the accommodative-feedback loop. It begins to develop as soon as the neonate opens her eyes and is well-developed by the third month (Hyvarinen & Lindstedt, 1981).

Position maintenance is heavily linked to the degree that the stimulus holds interest for the infant. In general, any object that has the contour of a human face is a highly captivating target. With a penlight inserted into the finger puppet, the examiner can flicker the target, which helps maintain or recapture attention.

Smooth Pursuit

The involuntary or reflex smooth pursuit component of OKN is present from birth. Voluntary smooth pursuit develops between the second and third month of age. At first it is limited to low velocity targets (Aslin, 1981). The examiner should therefore move the fixation target slowly with ample time for saccadic refixation. A target well-suited to this task is illustrated in Figure 3.1.

Saccades

The infant's saccadic eye movement system is functional at birth, but differs from the adult in latency (longer response time), hypometricity (a series of choppy saccades rather than a single ballistic movement), and extent of visual field covered (peripheral awareness usually limited to 30° off the midline) (Aslin, 1988). The developmental timetable for acquisition of adult saccade patterns is unknown at present.

Vergence

Infants less than six months old will not make the appropriate refixation saccade or vergence movements when prisms are placed in front of one eye (Hoyt, 1982). However, vergence response to approaching and receding targets such as finger

Table 3.3 Neonatal and infant visual reflexes

Reflex	Stimulus	Response	Age Range
Pupillary	Bright light	Constriction	8 months fetal through life
Visuo-palpebral	Bright light	Eyelid closure	6–7 months fetal through life
Eye-neck	Bright light in eye (head unsupported)	Opisthotonus	8–9 months fetal to 1–3 months
McCarthy's	Light touch above eyebrow	Homolateral blink	6–7 months fetal to 4 months
Naso-palpebral	Light touch on bridge of nose	Bilateral blink	6–7 months fetal to 4 months
Ciliary	Touch on eyelashes	Homolateral or bilateral blink	6–7 months fetal through life
Corneal	Touch on cornea	Homolateral blink	6–7 months fetal through life
Cutaneo-palpebral	Painful touch	Bilateral blink	6–7 months fetal through life
Cochleo-palpebral	Sharp sound	Bilateral blink	6–7 months fetal through life
Doll's eye	Passive head turning	Delay in eye movements following head	7–8 months fetal to 3 months
Defensive blink	Rapid approach of target	Blink	1–3 months through life

After RP Erhardt, Developmental visual dysfunction (Tucson: Therapy Skill Builders, 1990), p. 47.

puppets may be obtained as young as one month of age. Consequently for the infant under six months old, the presence but not the quantitative fusional range of convergence and divergence may be evaluated clinically.

Vestibulo-Ocular

The full range of eye movements can be elicited from the full-term neonate beyond seven days of age by use of the vestibulo-ocular reflex (VOR) (Eviatar et al, 1979). The infant is held by the examiner under the armpits at arm's length with its head tilted forward 30° toward the examiner's face (Figure 3.2). When the examiner spins in a continuous circle several times, labyrinthine induced nystagmus is noted with the slow (tonic) phase in the direction opposite rotation and the fast (jerk) phase in the same direction as the rotation. The absence of this reflex may indicate maturational delay of the medial longitudinal fasiculus (MLF), CNS damage, and brainstem or extraocular muscle abnormality.

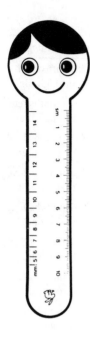

Figure 3.1 The face in this target elicits visual attention from the infant and serves as a stimulus for smooth pursuit movements (available from LVI, see Appendix A).

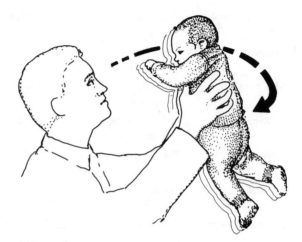

Figure 3.2 Procedure used for eliciting vestibulo-ocular reflex with infants.

Equally significant in the rotational nystagmus response is the time interval between the termination of spinning and the cessation of nystagmus. A sighted child inhibits the after-rotational nystagmus by refixating the examiner's face within 5 seconds after the examiner has stopped rotating. A blind child will persist in the nystagmus for up to 30 seconds until the labyrinthine-vestibular stimulation subsides because there is no visual refixation to block it (Hoyt, 1982).

When the infant has low muscle tone or is floppy, the examiner must provide extra support when tilting the child to perform the VOR spin procedure here described.

Optokinetic Nystagmus (OKN)

OKN is usually elicited from the infant by rotating a drum with stripes held closely enough to capture visual attention. This may have to be as close as five or ten centimeters. At first, the infant may prefer to fixate on the examiner's face as opposed to the drum, but with perseverance, the observation can usually be made. Pediatric OKN drums have bright pictures of animal faces (Figure 3.3) that help to elicit fixation and following responses. Horizontal OKN responses are one way to demonstrate integrity of the lateral and medial recti. OKN is considered a reliable index of visual resolution up to, but not necessarily including, the visual cortex. Consequently any infant with cortical damage or immaturity can be functionally blind yet show a brisk OKN response.

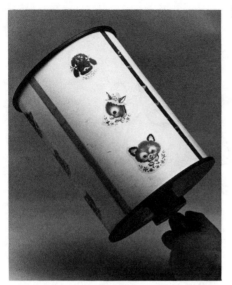

Figure 3.3   Pediatric OKN drum.

It has been established that monocular OKN is asymmetrical in newborns, being brisk when the stimulus is moved in the temporal to nasal direction and weak in the nasal to temporal direction (Braddick & Atkinson, 1983). By four months of age this asymmetry disappears. Persistence of asymmetry in the direction of OKN response beyond this age may indicate amblyopia or abnormal binocular development.

SYSTEM IV: VISUAL FIELD

The visual field may be probed by confrontation testing in which the examiner's face is used for central fixation and objects of interest such as finger puppets are moved in from the periphery (Keltner, 1977) (Figure 3.4). One puppet can be used to gain central fixation while the other puppet is moved in slowly from the periphery. Older infants will reach for the target when it is first sighted. When this fails, the visual threat response can be used, particularly for the older infant who seems unresponsive. If there is serious doubt about the infant's responsiveness to peripheral stimuli, a more formalized study of kinetic perimetry can be conducted using an arc perimeter (Schwartz et al, 1987). The development of the infant's visual field response is shown in Table 3.4.

SYSTEM V: BINOCULAR VISION
Alignment

The most practical method to determine the presence of binocular vision is observing symmetry of the Hirschberg corneal light reflection. It is particularly valuable in differentiating epicanthus (wide nasal skin folds), which simulates esotropia, from true esotropia (Figures 3.5; 3.6). The examiner shines a light source on the

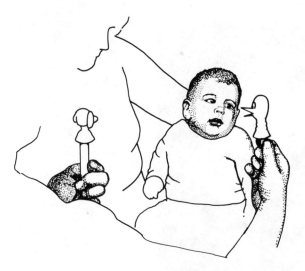

Figure 3.4 Procedure for conducting confrontation visual fields with infants.

midline at a fixation distance of 50 cm. A useful target is a Snoopy or similarly translucent finger puppet that collimates the light. The examiner notes if the relative position of the corneal light reflection is symmetrical or if one is displaced relative to the fellow eye. It is valid to assume that 1 mm of displacement is equal to 22 prism diopters in patients of all ages (Eskridge et al, 1988).

By 3 to 6 months of age, infants have an adequate refixation reflex to permit cover testing. The simplest technique is to grasp the infant's head lightly, allowing the thumb to drop down and serve as an occluder (Figure 3.7). The alternate or unilateral cover test can be performed in standard fashion with the same target as was described for generating the Hirschberg corneal light reflection. Cover testing should be done initially at 50 cm since the infant's primary visual world is at near. The furthest distance at which the examiner is likely to be able to maintain the infant's fixation for cover testing is 5 to 10 feet.

Table 3.4 Development of the infant's visual field in degrees

Quadrant	1 Month	3 Months	6 Months	12 Months	Adult
Up	20	30	40	60	60
Down	20	30	45	60	75
Left	35	40	65	85	105
Right	30	35	65	90	105

Adapted from G Mohn, J van Hof-van Duin. Development of the binocular and monocular visual fields of human infants during the first year of life, Clin Vision Sci 1986;1:51–64.

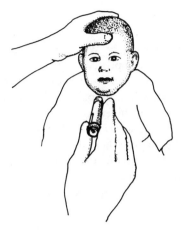 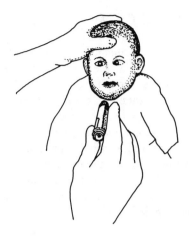

Figure 3.5 Symmetrical Hirschberg corneal light reflexes indicating binocular alignment.

Figure 3.6 Hirschberg corneal light reflex of left eye displaced temporal ward indicating left esotropia.

Vergence

Infants as young as one month of age can exhibit appropriate changes in convergence and divergence with advancing and receding targets. Target movement of approximately 10 cm/sec is the optimal rate of movement (Cron et al, 1986). Vergence responses are more accurate and consistent at three months of age, and vergence ranges in response to interposition of loose base-in or base-out prism can be demonstrated at six months of age.

Figure 3.7 Use of the examiner's thumb to serve as an occluder.

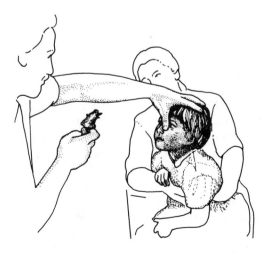

Special Tests for Binocular Function
The Bruckner Test

When an infant is uncooperative for cover testing or when the angle of strabismus is small, the detection of strabismus is aided by a procedure known as the Bruckner Test (Tongue & Cibis, 1981). The examiner sits at a distance of one meter opposite the infant in a dimly lit room and illuminates both pupils simultaneously with the beam of the direct ophthalmoscope. The examiner looks through the ophthalmoscope and judges the relative symmetry in color and brightness of the fundus (red) reflex. When strabismus is present, the fundus reflex of the nonfixating eye is a brighter or lighter yellowish color as compared with the normal red reflex. It should be borne in mind that asymmetry of the red reflex may stem from other causes such as differences in refractive state and pupil size as well as media opacities or posterior pole lesions.

Optokinetic Nystagmus

As was mentioned in Section III, monocular OKN is asymmetric in the normal infant until four months of age with the nasal to temporal direction relatively subdued. Asymmetry in OKN beyond this age is thought to be a direct consequence of midbrain deficiencies in binocular integration. The persistence of asymmetry in monocular OKN strongly suggests an early age of onset of a binocular vision anomaly (Westall et al, 1989).

Stereopsis

In recent years, behavioral as well as electrophysiological tests have demonstrated the onset of reliable stereopsis response in infants to occur between two and four months of age (Cron et al, 1986). Although there are not as yet any readily applicable clinical tests of stereopsis that can be administered to infants, it is conceivable that targets may soon become commercially available for use in a preferential looking format.

Visual Evoked Potential (VEP)

Binocular summation of the VEP has been advanced as an objective index of binocular visual function (Tsutusi et al, 1982). In clinical practice, this method is subject to artifacts and variation that tempers its usefulness as a quantifiable index of binocularity (Fulton & Robb, 1987).

SYSTEM VI: VISUAL ACUITY

Most clinical tests of infant acuity will give poorer results when they are conducted monocularly as compared with binocularly. This is because the infant is distracted by the presence of the patch. Consequently acuity testing should be done binocularly initially to make sure that the infant is responsive to the procedure itself.

Optokinetic Nystagmus

Numerous authors have raised caution in the equating of a positive OKN response with good vision (Glaser, 1975; Hoyt et al, 1982). Although experimental OKN studies were among the first used to assess acuity, the degree of resolution required to respond to the stimulus is questionable. As reviewed by Cron and associates (1986), it has been demonstrated that OKN is not affected by significant degrees of uncompensated refractive error. Moreover the targets used in clinical practice provide only a gross approximation of visual acuity (Campos & Chiesi, 1985).

The pediatric OKN drum, which has eight alternating columns of animals and stripes, is highly effective in gaining the infant's attention but has no correlation with Snellen acuity. The standard OKN drum, which has alternating columns of black and white stripes, has a theoretical Snellen equivalent based on the distance at which it is held. In order to obtain the infant's fixation, however, the target has to be held so close that it renders the acuity demand no greater than a gross index of resolution.

Visual Evoked Potential (VEP)

The landmark studies of Marg and colleagues (1976) and Sokol and Dobson (1976) have been used to demonstrate that, based on amplitude of the VEP, the capacity for adult-like levels of acuity develops early in infancy (Table 3.5). The VEP consistently shows a higher degree of visual potential in infants than is obtained through behavioral or psychophysical measures (Dobson & Teller, 1978). When the VEP latency is studied as an index of visual maturation, there is closer correlation with behavioral and psychophysical measures (Sokol & Moskowitz, 1985).

VEPs can be helpful in localizing important components of visual function. Cases of visual immaturity have documented where the electroretinogram (ERG) is normal but the VEP is not. As cortical maturation proceeded and the infants exhibited visual behavior, the VEPs showed less attenuation (Hoyt et al, 1983). The VEP is therefore an important diagnostic and prognostic tool for predicting the development of vision in premature or small for gestational age infants with generalized delays in motor development. At the opposite extreme, it is possible to obtain a normal VEP from a child who is functionally blind when the damage is localized to the cortical association areas (Bodis-Wollner et al, 1977).

Although VEP units are seldom found in private clinical practice, they are valuable in monitoring progress objectively when treatment has been implemented. The most common example is the increase in visual acuity anticipated with amblyopia therapy.

Preferential Looking (PL)

Originally introduced by experimental psychologists to study the looking behavior of infants (Fantz et al, 1962), PL has evolved into a valid measure of infant visual acuity. The infant is presented with a series of grating patterns with progressively smaller stripe widths. The gratings appear either to the left or right of the midline, and the examiner observes which side the infant prefers to look, hence the term *preferential looking*. At the point when the infant can no longer resolve the gratings, the side of the target containing the grating is indistinguishable from the opposite side. Since the infant cannot display a preference, the looking behavior to one side or the other should occur at the chance level.

Table 3.5 Development of visual acuity

Date	Investigator	Method	Birth to 1 Mo.	1 Mo.	2 Mos.	3 Mos.	4 Mos.	5 Mos.	6 Mos.	9 Mos.	1 Year
1962	Fantz et al	PV	20/800	20/800	20/400	20/400	20/200	20/200			
1962	Fantz et al	PV and OKN	20/800	20/800	20/800	20/400	20/400	20/200	20/200		
1962	Dayton et al	OKN	20/250–20/160						20/200		
1964	Dayton et al	OKN	20/440–20/150								
1973	Catford and Oliver	OKN						20/60			20/40
1976	Marg et al	VER		20/540	20/300	20/100	20/40	20/30	20/20		
1976	Sokol and Dobson	VER							20/20		
1978	Sokol	VER			20/150	20/80	20/80	20/50	20/30	20/20	
1980	Gwiazda et al	FPL	20/1000	20/1000		20/600	20/300	20/200	20/100	20/100	20/50
1986	McDonald et al (Teller Cards)	(F)PL	20/400–20/1200	20/300–20/1200	20/150–20/600		20/80–20/300		20/50–20/200		20/50–20/200

Modified from DC Lewerenz. Visual acuity and the developing visual system, J Am Optom Assoc 1978;49:1155–1160.

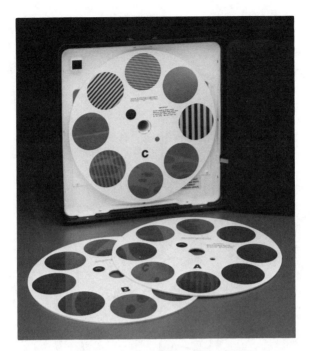

Figure 3.8 Testing wheel in the preferential looking paradigm of the PL 20/20 infant vision test device.

As originally introduced in the laboratories of Teller and associates (1974) and Held (Gwiazda et al, 1980), the methodology for PL was impractical for private practice settings. The technique has subsequently been streamlined in time as well as space and is now available in the form of cards (Dobson et al, 1986) as well as a testing wheel (Stebbins, 1986)(Figure 3.8). Ideally the examiner concentrates on the looking behavior of the child and an assistant records the results.

The optimum responses to this test are obtained between 3 and 12 months of age. From 9 months onward, infants do not sustain interest in the target due to habituation. The Teller Acuity Cards (see Appendix A) are available with an optional stage on which a reward such as a stuffed animal can appear when the infant correctly looks toward the grating (Figure 3.9). When cooperation is poor, the parent should take home a *practice sheet* containing stripes on one half and a blank circle on the other. The parent should condition the infant that stripes are preferable to look at as compared with the blank. One adult points to the stripes and says, "Hooray! Stripes!" while another claps and says, "Yay!"

Sheridan Tests for Young Children and Retardates (STYCAR)

The STYCAR are a series of pediatric vision tests developed by British ophthalmologist Mary Sheridan (1960). The portion of this test applicable to infants consists

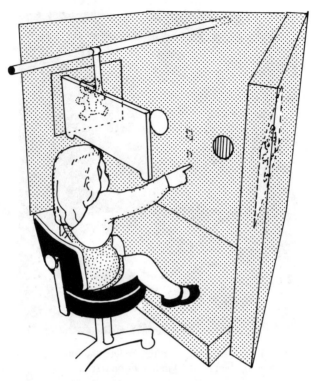

Figure 3.9 Operant conditioning procedure used with the
Teller Acuity Cards in the Vistech preferential looking paradigm.

of a series of Styrofoam balls of progressively smaller size. The examiner records the
smallest size ball the infant can fixate and follow at a distance of 10 feet (Figure 3.10).
The concept behind the test is valuable. Sheridan suggested that a white ball be used
against a black background, as the stark contrast maximizes the infant's attention to
the ball, but infants can spot the ball even under conditions of extreme blur. This bias
can be controlled by rolling the white ball on a neutral gray background (Press, 1982).

Toys and Common Objects

Visual acuity estimates obtained by using toys or other common objects can
create a false sense of security about visual resolution. The recognition of objects or
toys is a function of minimum observable acuity. In contrast, the resolution of
comparably sized letters on a Snellen chart is a function of minimum separable acuity
(Sheridan, 1976). Most toys to which infants are exposed are relatively large in overall
dimension. The infant can respond to favorite toys even with considerable uncompensated refractive error.

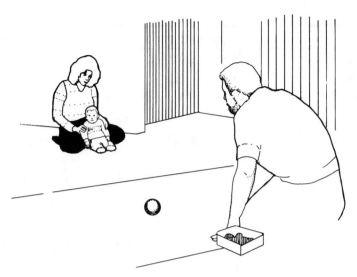

Figure 3.10 Examiner observing infant looking behavior toward a rolling ball as part of the STYCAR procedure.

Individuals who use rattles, keys, or similar noise-making objects to document a visual response have been observed. Fixation and following in this instance may be auditory-driven responses rather than visual ones.

A final assumption made is that resistance to occlusion of one eye compared to the fellow eye indicates amblyopia. Although this is true, the degree of acuity difference between the two eyes in order for this to occur is significantly greater than what can be detected by direct clinical measure. It is no longer acceptable in the contemporary practice of pediatric optometry to indicate on a record, "no resistance to occlusion of either eye," as the sole index of visual acuity.

SYSTEM VII: REFRACTIVE STATE
Retinoscopy

Retinoscopic evaluation may be conducted in either a cycloplegic or non-cycloplegic manner. Mohindra (1977) introduced a technique of noncycloplegic retinoscopy that correlates well with cycloplegic findings. The examining room is darkened, and the examiner maintains the retinoscope at a distance of 50 cm from the infant. For young infants, the best ways to scope are with the infant over the parent's shoulder or while the infant is being fed. Lens racks are used to neutralize the retinoscopic motion. An adjustment value of -1.25 is algebraically added to the neutrality value to determine the distance refractive state. As an example, if the motion is neutral with a $+1.25$ lens in place, the infant is emmetropic. The data compiled in Table 3.6 are extracted from Mohindra's developmental inventory for infants and young children (Mohindra, 1979).

Table 3.6 Infant refraction

Age	Sphere/SD	Cylinder/SD
0–1 month	−0.90D / ± 3.17	−2.20D / ± 1.43 (31%)
2–3 months	−0.47D / ± 2.28	−2.02D / ± 1.17 (50%)
4–6 months	+0.00D / ± 1.31	−2.20D / ± 1.15 (44%)
6–9 months	+0.50D / ± 0.99	−2.20D / ± 1.15 (44%)
9–12 months	+0.60D / ± 1.30	−1.64D / ± 0.62 (34%)
12–15 months	+0.60D / ± 1.30	−1.25D / ± 0.62 (19%)
15–18 months	+0.60D / ± 1.30	−1.44D / ± 0.77 (19%)
18–24 months	+0.60D / ± 1.30	−1.44D / ± 0.77 (19%)
24–36 months	+1.96D / ± 0.40	−1.00D (4%)

From I Mohindra. Developmental inventory for infants and young childen. Optom Monthly 1979;70: 505–509.

Recently, Wesson and colleagues (1990) suggested caution in substituting the Mohindra near retinoscopy technique for cycloplegic refraction using an adjustment value. They found significant differences between the two techniques in both sphere and cylinder power. In citing two other recent studies on the subject, they concluded that research on larger samples of infants must be done to arrive at a valid correlation between the two techniques. Mohindra retinoscopy is adequate for infants who do not exhibit esophoria or esotropia. When either of these conditions exists, uncovering the full amount of latent hyperopia is imperative. In addition, the numerous instances in which dilation is desirable provides an opportunity to compare cycloplegic with noncycloplegic findings.

Cycloplegic retinoscopy of infants is usually accomplished with 0.5 percent cyclopentolate. This is usually instilled with 2.5 percent neosynephrine and 0.5 percent tropicamide since fundoscopy will be performed as well. An adjustment value is algebraically added to allow for tonus of the ciliary muscle (Amos, 1989). Guidelines for prescribing are given in Chapter 5.

Photorefraction

Photorefraction is a procedure that uses adapted photographic equipment to evaluate the refractive status of the eye (Duckman, 1990). Although it holds great promise as a screening and diagnostic tool, it requires extensive skill and training to interpret the photographic crescents. The cost of the commercially available apparatus necessary for this procedure is prohibitive for most practices. Duckman (1990) includes a description of his set-up for those interested in exploring the procedure further.

SYSTEM VIII: INTERNAL OCULAR HEALTH

The internal structures must be inspected ophthalmoscopically. The ideal time for inspection is when the infant is drowsy or being bottle fed. Either of these states places the infant in a sedate condition. This makes it possible for the examiner to inspect various regions of the posterior segment. An alert, attentive infant will stare directly into the light, making it difficult to observe anything other than the macular area. The monocular indirect ophthalmoscope affords the best composite view of the fundus. It is best to instruct the parent to hold the infant in the crook of the arm. When the infant is uncooperative, restraint may be necessary. This is usually accomplished by having the parent hold the arms and legs while the examiner controls the infant's head.

When doing binocular indirect ophthalmoscopy, a yellow condensing lens reduces the discomfort of the bright light. The infant's direction of gaze can be changed by the movement of a finger puppet held by an assistant in view of the opposite eye.

When ophthalmoscopy must be performed but the infant is uncooperative, the examination may need to be performed under sedation. One method for accomplishing this is chloral hydrate sedation. A disposable syringe may be loaded with the solution and squeezed into the infant's mouth (Press et al, 1982). This procedure can only be done in consultation with a physician and is reserved for circumstances in which the fundi cannot be viewed in any other manner.

With parental assistance, most infants can be propped up for biomicroscopic evaluation (Figure 3.11). Hand-held slit lamps are available that facilitate biomicroscopy and gonioscopy on infants (see Appendix A). Procedural considerations are similar to those discussed above. Tonometry is best performed with portable applanation tonometers. Models are available that provide valid readings when the infant is applanated on the sclera rather than requiring apical corneal pressure.

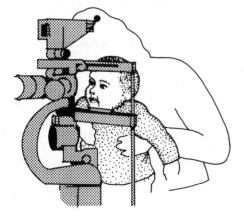

Figure 3.11 Infant propped up by parent for biomicroscopic evaluation.

REFERENCES

Amos D. Cycloplegic refraction. In Bartlett JD, Jaanus SD, eds. Clinical ocular pharmacology, 2d ed. Boston: Butterworth–Heinemann, 1989;426.

Aslin RN. Development of smooth pursuit in human infants. In: Fisher DF, Monty RA, Senders JW, eds. Eye movements: Cognition and visual perception. Hillsdale, N.J.: Lawrence Erlbaum Associates, 1981;31–51.

Aslin RN. Anatomical constraints on oculomotor development: Implications for infant perception. In Yonas A, ed. Perceptual development in infancy. The Minnesota symposia on child psychology, vol. 20. Hillsdale, N.J.: Lawrence Erlbaum Associates, 1988;67–104.

Banks MS. The development of visual accommodation during early infancy. Child Devel 1980;51:646–666.

Behrman RE, Vaughan VC. Nelson textbook of pediatrics, 12th ed. Philadelphia: W.B. Saunders, 1983;19.

Bodis-Wollner I, Atkin A, Raab E, et al. Visual association cortex and vision in man: Pattern-evoked occipital potentials in a blind boy. Science 1977;198:629–631.

Braddick O, Atkinson J. The development of binocular function in early infancy. In Hyvarinen L, Lindstedt E, eds. Early visual development: Normal and abnormal. Acta Ophthalmol 1983;(suppl)157:27–35.

Campos EC, Chiesi C. Critical analysis of visual function evaluating techniques in newborn babies. Intnl Ophthalmol 1985;8:25–31.

Cron MJ, Garzia R, Richman J. Infant visual development. J Optom Vis Devel 1986;17(1):6–18.

Dobson V, McDonald MA, Kohl P, et al. Visual acuity screening of infants and children with the acuity card procedure. J Am Optom Assoc 1986;57:284–289.

Dobson V, Teller DY. Visual acuity in infants: A review and comparison of behavioral and electrophysiological studies. Vision Res 1978;18:1469–1483.

Duckman R. Using photorefraction to evaluate refractive error, ocular alignment, and accommodation in infants, toddlers, and mentally handicapped children. In Scheiman MM, ed. Problems in optometry: Pediatric Optometry, 1990;2:333–353.

Erhardt RP. Developmental visual dysfunction. Tucson: Therapy Skill Builders, 1990;47.

Eskridge JB, Wick B, Perrigin D. The Hirschberg test: A double-masked clinical evaluation. Am J Optom Physiol Opt 1988;65:745–750.

Eviatar L, Miranda S, Eviatar A, et al. Development of nystagmus in response to vestibular stimulation in infants. Ann Neurol 1979;5:508–514.

Fantz RL, Ordy JM, Udelf MS. Maturation of pattern vision in infants during the first six months. J Compar Physiol Psych 1962;55:907–917.

Fulton AB, Robb RM. Special diagnostic and therapeutic modalities in pediatric ophthalmology. In Martyn LJ, ed. The pediatric clinics of North America: Pediatric Ophthalmology 1987;34:1543–1553.

Gesell A, Ilg FL, Bullis GE. Vision: Its development in infant and child. New York: Harper and Brothers, 1949.

Glaser JS. Missed diagnoses in pediatric neuro-ophthalmology. Am Orthop J 1975;25:18–26.

Gwiazda J, Brill S, Mohindra I, et al. Preferential looking acuity in infants from two to fifty-eight weeks of age. Am J Optom Physiol Opt 1980;57:428–432.

Hoyt CS, Jastozebski G, Marg E. Delayed visual maturation in infancy. Br J Ophthalmol 1983;67:127–130.

Hoyt CS, Nickel BJ, Billson FA. Ophthalmological examination of the infant: Developmental aspects. Surv Ophthalmol 1982;26:177–189.

Hyvarinen L, Lindstedt E. Assessment of vision in children. Stockholm: SRF Tal and Punkt, 1981;17.

Keltner JL. Neuro-ophthalmology for the pediatrician. Ped Annals 1977;6:78–127.

Lewerenz DC. Visual acuity and the developing visual system. J Am Optom Assoc 1978;49:1155–1160.

Marg E, Freeman DN, Peltzman P, et al. Visual acuity development in human infants: Evoked potential measurements. Invest Ophthalmol 1976;15:150.

Martin LJ. The pupil. In Isenberg SJ, ed. The eye in infancy. Chicago: Year Book Medical Publishers, 1989;362.

Mohindra I. Developmental inventory for infants and young children. Optom Monthly 1979;70:505–509.

Mohindra I. Comparison of near retinoscopy and subjective refraction in adults. Am J Optom Physiol Opt 1977;54:319–322.

Mohn G, van Hof-van Duin J. Development of the binocular and monocular visual fields of human infants during the first year of life. Clin Vision Sci 1986;1:51–64.

Press LJ. STYCAR ball acuity in relation to contrast and blur. Am J Optom Physiol Opt 1982;59:128–134.

Press LJ, Cummings RW, Siegfried JB, et al. Electrodiagnostic testing of visually impaired children under sedation. J Vis Impairment and Blindness 1982;76:129–132.

Riordan-Eva P. Special subjects of pediatric interest. In Vaughn D, Asbury T, Tabbara KF, eds. General ophthalmology, 12th ed. Norwalk, Conn.: Appleton and Lange, 1989; 330.

Saint-Anne Dargassies S. The neuro-motor and psycho-affective development of the infant. Amsterdam: Elsevier, 1986;95.

Schwartz TL, Dobson V, Sandstrom DJ, et al. Kinetic perimetry assessment of binocular visual field shape and size in young infants. Vision Res 1987;27:2163–2175.

Sheridan MD. STYCAR vision. Windsor, Eng.: NFER-Nelson, 1976;32–34.

Sheridan MD. Vision screening of very young or handicapped children. Br Med J 1960; 2:453–456.

Sokol S, Dobson V. Pattern reversal visually evoked potentials in infants. Invest Ophthalmol 1976;15:58.

Sokol S, Moskowitz A. Comparison of pattern VEP's and PL behavior in 3 month-old infants. Invest Ophthalmol Vis Sci 1985;26:359–365.

Stebbins A. Clinical assessment of the PL 20/20 infant vision tester. J Am Optom Assoc 1986;57:465–469.

Teller DY, Morse R, Borton R, et al. Visual acuity for vertical and diagonal gratings in human infants. Vision Res 1974;14:1433–1439.

Tongue AC, Cibis GW. Bruckner test. Ophthalmology 1981;88:1041–1044.

Tsutusi J, Kimura H, Fukai S. Binocular facilitation of VECP and binocular disparity. Doc Ophthalmol 1982; (Proc Series) 31:399–405.

Vurpillot E. The visual world of the child. New York: International Universities Press, 1976;274.

Wesson MD, Mann KR, Bray NW. A comparison of cycloplegic refraction to the near retinoscopy technique for refractive error determination. J Am Optom Assoc 1990;61:680–684.

Westall CA, Woodhouse JM, Brown VA. OKN asymmetries and binocular function in amblyopia. Ophthal Physiol Opt 1989;9:269–276.

Woodruff ME. A systems examination of the infant's visual function. J Am Optom Assoc 1973;45:410–415.

4

Examination of the Preschool Child

Leonard J. Press

In the course of examining the preschool child, defined for purposes of this text as being between the ages of 3 and 6 years, the patient's subjective awareness can be studied. Case history is still conducted principally through a parent or guardian, however, as reviewed in Chapter 1.

The pediatric optometrist should take measures to insure that the child's initial visit to the office is an enjoyable experience (McMonnies, 1979). It is prudent not to bring the child directly in to the doctor; rather, have a distinct children's pretesting room, discussed in detail in Chapter 21, with an assistant who greets the child and says, "Hi Joey, my name is Evelyn. We have a special room for you to play some games in; would you like to see it?"

The pretesting involves a station for random dot stereopsis, Farnsworth D-15 color caps, and the Keystone Peek-A-Boo Telebinocular Series for eye coordination and fusion. After the assistant's initial contact is completed, review the results as well as the history sheet completed by the parent. The assistant then introduces the child to the doctor.

It is generally preferable for the parent or guardian to accompany the child into the examination room. The decor of the examination room should be inviting and warm to children. A child's booster chair should be placed onto the examination chair. The doctor should greet the child and say: "Hi Joey, my name is Dr. Press, and we're going to play some games today. We have a special chair for you to sit in over here!" If the child is hesitant, have him sit in mother's lap.

The balance of this chapter will follow a systems approach to examination similar to that found in Chapter 3. The sequencing of the exam follows a procedure more like that used for adults in which visual acuity is assessed immediately on completion of the case history.

SYSTEM I: VISUAL ACUITY

Acuity testing generally begins under binocular conditions. When proceeding to monocular testing, the child may resist being occluded. To allay concerns about the object that is approaching their face, refer to the occluder as a lollipop or soup spoon. If the child continually peeks, the elastic band patch is used. Another way to accomplish occlusion is by putting on the "magic red and green glasses." The examiner can then insert a red filter on the green side to achieve cancellation.

There are many visual acuity tests available for use with preschoolers. The results obtained with the various tests are not directly comparable but may be loosely subdivided into three categories: resolution, detection, or recognition acuity (Richman, 1990). Attempt some measure of resolution acuity with letters or numbers as the optimal goal. Since the advent of the television program, "Sesame Street," a surprising number of preschoolers have reliable knowledge of the alphabet. Ask the parent if the child is familiar with alphabet letters. If there is any doubt, proceed to the Lighthouse Picture Cards.

The thought process in the preference for test selection also follows the suggestion by Marsh-Tootle (1991) to categorize acuity tests according to cognitive abilities as basic, medium, or advanced. Begin with advanced tests and retreat to more basic tests if it is apparent that the child does not understand the more advanced tests. When the child is insecure, basic tests may be selected first to make the child more at ease. When monitoring amblyopia, a combination of tests is desirable and should be used consistently to monitor acuity so that *apples are compared to apples.*

Bock Candy Bead Test

The use of candy beads provides a gross estimate of visual acuity at nearpoint (Bock, 1960). It is a task that one can administer when preferential looking and picture cards are unsuccessful. Candy bead cake decorations (nonpareils) are commercially available in food stores (Figure 4.1). The examiner places a couple of beads in one palm, leaving the other palm empty. The examiner extends both palms and asks the child if he would like some candy. By the age of 18 months, the child who can resolve the candy bead will reach for it with pincer grasp. Be less concerned with the

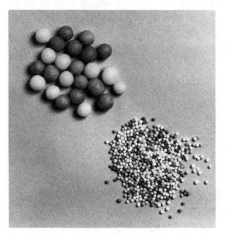

Figure 4.1 Candy beads, commercially available in food stores, used for visual acuity testing.

accuracy of the motor movement and more interested in the visual confirmation that the beads were seen. If vision is poor, the child will look toward one or both palms with equal disinterest.

It has been estimated that candy beads held at 40 cm approximates a Snellen equivalent of 20/285 (Frenkel & Evans, 1980; Richman & Garzia, 1983), rendering this an insensitive but useful test of acuity. To extend the procedure and to further differentiate between the two eyes, one can obtain different size beads from a candy shop. With the parent's permission, a bead that is spotted can be given to the child to eat as an operant conditioning procedure.

Dot Acuity Test

This test is a more sophisticated version of the Bock Candy Bead Test. Introduced by Kirschen and colleagues (1983), it is similar to the Solo Dot Test developed by Sheridan (1976) as part of the Sheridan Tests for Young Children and Retardates (STYCAR) battery of vision tests. It consists of isolated dots in progressively smaller sizes to which children point.

STYCAR Miniature Toys

As was reviewed in Chapter 3, STYCAR consists of toys familiar to preschoolers—a series of chairs, dolls, airplanes, and silverware (Figure 4.2). Sheridan (1969) estimated that differential resolution of the larger fork and spoon at 10 feet is equivalent to 20/30 acuity. The STYCAR series of pediatric vision tests is an excellent clinical tool that is underused in the United States in part because its distribution is limited to a source in England (see Appendix A).

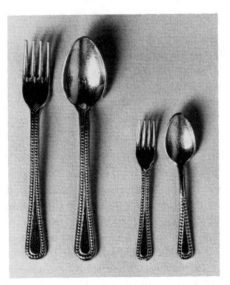

Figure 4.2 Two different-sized sets of toy silverware as used in the STYCAR battery for visual acuity testing.

Lighthouse Picture Cards

This series consists of three pictures, an apple, a house, and an umbrella (Figure 4.3). A key feature of these cards is that they are universally recognized by this age group. Each picture appears in a Snellen subtense ranging from 20/200 to 20/10. The Snellen fraction on the card is designed for 20 feet although the test is usually administered at 10 feet to maximize the child's attention. If the card is moved inward for the child to identify it, the test distance becomes the numerator. For example, if the card marked 20/50 is identified at 5 feet, the acuity should be recorded as 5/50 (20/200 Snellen equivalent).

The use of isolated symbols tends to mask amblyopia. Although the experienced examiner can sense a difference in the speed or reliability of response between the two eyes, some may prefer to use a setup such as the Goodlight box which houses the Lighthouse Picture Symbols in a whole chart format yet permits isolation of lines or symbols.

Allen Picture Symbols

Allen symbols are similar to the Lighthouse pictures but are abstract and require visual closure. When the child's response is poor, one must take into consideration the degree to which the perceptual skill involved is too demanding for the child's cognitive ability. There are many other commercially available picture tests, as reviewed by Fern and Manny (1986).

Mayer and Gross (1990) introduced a simple modification of the Allen pictures that induces contour interaction similar to Snellen acuity. This is accomplished by the symmetrical placement of bars in octagonal configuration surrounding the picture symbol.

Bailey-Hall Cereal Test

This picture card test is designed primarily for use with children between 18 months and 3 years of age (Bailey & Hall, 1984). At each acuity level, there is a matched pair of cards, one with a round piece of cereal and the other with a square box (Figure 4.4). Operant conditioning can be employed by allowing the child to eat a Cheerio or Froot Loop when he points to the correct cereal card.

Broken Wheel Test

Richman and associates (1984) introduced a combination picture card/Landolt "C" test, where the Landolt "C"s are in the form of *broken wheels* on a car (Figure 4.5). The test is designed to be administered at 3 meters (10 feet). The range of acuity tested is 20/100 to 20/20. For each Snellen-equivalent card with broken wheels, there is a paired card with good wheels. Beginning with the 20/100 card, the examiner holds the pair and asks the child to point to the car with the broken wheels. Children begin to respond well to this test at 3 years of age (McDonald and

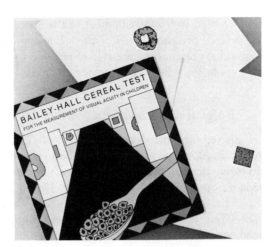

Figure 4.3 One of the pictures used in the Lighthouse acuity card series, each with a Snellen designation for use at a 10-foot test distance.

Figure 4.4 The Bailey-Hall cereal test. Beyond the limit of resolution, the card with the cereal is indistinguishable from the card with the box.

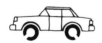

Figure 4.5 The broken wheel test. Beyond the limit of resolution, the gap in the broken wheel cannot be differentiated from a paired card containing a car with unbroken wheels.

Chaudry, 1989). It is more sensitive than other picture cards in detecting subtle differences in acuity between the two eyes as well as in determining if prescriptive lenses improve acuity.

Tumbling E

The Tumbling E is a widely used acuity test for preschoolers though acknowledged to be confounded by the requirement of directional knowledge. Even when using a plastic demonstrator "E," some children lack the dexterity or cognition to match directional orientation in space. It is helpful to have the parent practice this at home with the child before an office visit. There are several similar directional tests, one using a hand, another using the Landolt "C." Among preliterate acuity tests, results with directional tests are relatively inconsistent (Schmidt, 1991).

STYCAR Letter Chart

To establish developmental trends, Sheridan (1963) investigated the early letter identification patterns among thousands of preschoolers. She noted a relationship between graphomotor skills and the earliest letters children could reproduce (Table

4.1). This led to the development of the Sheridan-Gardner HOTV chart, the most widely used preschool letter chart in England and the United States. An additional reason that preschoolers are able to respond to this test at a young age is that there is no confusion when the letters are reversed.

B-VAT II (Binocular-Visual Acuity Tester)

A recently introduced device, the B-VAT II (marketed by Mentor, Inc., see Appendix A), seems to combine the best features of all the just described tests. This electronic device operates through a hand-controller that instantaneously changes pediatric optotypes on a video monitor. The optotypes include four alternative forced choice bar gratings, Allen symbols, tumbling Es, an "O"/"C" version of the Broken Wheel Test, numbers, HOTV letters, and contour interaction bars. In addition, the hand controller has an LED (light emitting diode) that allows the examiner to know what is on the screen yet remain facing the child. This is a distinct advantage when trying to monitor the child who peeks when monocularly occluded. Moreover the randomization in presentation of optotypes prevents the child from memorizng the presentations. It is easy to direct children's attention to a TV screen, but the ability to interpose an animated fixation bear on the screen quickly helps maintain interaction even with children who are attention deficient. This is a very efficient system as well as a good practice management tool.

Contrast Sensitivity

Contrast sensitivity testing has become more common with adults but has yet to be extended to the routine testing of children. Several tests hold promise in this regard. The Horse and Zebras Test (Maione et al, 1983) is a forced-choice test similar to the Bailey-Hall Cereal Test. The stripes of the zebra serve as the contrast sensitivity pattern. When the stripes can no longer be resolved, the zebra is indistinguishable from the horse. More recently, Regan (1988) modified visual acuity charts for children to allow low contrast visual acuity testing. The B-VAT II system includes options for contrast sensitivity testing.

Table 4.1 Sheridan's developmental timetable of graphomotor skills

Graphomotor Skill	Letters	Age (years)
Vertical stroke	—	2
Horizontal stroke	L,H,T	2.5
Copies a circle	O,C	3
Copies a cross	X	4
Copies a square	U	5
Copies a triangle	A,V	5.5

MD Sheridan, STYCAR Vision, Windsor, Eng.: NFER-Nelson, 1976.

SYSTEM II: REFRACTIVE STATE
Keratometry

The child is advised that when he peeks inside the hole he will magically see a picture of his eye. This usually reassures the child that nothing uncomfortable will happen from use of this ominous instrument. Most older children find this fun although some describe the view as "gross."

Retinoscopy
Distance
Use of a video cassette player/television setup in the examination room with cartoons or films of interest is helpful in maintaining distance fixation (Fisher, 1981). A sample of the banter is, "Daniel, do you know who's out there in the TV set? That's right—it's Big Bird! I can't see when Big Bird finds Snuffalufagus because my back is turned. Will you let me know as soon as you see him?" Lens racks can be used as they are with infants, but many preschoolers are ready to sit behind the phoroptor.

Nearpoint
One can begin to obtain additional information from the variety of nearpoint retinoscopies at these ages by using appropriate nearpoint targets (Kenitz, 1987). The MEM cards contain Allen picture symbols for preschoolers. Procedures for MEM retinoscopy are reviewed in detail in Chapter 5. Book retinoscopy can be done with comic or picture books. Apell and Lowry (1959) differentiated characteristic responses of children from two to five years of age (Table 4.2).

Subjective Refraction

The examiner must learn to communicate using the vocabulary that preschoolers use. As an example, most preschoolers do not have the word *blur* in their vocabulary but understand the concept of *fuzzy*. After having done retinoscopy, the appropriate lenses are placed in a trial frame. A convenient and comfortable arrangement for loose lenses is to cut the bottom of a P-3 zyl frame (Figure 4.6). Insert + 2.00 lenses in excess of the retinoscopy value; instruct the child to look into the distance and say, "Do you see what this looks like now? That's what we mean by *fuzzy*. If the pictures look fuzzy, let me know." Many children do not react to blur, but simply hesitate or stop responding when things are not clear. Suggested guidelines for prescribing based on the refraction are discussed in Chapter 12.

SYSTEM III: OCULAR MOTILITY

Eye movements may be subdivided into six essential categories: (1) position maintenance, (2) smooth pursuit, (3) saccadic, (4) vergence, (5) vestibulo-ocular, and (6) optokinetic nystagmus. The clinical investigation of these functions is discussed in

Table 4.2 Developmental characteristics of book retinoscopy

Age (years)	Motion	Range	Release
2	Against of − .25 to − .50 when searching	− .25 to − .50	With motion when looks to examiner
2.5	Against of − .50 to − .75 when searching	− .50 to − .75	With motion when looks to examiner
3	Against of − .25 when searching; more against with pointing	− .25 to − 1.00	With motion + .50 to + 1.00 when looks to examiner
3.5	More against when searching; less against when finding	Nonspecific	Poor with motion when looks to examiner
4	Less against when searching; more against when pointing	− .25 to − .75	Plano to + .50 when looks to examiner
5	With or slow transition to against	− .25 to − .75	May not release to examiner

After RJ Apell, RW Lowry, Preschool vision (St. Louis: American Optometric Association, 1959).

Chapter 3, and applies equally to preschoolers. The two categories bearing amplification in this age range are position maintenance and smooth pursuit.

Position Maintenance

In addition to a finger puppet, accurate fixation can be attained by asking the child to "blow out the light" of a penlight. A variation of this technique, which also serves as an icebreaker if the child is poorly responsive, is to press the penlight onto your finger from behind. This illuminates your cuticle. After demonstrating this to the

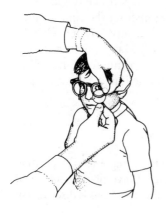

Figure 4.6 A P-3 zyl that has been cut at the bottom to allow insertion of loose trial lenses.

child, say, "Look how I made my finger light up like magic, Johnny; can you make yours light up too?" Intense fixation can be observed as the child reaches to touch the light with his finger and make it glow.

Position maintenance can also be determined by the same technique used to investigate fixation status in amblyopia. Using the Welch-Allyn ophthalmoscope, the examiner shines the target containing the hole inside the grid onto his palm and says, "Do you see this hole inside my hand? Touch it. Good! When I shine this light into your eye, I want you to aim your eye into the middle of that hole and keep it as still as you can, just like you were pointing to it." Often a fine nystagmus can be detected in this manner that escapes detection otherwise.

Smooth Pursuits
Penlight pursuits follow a developmental continuum in behavior (Apell & Lowry, 1959; Getman, 1987). This is outlined in Table 4.3.

SYSTEM IV: BINOCULAR VISION
Heterophoria

One can obtain a measurement of the phoria by using a combination Risley rotary prism and red Maddox rod (Bernell Corp., see Appendix A). Shine a penlight on the midline with the rotary prism/Maddox rod held before one eye and ask, "Do you see a white ball and a red stick? Good. Is the stick touching the ball?" If the answer is yes, orthophoria is indicated. If it is no, the examiner rotates the prism until the child first reports that the stick is touching the ball. This should be done at distance as well as near and in the vertical as well as the horizontal direction.

Table 4.3 Developmental characteristics of penlight pursuits

Age 2 years
Follows briefly with eyes leading head and releases. May be aware of light w/o looking directly at it.

Age 2.5 years
Eyes lead head and may follow up to ½ circle.

Age 3 years
Follows best in horizontal and vertical meridians. Follows a ½ cycle and releases to examiner. Cannot inhibit head movements.

Age 3.5 years
May be tense and momentary like 2.5 yrs. or more sustained like 4 years.

Age 4 years
Follows ½ to 1 cycle with eyes leading head. Inhibits head movement.

Age 5 years
Horizontal and vertical meridians are good, Oblique meridians done in stairstep fashion.

After RJ Apell, RW Lowry, Preschool vision (St. Louis: American Optometric Association, 1959).

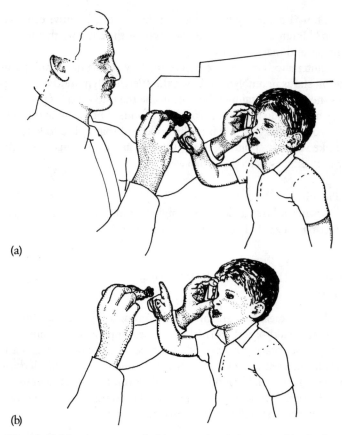

(a)

(b)

Figure 4.7 (a) Child points to actual object as prism is interposed in the front of one eye. (b) Child points toward upper diplopic image of target created by base down prism.

Vergence Range

The prism bar is used to determine the limits of convergence and divergence. It is helpful to use an illuminated fixation target so that one can observe corneal light reflexes. Before introducing the prism bar, place a loose vertical prism of 20 diopters in front of one eye to confirm that the child understands what it means to see double. If he does not have the ability to confirm that he sees two verbally, ask him to touch both targets (Figure 4.7) or watch as he looks back and forth to check out each image. Any of these observations will suffice in determining that the limit of fusion has been reached as the prism bar is moved in base-in and base-out directions.

Nearpoint of Convergence

The convergence nearpoint (CNP) can be elicited easily with a target of interest. A finger puppet can be used, and the examiner says, "Watch Big Bird—he's going to come closer and kiss your nose." As you touch the bridge of the nose with the puppet, make a kiss sound.

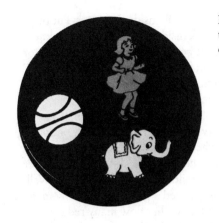

Figure 4.8 Bernell 3-figure anaglyphic flashlight target. The basketball is white, the girl is red, and the elephant is green.

Suppression

There are numerous ways to monitor suppression specifically adapted to pre-schoolers. One simple anaglyphic test is the Bernell 3-Figure flashlight, which is a pediatric version of the Worth-4-Dot (Figure 4.8). It contains a white ball, red girl, and green elephant. Another suitable target is the Mother Goose polarized vectogram. Lastly there are several stereoscope test series for preschoolers such as Keystone's Peek-A-Boo cards and Bernell's kindergarten set (see Appendix A).

Stereopsis

At present, the most commonly used tests of stereopsis are the Random Dot E (RDE) and the Titmus Stereo Fly. The stereograms that do not employ the random dot principle have a drawback in that they can be identified even when the child has small angle strabismus. Their advantage lies in the ease of gaining a response to the test by pointing. The random dot tests are potentially confounded by the fact that they require figure-ground capabilities.

Rosner and Rosner (1990) have an excellent discussion on the clinical administration and interpretation of stereoacuity testing with young children. The TNO random dot test is very good. The higher stereoacuity values are represented by a Pac-Man figure. The child can be asked which way Pac-Man's mouth is going. A demonstrator card comes with the binder that the child can use in a matching response format. As will be discussed in Chapter 20, this game is an integral part of our pretesting routine. A useful guide for normative clinical values of stereopsis is 150 seconds of arc at 3 to 4 years, 70 seconds at 4 to 5 years, and 40 seconds at 5 to 8 years (Reading, 1983).

SYSTEM V: OCULAR HEALTH
Dialogue for Ophthalmoscopy

The inspection of ocular health in preschoolers mirrors the procedure of infants but differs in the extent to which the child can be a cooperative subject. It is an awkward feeling for young children to have someone look inside their eyes. Put them at ease by using banter like, "Tanya, I'm going to look inside your eye—and you know what? If you look at the cake across the room, I'll be able to tell what you had for breakfast today. There it is—I think I see it! Did you have cereal for breakfast today?"

Another technique to engage distance fixation during ophthalmoscopy makes use of the birthday cake on the American Optical (AO) picture chart. Project the 20/200 birthday cake split with the bichrome slide into half red and half green. Proceed with, "Janie, I'm going to ask you a tricky question. Are you ready? Look at the cake and tell me—how candles you see out there? Good! There are three. Now comes the tricky part. How many red candles are there? [Most children will answer 'two'.] How many green candles are there? [Most children will answer 'one'.] Well, that's what I used to think. But once upon a time I asked a girl your age how many candles there were, and she said 'three.' And then I asked her how many red candles, and she said 'none;' and I asked her how many green candles there were, and she said 'none.' So I said—wait a minute! You told me there were three candles out there. How could there be no red or green candles? And do you know what she said? All the candles are black!" This technique procures all the time you'll need for distance fixation.

Dialogue for Biomicroscopy

A good number of preschoolers are cooperative for biomicroscopy. If you have handles on the side of the vertical bars that center the chin rest, tell the child to hold onto the handle bars and make believe that he is riding a bike. It is helpful to have the child sit on his knees so that his head can be gently held forward against the head rest.

SYSTEM VI: VISION DEVELOPMENT

Vision develops in a continuum through the integration of central visual processing (perceptuocognitive function) with peripheral visual processing (ocular-motor performance). The earlier systems in this chapter are predominantly peripheral in nature. This section deals with vision development predominantly central in nature. Specifically it addresses the acquisition and use of visual skills in the context of the child's behavioral growth.

General Development

Among the many developmental screening tests introduced, one of the more popular ones remains the Denver Developmental Screening Test (see Appendix A). There are four sections in this test, Personal/Social, Fine Motor/Adaptive, Language, and Gross Motor. The Fine Motor/Adaptive section contains items that are of interest in rating the child's level of visual development (Table 4.4).

This test is useful not only because it gives the optometrist a percentile metric for developmental milestones but also because it affords a common language with pediatricians and allied developmental practitioners.

Table 4.4 Fine-motor adaptive development in the DDST

	Age Level
Ocular pursuit	
Follows to the midline	1 month
Follows past the midline	2 months
Follows 180 degrees	3 months
Visual-motor	
Grasps rattle	4 months
Passes cube hand to hand	6 months
Bangs two cubes together	10 months
Eye-hand coordination	
Pincer grasp of raisin	12 months
Scribbles spontaneously	15 months
Tower of two cubes	17 months
Tower of four cubes	20 months
Imitates vertical line	24 months
Tower of eight cubes	26 months
Imitates bridge	3.0 years
Copies a circle	3.0 years
Picks longer of two lines	3.5 years
Draws man—3 parts	4.5 years
Draws man—6 parts	5.0 years
Copies a square	5.5 years

Age level indicates times at which 75 percent of children attain function.

Visual-Motor Development

The visual-motor model of development leads one to clinically probe the balance between vision and development throughout childhood. Although speech and language play a role in this model, it has become labelled a visual-motor model. Getman was a pioneer in this field and delineated the developmental hierarchy in which early movement patterns are integrated with vision (Getman, 1987) (Table 4.5).

1. Hand
2. Hand-eye
3. Motor-visual (motor predominates)
4. Motor-visual
5. Visual-motor

Table 4.5 Profile of clinical tests to follow visual-spatial development ages 2–9

Factors	Area Probed	Clinical Tests
Body knowledge and control	Relative integrity of the invariant (egocentric localization)	Standing angels Chalkboard circles 3:3 alternate hop Draw-a-person test
Bimanual integration and/or ability to cross midline	Knowledge of oneself as a bilateral being	Circus puzzle Pegboard test copy forms
Form matching or reproduction	Spatial organization and manipulation	Circus puzzle Pegboard test Copy forms
Visualized reversals	Rotation of space	Pegboard test
Organization	Visual planning in a defined spatial area	Copy forms
Visual-motor hierarchy	Transition from ego to oculocentric localization	Circus puzzle Pegboard test Copy forms

Adapted from IB Suchoff, Visual spatial development in the child: An optometric theoretical and clinical approach (New York: State University of New York, State College of Optometry, 1975).

6. Visual-motor (visual predominates)
7. Visual-language-action (visual predominates)

Getman elaborated this developmental continuum with renewed emphasis on retinoscopic observations of the visual response. This model relies heavily on qualitative observations to the point that it almost eschews quantitative, age-related normative data (Figures 4.9, 4.10, and 4.11). One should not make the mistake, however, of thinking that evaluative criteria based on qualitative observations are less significant than are quantitative observations.

Visual-Spatial Development

Suchoff (1975) first called attention to the fact that studies investigating the looking preference of infants created the need for distinction between stimuli that reflexively captures the infant and the later, purposeful use of vision in the process of conceptualization. Incorporating the principles of Piagetian development, he developed a clinical approach to visual-perceptual development relying heavily on motoric and cognitive skills (Table 4.5). The areas of evaluation probe the relative state of the invariant (egocentric localization), the body schema, and the ability to organize and manipulate visual space (oculocentric localization).

The Getman and Suchoff approaches share much in common. The reader is encouraged to obtain copies of their monographs (referenced at the end of this

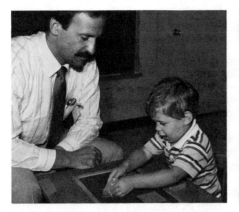

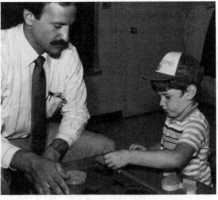

Figure 4.9 The three-figure form board. Placement of the triangle, square, and circle can be accomplished by age two. Observations include the use of one or both hands, visual versus tactile placement, and crossing of the midline.

Figure 4.10 The six-figure form board. Placement of the forms can be accomplished by age three. The divided form board in which each figure comes in two parts can be accomplished by age six.

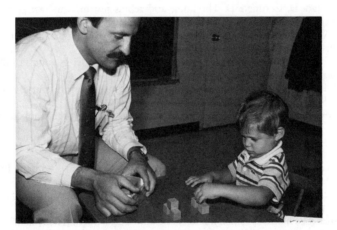

Figure 4.11 One-inch cube used to build a bridge. The three-cube bridge is accomplished by age three.

chapter). They offer loose normative data that are very useful for evaluating visual development in the preschool years. Getman relies more heavily on qualitative retinoscopic data to infer the visual response. The individual pediatric optometrist will adopt one of these approaches to enable the analysis of ocular-motor and refractive data to be coupled with a visual-perceptual profile. This becomes paramount in following the child's development into the school age years (see Chapter 5) and in considering the interrelationship of vision and school performance (see Chapter 6).

REFERENCES

Apell RJ, Lowry RW. Preschool vision. St. Louis: American Optometric Association, 1959.

Bailey IL, Hall AP. New visual acuity tests for children. Am J Optom Physiol Opt 1984;61:962–965.

Bock RH. Amblyopia detection in the practice of pediatrics. Arch Pediatr 1960;77:335–339.

Fern KD, Manny RE. Visual acuity of the preschool child: A review. Am J Optom Physiol Opt 1986;319–345.

Fisher NF. An audio-visual distant fixation system for infants and children. J Ped Ophthalmol Strab 1981;18:41–43.

Frenkel M, Evans LE. The nonpareil test of visual acuity in the young and retarded. Ann Ophthalmol 1980;12:811.

Getman GN. Developmental optometry: The optometric appraisal of vision development and visual performance. White Plains, Md.: Research Publications, 1987.

Kenitz S. Examination of the younger pediatric patient. J Wisconsin Optom Assoc 1987;31(2):4–6.

Kirschen DG, Rosenbaum AL, Ballard EA. The dot visual acuity test—a new acuity test for children. J Am Optom Assoc 1983;73:1055–1059.

McDonald M, Chaudry NM. Comparison of four methods of assessing visual acuity in young children. Optom Vis Sci 1989;66:363–369.

McMonnies CW. Optimum conditions for examining children. Aust J Optom 1979;62:368–373.

Maione M, Berfadi D, Cerimele D. The horse and zebras test in visual acuity and contrast sensitivity assessment. Ophthal Ped and Genetics 1983;2:149–152.

Marsh-Tootle WL. Clinical methods of testing visual acuity in amblyopia. In: Rutstein RP, ed. Problems in optometry: Amblyopia 1991; 3(2):208–236.

Mayer DL, Gross RD. Modified Allen pictures to assess amblyopia in young children. Ophthalmology 1990; 97:827–832.

Reading RW. Binocular vision: Foundation and applications. Boston: Butterworth–Heinemann, 1983:199.

Regan D. Low-contrast visual acuity test for pediatric use. Can J Ophthalmol 1988;23:224–227.

Richman JE. Assessment of visual acuity in preschool children. In Scheiman MM, ed. Problems in optometry: Pediatric optometry 1990;2:319–332.

Richman JE, Garzia RP. The bead test: A critical reappraisal. Am J Optom Physiol Opt 1983;60:199–203.

Richman JE, Petito GT, Cron M. Broken wheel acuity test: A new and valid test for preschool and exceptional children. J Am Optom Assoc 1984;55:561–565.

Rosner J, Rosner J. Pediatric optometry. 2nd ed. Boston: Butterworth–Heinemann, 1990;175–203.

Schmidt PP. Comparisons of testability of preliterate visual acuity tests in preschool children. Binoc Vis Quarterly 1991;6:37–42.

Sheridan MD. STYCAR vision. Windsor, Eng.: NFER-Nelson, 1976.

Sheridan MD. Vision screening procedures for very young or handicapped children. In Gardiner P, Mackeith R, Smith V, eds. Aspects of developmental and pediatric ophthalmology. Clinics in Developmental Medicine, No. 32. London: Spastics International Medical Publications, 1969;39–47.

Sheridan MD. Diagnosis of visual defect in early childhood. Brit Orthopt J 1963;20:29–36.

Suchoff IB. Visual spatial development in the child: An optometric theoretical and clinical approach. New York: State University of New York, State College of Optometry, 1975.

5

Examination of the School-Aged Child

Leonard J. Press

Much of the procedural strategy adopted in Chapter 4 on preschoolers can be extended to school-aged children. Major differences that occur are that the child is expected to sit behind the phoroptor and that more specific information can be obtained. This extends to tests of visual-motor performance as well. Another major difference lies in case history and how it steers the course of the examination. Concern about inadequate performance in school will prompt a more extensive investigation of the child's visual-perceptual skills than will concern over failure of an acuity screening in school as was elaborated in Chapter 1. This chapter will follow the systems approach adopted in Chapters 2 and 3.

SYSTEM I: VISUAL ACUITY

For the younger patient, the child's familiarity with the alphabet should be corroborated with the parent before testing begins. It is not uncommon for some children to need a "warm-up." If acuity is better with the second eye tested, the examiner should return briefly to the first eye to recheck acuity.

Some younger children seem unwilling to read beyond a certain line on the Snellen chart. If the child breezes through to the 20/40 line, then stops and says she can't see anything else, the examiner should coax the child, "Come on Susie. You did so well with the other lines. I'll bet you can see some of these letters if you take your time. You can even guess—there's no extra charge!"

SYSTEM II: REFRACTIVE STATE

While the majority of children entering school are hyperopic, there is a shift toward myopia as the child progresses through school (Hirsch & Weymouth, 1991). This is probably due in part to intrinsic anatomic growth factors, in part to genetic programming, and in part to extrinsic environmental forces. This subject is discussed further in Chapter 17 on progressive myopia.

As more practices gravitate toward the use of technicians and assistants, the practitioner will have autorefractor findings available on older children before conducting retinoscopy. Refraction may be conducted under cycloplegic or noncycloplegic conditions. In either event, use of a video player to engage distance fixation during retinoscopy is helpful.

The pharmaceutical agent of choice for school-aged children is 1 percent cyclopentolate preceded by 0.5 percent proparacaine to aid ocular absorption. When the child is averse to drops, forego the proparacaine, and let the child rub the eyes to facilitate absorption. Children with dark pigmentation of the iris as well as those with excessive body weight may require an additional drop within five minutes to allow adequate cycloplegia. Cycloplegic findings are desirable in all instances of esotropia, convergence excess, accommodative spasm, and moderate hyperopia and when reliable findings cannot be obtained in the dry state.

In cases of hyperopia, certain rules of thumb have been proposed for reducing the amount of plus prescribed as compared with the cycloplegic findings (Amos, 1989). As a general rule, more plus is reduced in the distance prescription with higher amounts of hyperopia or if the child is older (Table 5.1).

SYSTEM III: OCULAR MOTILITY

Eye movement control takes on a greater significance with school-aged children because of its potential association with mechanical errors in reading and fine-motor tasks such as copying from a book or blackboard. The two areas of concern are saccadic fixations and pursuits.

Table 5.1 Plus lens correction prescribed for latent hyperopia

Manifest Refraction (D)	Cycloplegic Refraction		
	1.00	2.50	5.00
	Age 5 years		
Plano	0.50	1.25	2.50
1.00	1.00	1.50	2.50
2.00	n/a	2.25	3.00
	Age 12 years		
Plano	0.50	1.00	2.00
1.00	1.00	1.50	2.50
2.00	n/a	2.25	2.75

Modified from DM Amos, Cycloplegic refraction. In D Bartlett, SD Jaanus, eds. Clinical ocular pharmacology, 2d ed. Boston: Butterworth–Heinemann, 1989;428.

Saccadic Fixations

Saccadic fixations are the definitive eye movements used in reading and show clear developmental trends. Saccades are patterns of movement made between fixational pauses as a reader moves along a line of print. Immature readers make more pauses and therefore execute more saccadic fixations per line than do mature readers. The duration of a saccade is approximately 25 msecs. The duration of a fixation is 250 to 350 msecs, increasing progressively throughout childhood. No meaningful information is taken in during the saccade. It is now believed that the function of the saccade is to backward mask the trail of visible persistence from the next fixation. This is considered an interplay between the transient properties of the saccade and the sustained properties of the fixation. Poor readers may see print run together because of an inefficient saccadic mechanism as will be discussed in detail in Chapter 6.

Objective Recording

The definitive instrument to measure saccades objectively is an Eye-Trac (Winter, 1974). This photoelectric device is costly, difficult to maintain, and no longer manufactured. It is unparalleled, however, in its ability to document the nature of saccades and fixational pauses during the act of reading. In addition to the Eye-Trac or its updated counterpart the Vis-A-Graph (Maino & Press, 1988), several clinical tests can be used to test saccades.

The saccades used in reading have been termed *stimulus generated*, whereas the saccades used in near-to-far fixation, as when copying from the board, are considered *voluntary saccadics* (Steele, 1990).

Voluntary Saccades

Wolff wands (Vision Extension, Inc., see Appendix A) are used to probe the accuracy of large-angle saccades. These wands consist of two sticks with a metallic gold ball on the tip of one and a silver ball on the tip of the other (Streff et al, 1985). The wands are held at a distance of 40cm outward from the child's eyes and separated from one another by 40cm held equidistant from the midline. The child is instructed to switch fixation from the gold ball to the silver ball on command approximately ten times. The examiner makes empirical note of the number of times that the child's fixation falls short of the target (undershoots) or beyond the target (overshoots). The scoring systems for saccadic fixations are listed in Table 5.2. Alphabet pencils may be used that are identical to the Wolff wand procedure, with the exception that the child calls out the letters on each pencil. These tests probe voluntary saccadic movement.

Stimulus-Generated Saccades

The Pierce Saccade Test (Bernell Corp., see Appendix A) is similar in concept to the alphabet pencils, but it moves the task from a spatial demand to the plane of the printed page. In addition, the spacing of the numbers becomes progressively tighter on each of the test levels, simulating the progression to smaller print with increasing grade levels. A limitation of these tests is that they only test wide-angle saccades, simulating eye movements that occur when moving from the end of one line to the

Table 5.2 Comparative scoring systems for saccadic fixations

NSU*	SCCO†	Marcus	Heinsen/Schrock
5 Completes 5 round trips with no over shooting or body motion	4+ Smooth and accurate	5 Accurate fixation in all meridians	10 point maximum scale as follows: 3 points possible for quality of head movement
4 Completes 4 round trips with slight over/under shooting or body motion	3+ Slight undershoot	4 Fair landings but slight corrective movements	2 points possible for accuracy
3 Completes 3 round trips with consistent over/undershoot or body motion	2+ Gross undershoot or overshoot or increased latency	3 Accurate fixations on X/Y axis; breaks down on z-axis	2 points possible for automaticity
2 Completes 2 round trips with large over/undershoot or body motion	1+ Inability to do task or increased latency	2 Inequality of fixation performance between the two eyes	2 points possible for stability (20 seconds duration)
1 No attempt made to perform the task to 1 round trip; gross over/undershoot or body motion		0 No rapport with the target	1 point possible for stamina

Adapted from WC Maples, TW Ficlin, A preliminary study of the oculomotor skills of LD, gifted, and normal children. J Optom Vis Devel 1989;20:9–14.
*NSU = Northeastern State University, College of Optometry
†SCCO = Southern California College of Optometry

beginning of the next line (Griffin, 1982). To address this limitation, the King-Devick Test (Bernell Corp., see Appendix A) introduced random spacing of numbers across the line to simulate the fixational pauses that occur with word strings of varying length (Lieberman et al, 1983). These tests are probes of stimulus-generated saccadic movement.

Although the King-Devick Test remains the most commonly used clinical measure of saccades, the entire applicability of tests such as these to saccadic function has been called into question. Claiming that such tests are more related to the developmental skill of rapid automatic naming of numbers than to saccadic function,

Garzia and colleagues (1990) introduced a test to account for this factor, known as the test for developmental eye movements (DEM). By obtaining a ratio between the horizontal and vertical columnar arrangement of numbers, one can differentiate saccadic dysfunction (high ratio) from poorly developed automaticity in number naming (normal ratio).

Pursuits

Pursuits are not as relevant to reading or learning as are saccades. They have more relevance to skills outside the classroom such as gross-motor performance in general and athletic performance in particular. As with saccades, pursuit tasks may be subclassified as stimulus-generated or voluntary. Stimulus-generated pursuits are elicited when the child is instructed to follow a moving target. Voluntary pursuits are elicited when the child is instructed to track a stationary path.

The most commonly used procedure for eliciting stimulus-generated pursuit movement is to ask the child to follow a penlight or a bright object. Movements are done in five axes (Streff et al, 1985): (1) horizontal, (2) vertical, (3) diagonal, (4) rotational, and (5) in-out (z-axis). The examiner notes how accurately the child tracks the target and if the pursuit movement breaks down into anticipatory saccades. Qualitative observations about head movement should be made as well as indications of motor overflow such as tongue movement or postural alteration.

The most commonly used clinical test for voluntary pursuit movement is Groffman Visual Tracings (Mast-Keystone, see Appendix A). This test, in which the child must trace a path visually between a letter on one side of the page and a number on the opposite side of the page, involves a significant degree of visual-perceptual skill in the figure-ground and visualization areas.

SYSTEM IV: BINOCULAR VISION

Depending on the age of the child, more sophisticated tests of binocular vision can be incorporated. Most of the standard tests done through the phoroptor can be administered to school-aged children. Areas probed should include phoria, vergence range, vergence facility and stamina, vergence amplitude (NPC), suppression, and stereopsis.

Heterophoria

The instructional set for lateral phoria is: "I want you to say stop as soon as these two letters are lined up under each other just like buttons on a shirt." For vertical phoria, the instructional set is: "I want you to stay stop as soon as these two letters are lined up side-by-side just like headlights on a car." Younger children and shy ones are slower to respond in which case you must turn the Risley prisms more slowly. On occasion, you will get no response at all in which case you should swing the phoroptor away to demonstrate the procedure. Make two circles with your fingers, hold one above the other, and show the child what it will look like when the two circles are one under the other. If he is unable to tell you when to stop in free space, discontinue the test.

Vergence Range

Procedures are generally the same as they are with adults. Again the Risley prisms should be turned slowly enough to allow time for the child to respond. With younger children, the blur portion of the response will be difficult to elicit.

Vergence Facility and Stamina

This function is the vergence analog of accommodative facility and stamina. As opposed to the slow, sustaining changes of Risley prisms, it measures the accuracy and ability to sustain binocularity when the child changes fixation from the blackboard to the desk and vice versa. It is sometimes difficult for a child to report seeing double. Demonstrate this by holding a vertical prism of 10 diopters that cannot be fused, and reminding the child, "This is what you might see—two pencil tips instead of one, except they'll be side-by-side instead of up and down." Normative values for children have been established (Table 5.3).

Convergence Nearpoint

Many children will find it difficult to maintain convergence inward even though they are capable of doing so. Notice that at several inches from the nose they lose interest in the target and look from the target to your eyes. Remind the child not to

Table 5.3 Vergence facility rates for children on 4 BI/16 BO

Age (yr/mo)	Flips/Min
5/5	7.63
6/6	8.16
7/7	7.49
8/8	9.52
9/9	10.65
10/10	10.97
11/11	11.85
12/12	13.00
13/13	11.63

A Buzzelli, Vergence facility: Developmental trends in a school age population. Am J Optom Physiol Opt 1986;63:351–355.

look anywhere except at the target. In addition, children tend to look away from the target after a breakpoint is elicited and must be reminded to keep looking at the target while it is pulled back out until it snaps back into one.

Suppression

The Worth-4-Dot is the simplest tool to document suppression as well as the easiest with which to demonstrate suppression to the parent. In addition, the interpretation of the response is relatively unequivocal, a key element when testing children. Another convenient target is the Bernell #9 acuity suppression slide (Bernell Corp., see Appendix A) that has one line of print seen exclusively by the right eye and another line exclusively seen by the left eye.

Stereopsis

School-aged children should be capable of performing any of the clinical tests of stereopsis available. Some of the younger children may still need to be given a forced-choice paradigm. Consideration of several tests of stereopsis was given in Chapter 4.

SYSTEM V: ACCOMMODATION
Amplitude

Amplitude is determined clinically by either push-up or minus lens to blur method. Using a modification of the minus lens method, Woodruff and associates (1987) determined representative values for children between the ages of 3 and 11 (Table 5.4). The association between early stages of juvenile onset diabetes and reduced amplitude of accommodation warrants routine testing of amplitude in children (Moss et al, 1987).

Lag

The lag of accommodation can be considered an index of accommodative accuracy. It is principally determined by the monocular estimate method (MEM) of nearpoint retinoscopy. While the child reads the words binocularly on a target clipped onto a retinoscope, the examiner interposes lenses briefly in front of one eye to confirm the estimate of the motion. The mean lag in an elementary school population is +0.35 diopter (Rouse et al, 1984). It is helpful to have MEM flippers available with the four cells comprised of the most commonly expected values, +0.25 through +1.00.

There are many variations of nearpoint retinoscopy. Book retinoscopy (Getman, 1960) is essentially the same as MEM except that the examiner is noting the response as the child continues to read a story. In addition to motion, the brightness and color

Table 5.4 Minimum normal accommodative amplitudes for children

Age (years)	Minus Lens Amplitude (D)*	Hofstetter's Formula†
3	7.7	14.25
4	7.9	14.00
5	8.1	13.75
6	8.3	13.50
7	8.5	13.25
8	8.6	13.00
9	8.8	12.75
10	8.9	12.50
11	8.9	12.25

*ME Woodruff, JV Lovasik, MM Spafford, Ocular accommodation in juvenile diabetics: A preliminary report. Can J Optom 1987;45:146–149.
†J Cooper, Accommodative dysfunction. In JF Amos, ed. Diagnosis and management in vision care. Boston: Butterworth–Heinemann 1987;431–459.

of the reflex lend significance to the response. Brightness signifies the child's readiness to participate. White indicates maximum processing with pink being intermediate and brick red indicating limited processing.

Bell retinoscopy, in which the examiner watches the change in reflex as a silvered bell is brought close to the child and is then receded, is the spatial analog of NRA/PRA. Movement of the target along the z-axis is the parallel of 0.25 diopter changes in the phoroptor. Neutrality should straddle the child's Harmon distance, the distance from the child's first midknuckle to the elbow. With motion should be noted outside the Harmon distance, neutral around the Harmon distance, and against motion inside the Harmon distance.

Facility and Stamina

This test is done with $+/-2.00$ lens flippers and 20/30 numbers. Schlange and Terranova (1986) differentiated normative values for larger size characters. The number of cycles of lens flips per minute that can be cleared is greater when the print is larger. Bernell distributes an Accommodative Rock Card with different-sized letters for this purpose (see Appendix A). Scheiman and colleagues (1988) recorded normative values for monocular and binocular facility for elementary schoolchildren (Table 5.5). The Bernell #9 acuity suppression slide should be used to monitor suppression. Some children hesitate, lose their place, or start again from the beginning of the line as soon as the flippers are turned for reasons unrelated to accommodative demand. These children are simply distracted by the process of flipping rather than by blur, diplopia, or shifting of the letters.

Table 5.5 Normative values for accommodative facility in children

Age (years)	Monocular		Binocular	
	Mean (cycles/min)	SD	Mean (cycles/min)	SD
6	5.5	+/−2.5	3	+/−2.5
7	6.5	+/−2.0	3.5	+/−2.5
8–12	7.0	+/−2.5	5.0	+/−2.5

Haynes (1979) presented preliminary normative data in elementary schoolchildren for near-to-far rock, a crossover between accommodative facility and saccadic fixation. As with lens flippers and most ocular performance tests, the results show an increase in speed that follows a developmental curve, increasing in speed and topping out at the sixth-grade level. The average response time for a near-far-near cycle is 4.5 seconds for grade one, 3.5 seconds for grade three, and 2.5 seconds for grade five. Since this procedure is used in near-to-far Hart charts, a commonly used accommodative rock therapy procedure, normative data is useful.

SYSTEM VI: VISUAL SKILLS AND PERFORMANCE

There are a constellation of findings that do not fall neatly within the 21-point analytical sequence or the systems here outlined, but that are integral to, or useful in, the examination of the school-aged child. Stereoscope screening tests such as the Keystone Visual Skills (Mast-Keystone, see Appendix A) yield important qualitative information not otherwise attainable.

Visual-Spatial Mismatch

After positioning their heads in the stereoscope, some children can be observed to pull their heads out of the instrument to look at the target. This is most often due to their initial inability to resolve the mismatch between the known location of the target in space and the perceived location of the target in the instrument.

Stability and Binocularity

When the child is asked to tell which number the arrow is pointing to, the examiner should inquire if the arrow is still or if it wiggles a lot. The child who reports the arrow floating between several numbers has an instability of fusion that may be difficult to elicit from other tests.

Van Orden Binocular Behavior Pattern

The Van Orden (VO) Binocular Behavior Pattern (Mast-Keystone, see Appendix A) is the VO-2 target in the Keystone Series administered in the Correct-Eye-Scope. The child is instructed to draw a line from the symbol on the side of the sheet to the center of the target. Remind the child to stop when the pencils first look like they touch, not when they feel like they touch. This task not only probes accuracy and stability of binocular projection, but it also presents a complex bilateral integration task of eye-hand coordination.

Cheiroscopic Tracing

This interocular transfer task involves an object seen by one eye being traced onto the paper as guided by the fellow eye. As with the VO pattern, it is sensitive to vertical as well as lateral fusion imbalance. These tests are particularly useful in demonstrating performance of the child to the parent.

SYSTEM VII: COLOR VISION

Much ado has been made of the importance of testing color vision in children. There are three reasons typically given for the routine testing of color vision: (1) early identification of defects to enable alternative instruction in color-coded school materials (Olsen & Harris, 1989), (2) career counseling to educate the older child about occupations that may prove difficult based on the need for fine color discrimination, and (3) early diagnosis of ocular diseases or systemic diseases with ocular manifestations reportedly associated with changes in color perception (Hagerstrom-Portnoy, 1990).

The emphasis on early identification of color vision anomaly is based more on intuition than on comprehensive study. Indeed, studies to date have not supported the notion that color vision deficiency is an educational handicap (Fletcher & Voke, 1985) or that it exists to any greater degree in students manifesting reading or learning disorders (Bleeker & Robertson, 1986). Nevertheless school vision screenings and report forms continue to feature color vision testing.

From a clinical standpoint, school-aged children can respond readily to the Farnsworth D-15 (Bernell Corp., see Appendix A) when it is made into a game. Some children have difficulty placing the color caps in proper order, not because they have a color deficiency but because they are poor perceptually with visual sequential processing. The Ishihara Color Plates (Bernell Corp., see Appendix A) are often administered to children, though not giving as specific a profile of color deficiency as does the Farnsworth D-15. With younger children who may have difficulty with the two-digit number, cover one side of the page so that they can report the single digit. If the figure-ground nature of the task presents difficulty, the child can be given a thin paint brush with which to trace over the number. The child can also be asked to point to specific color dots. Haegerstrom-Portnoy (1990) reviews other color vision tests as well as suggestions for compensation in the classroom when the child is color deficient.

SYSTEM VIII: PERCEPTUAL-MOTOR DEVELOPMENT

In selecting perceptual tests to administer to the school-aged child, the examiner is guided by concerns raised during the taking of the case history or by observations made during prior testing. There are instances where the initial history is unremarkable, but it becomes apparent during testing that the child is lacking in basic perceptual skills. As an example, directional confusion can be noted by handing the child an occluder with instructions to cover the right eye. Children with poor directional skills can be observed to equivocate.

In chapter 4, the concept of vision development in the context of visual-motor and visual-spatial development was addressed. This supplies a foundation that must be extended into a standardized battery of clinical tests. Hoffman (1979) formalized a developmental inventory of perceptual skills predicated on standardized testing that has proven useful in clinical settings. Discussion of the statistical application of tests and measurements is beyond the scope of this section and is fully treated elsewhere (Solan & Suchoff, 1991). When documenting the developmental level of the child's perceptual skills, at least one test should be administered in each of the following principal categories:

1. Gross-motor control and bilateral integration
2. Visual-motor integration and organization
3. Visual-perceptual discrimination and attention
4. Auditory-perceptual discrimination and integration

Gross-Motor Control and Bilateral Integration

The most widespread test of gross-motor performance, common to virtually all developmental profiles, is standing balance. The norms given in Table 5.6 are for the Standing Balance: Eyes Open (SBO) and Eyes Closed (SBC) tests, which are part of the Southern California Sensory Integration Tests developed by Ayres (Western

Table 5.6 Normative values (in secs) for standing balance eyes open (SBO) and eyes closed (SBC)

	Age Level (yrs/mos)				
	4.0–4.5	*4.5–4.11*	*5.0–5.5*	*5.6–5.11*	*6.0–6.5*
SBO	13.7	18.7	24.0	34.4	44.4
SBC	3.3	4.3	5.1	6.5	7.4
	6.6–6.11	*7.0–7.5*	*7.5–7.11*	*8.0–8.5*	*8.6–8.11*
SBO	60.8	75.2	73.1	86.5	113.2
SBC	9.3	9.7	11.3	11.2	12.8

Psychological Services, see Appendix A). The child is asked to stand with arms folded across the chest and then instructed to raise one leg. The examiner scores the number of seconds that the subject can stand on each foot. The total number of seconds recorded for the right and left foot constitutes the score for the test. This is repeated with the child instructed to keep eyes closed. The fact that SBO is significantly greater than SBC underscores the role that vision plays in balance.

Visual-Motor Integration and Organization

The number of tests in this area is legion, but one that has high test-retest reliability is the Beery-Buktenica Developmental Test of Visual-Motor Integration (VMI), widely used and similar in nature to the Winterhaven (Gesell) Copy Forms (Vision Extension, see Appendix A). Both involve the graphomotor task of copying geometric designs. An advantage of the VMI is that its norms are extended to a greater age range than are those of the Copy Forms. A disadvantage of the VMI is that its forms are reproduced within a prescribed space. The copy forms are reproduced onto a blank sheet of paper, and inferences are made based on the pattern of organization with which the child reproduces the forms. As an example, organizing the responses in a vertical row signifies a lower developmental level than does organizing the responses in horizontal rows (Figure 5.1).

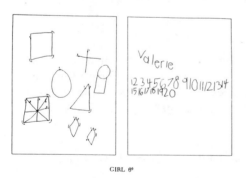

GIRL 6°

Figure 5.1 Samples of on-age performance of Gesell Copy Forms figures. (Used with permission of the publisher from School readiness: Behavior tests used at the Gesell Institute. New York: Harper & Row, 1972.

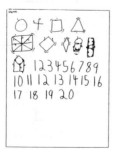

BOY 7ᴬ

There are several other notable tests in the *pencil-and-paper* category. Rosner is a strong proponent of the Test of Visual Analysis Skills (TVAS). This is an updated version of the Visual Analysis Test (Rosner & Fern, 1983), itself an outgrowth of Rosner's Perceptual Skills Curriculum. It is essentially a series of increasingly complex dot-to-dot patterns, closely related to primary grade achievement (Rosner, 1976).

Direct insight into classroom performance can be gained through the Wold Sentence Copy Test. Wold (1970) devised a sentence consisting of 110 letters that the child is instructed to copy. The rate of handwriting in letters per minute is therefore calculated as 6600 divided by the time (in seconds) it takes the child to copy the letters (Table 5.7). In addition, qualitative observations about performance are made (Table 5.8).

Visual-Perceptual Discrimination and Attention

The Motor-Free Visual Perception Test (MVPT) is representative of tests in this category. It probes the areas of spatial orientation, figure-ground, size and shape constancy, visual memory, and visual closure. Its only drawback is that normative data is available only for the overall score and not for the individual subcategories. A standardized test that enables the examiner to generate scores for the individual categories of the MVPT is the Morrison-Gardner Test of Visual-Perceptual Skills (TVPS) (Bernell Corp., see Appendix A). Due to the length of time required to administer the TVPS, the MVPT should be regarded as a screening test and the TVPS as an in-depth analysis of specific subcategories.

The concept of left-right awareness should be addressed directly if persistent reversals and/or directional confusion are among the chief complaints reported by the parent. Among the more useful tests to probe these areas are the Piaget Test of

Table 5.7 Rate of handwriting

Grade	Freeman Letters/minute	Ayres Letters/minute (speed and legibility)
2	30	39.7
3	40	42.0
4	50	45.8
5	60	50.5
6	67	54.5
7	74	58.9
8	80	62.8

From RM Wold, Screening tests to be used by the classroom teacher. Novato, Calif.: Academic Therapy Publications, 1970;4–5.

Table 5.8 Observations during sentence copy test

Factors	Observations
1. Posture	Pencil grip; initial working distance; proximity of working distance overtime; head posture; rotation of paper; motor overflow
2. Number of fixations	Method of reproduction: memory of words or phrases versus frequent refixation to individual letters; ability to keep place while copying.
3. Spacing (figure-ground)	Spacing of letters; sequencing of letters and words.
4. Vocalization or subvocalization	Is each letter or word said aloud while copying?
5. Concentration, attention, and fatigue	Distractibility and on-task time.
6. Formation	Are letters formed correctly?
7. Frustration level	Erasures; self-assessment; neatness over time.
8. Speed	Per formula: Rate of letters per min = 6600/# of secs (see Table 5.7 for grade level resultant).

From RM Wold, Screening tests to be used by the classroom teacher. Novato, Calif.: Academic Therapy Publications, 1970;4–5.

Left-Right (L-R) Concepts and the Jordan Reversal Frequency Test (both are marketed by Bernell Corp., see Appendix A). The Piaget L-R Test investigates the child's ability to differentiate left from right on herself in a mirror-image and as projected onto objects in space (Table 5.9). The Jordan Reversal Frequency Test documents reversal tendency on individual letters and numbers as well as transpositions or reversal of individual letters within words or of words within sentences.

Auditory-Perceptual Discrimination and Integration

There are two primary tests used clinically. The Birch-Belmont Test of Auditory Visual Integration (AVI) (Vision Extension, see Appendix A) is a Morse code-like test in which the child must match a sequential pattern of taps to its pictorial representation (Figure 5.2). Performance is strongly linked to the child's strength in simultaneous versus successive processing skills, a subject more thoroughly explored in Chapter 6.

The Test of Auditory Analysis Skills (TAAS) is a phonics test in which the child is asked to listen to a word, then repeat it with part of the word deleted. As an example the child is instructed to say "stale" and then to repeat the word without the *t*. This ability involves a high level of integration between phonics and visualization. Normative data is available for children between grades K through 3.

Table 5.9 Piaget L-R Test

Administration of test

Section 1: Subject's designation of own parts

Child is asked to show examiner in succession his own: right hand, left leg, right ear, left hand, right leg, left ear.

Section 2: Subject's designation of examiner's parts

Child is asked to show examiner in succession examiner's: left hand, right ear, left leg, right hand, left ear, right leg.

Section 3: Relative position of three objects

A wooden block, plate, and pencil are arranged in that order from left to right on a 21 × 25 cm sheet of paper. The child is asked the following in succession:
 a. Is the pencil to the left or to the right of the plate?
 b. Is the plate to the left or to the right of the block?
 c. Is the block to the left or to the right of the pencil?
 d. Is the pencil to the left or to the right of the block?
 e. Is the plate to the left or to the right of the pencil?
 f. Is the block to the left or to the right of the plate?

Scoring criteria

(Credit is given for systematic reversals, that is, consistently naming *right* parts or objects as *left* and *left* as *right* within a given section; all six questions must be answered correctly to obtain credit for a section.)

Stage 1a (Age 6)	Either section 1 or section 2 completely correct. May get end position objects on section 3 but not relativity of middle object.
Stage 1b (Age 7)	Section 1 always correct; section 2 incorrect; may get end position objects section 3 but not relativity of middle object.
Stage 2 (Age 9)	Sections 1 and 2 correct; typically misses b and e in section 3.
Stage 3 (Age 12)	All sections correct.

After Laurendeau M, Pinard A. The development of the concept of space in the child. New York: International Universities Press, 1970.

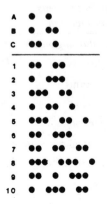

Figure 5.2 Samples of auditory tap patterns used in the Birch-Belmont Auditory Visual Integration Test.

SYSTEM IX: VISUAL THINKING AND COGNITIVE PROCESSING

Rather than comprising a separate entity of testing, this system presents a manner in which to analyze visual, auditory, and perceptual-motor tasks. In recent years, the concept of a dual system of cognitive processing has taken hold in psychology and education (Groffman & Press, 1989). This theory, based on ideas developed by Luria (1966), holds that humans process information either simultaneously or sequentially.

Simultaneous Processing

Simultaneous processing is the processing of information that arrives in the brain spatially so that all parts of the coded information are available. It is considered a right hemisphere function. Examples include copying geometric forms, visual closure, spatial visualization, spatial memory, most mathematics activities, and reading comprehension.

Sequential Processing

Sequential processing is the processing of information arriving in the brain in serial and successive order. The stimuli are temporal in nature and not totally surveyable at any point in time. It is considered a left hemisphere function. Examples include following a route on a map, remembering a series of unrelated facts, doing complex motoric activities, or analyzing the phonic structure of words.

Table 5.10 Sequential versus simultaneous profile of selected optometric developmental tests/activities

Areas Principally Involving Sequential Processing	Areas Principally Involving Simultaneous Processing
Gross-motor control	Visual-motor integration/organization
Angels in the snow	Beery-Buktenica VMI
SBO/SBCT (standing balance eyes open/closed)	Winterhaven Copy Forms
Slap/tap or ball bounce sequences	Groffman Visual Tracing
Auditory-visual integration	Motor-free visual perception
TAAS (auditory analysis skills)	MVPT (motor-free visual perception)
Birch-Belmont	TVPS (visual-perception skills)
Metronome	Peripheral awareness

Differential Diagnosis

The Kaufman Assessment Battery for Children (K-ABC) test was specifically developed to diagnose simultaneous versus successive processing deficits differentially (Kaufman & Kaufman, 1983). One can diagnose strengths and weaknesses in these areas, however, by categorizing the tests of the Hoffman-Richman Developmental Inventory of Perceptual Skills appropriately as presented in System VIII as weighted toward simultaneous or successive processing tasks (Table 5.10).

A deficit in either system will produce academic and other dysfunctions and warrants perceptuocognitive therapy. Cognitive processing can be improved through training, and the improvement is transferred to academic tasks (Krywaniuk & Das, 1983; Kaufman & Kaufman, 1983). The impact of these areas on school performance is discussed in Chapter 6, and procedures for vision therapy are addressed in Chapter 16.

REFERENCES

Amos DM. Cycloplegic refraction. In Bartlett D, Jaanus SD, eds. Clinical ocular pharmacology, 2d ed. Boston: Butterworth–Heinemann, 1989;428.

Bleeker GA, Robertson K. Color vision deficiencies and learning disorders. J Optom Vis Devel 1986;17:12–17.

Buzzelli A. Vergence facility: Developmental trends in a school age population. Am J Optom Physiol Opt 1986;63:351–355.

Cooper J. Accommodative dysfunction. In Amos JF, ed. Diagnosis and management in vision care. Boston: Butterworth–Heinemann, 1987;431–459.

Fletcher R, Voke J. Defective color vision: Fundamentals, diagnosis, and management. Boston: Adam Higler, 1985.

Garzia RP, Richman JE, Nicholson SB, et al. A new visual-verbal saccade test: The Developmental Eye Movement test (DEM). J Am Optom Assoc 1990;61:124–135.

Getman GN. Techniques and diagnostic criteria for the optometric care of children's vision. Duncan, Okla.: Optometric Extension Program, 1960.

Griffin JR. Binocular vision anomalies: Procedures for vision therapy, 2d ed. Chicago: Professional Press, 1982;353.

Groffman S, Press LJ. Computerized perceptual therapy programs: Part I. Santa Ana, Calif.: Optometric Extension Program, Curr II, 1989;61:387–393.

Hagerstrom-Portnoy G. Color vision. In Rosenbloom AA, Morgan MW, eds. Principles and practice of pediatric optometry. Philadelphia: Lippincott, 1990;449–466.

Haynes HM. The distance rock test—a preliminary report. J Am Optom Assoc 1979;50:707–713.

Hirsch MJ, Weymouth FW. Prevalence of refractive anomalies. In Grosvenor T, Flom MC, eds. Refractive anomalies: Research and clinical applications. Boston: Butterworth–Heinemann, 1991;15–38.

Hoffman LG. An optometric learning disability evaluation—part 2. Optom Monthly 1979;70:201–205.

Kaufman AS, Kaufman NL. K-ABC: Interpretive manual. Circle Pines, Minn.: American Guidance Service, 1983; 25–33.

Krywaniuk LW, Das JP. Cognitive strategies in native children: Analysis and intervention. Alberta J Educat Res, 1976.

Laurendau M, Pinard A. The development of the concept of space in the child. New York: International Universities Press, 1970.

Lieberman S, Cohen AH, Rubin J. NYSOA K-D test. J Am Optom Assoc 1983;54:631–637.

Luria AR. Higher cortical functions in man. New York: Basic Books, 1966.

Maino D, Press LJ. The visagraph eye movement recording system. OEP Curr II 1988;60:391–395.

Maples WC, Ficlin TW. A preliminary study of the oculomotor skills of LD, gifted, and normal children. J Optom Vis Devel 1989;20:9–14.

Moss SE, Klein K, Klein BEK. Accommodative ability in younger-onset diabetics. Arch Ophthalmol 1987;105:508–512.

Olsen MM, Harris KR. Color vision deficiency and color blindness: An introduction to the problem. Eugene, Ore.: Fern Ridge Press, 1989;9–15.

Rosner J. Criterion referenced testing of visual-motor development: The visual analysis test. In Greenstein T, ed. Vision and learning disability. St. Louis: American Optometric Association, 1976;159–177.

Rosner J, Fern K. A new version of the TVAS: A validation report. J Am Optom Assoc 1983;54:603.

Rouse MW, Hutter RF, Shiftlett R. A normative study of the accommodative lag in elementary school children. Am J Optom Physiol Opt 1984;61:693–697.

Scheiman M, Herzberg H, Frantz K, et al. Normative study of accommodative facility in elementary schoolchildren. Am J Optom Physiol Opt 1988;65:127–134.

Schlange DG, Terranova F. The accommodative rock card series: Clinical value in treating accommodative disorders. Am J Optom Physiol Opt 1986;63:77P.

Solan HA, Suchoff IB. Tests and measurements in behavioral optometry. Santa Ana, Calif.: Optometric Extension Program, 1991.

Steele GT. The diagnosis, treatment, and management of ocular motility dysfunction. In Cohen A, ed. The management of nonstrabismic binocular vision problems in a primary care practice. St. Louis: American Optometric Association, 1990;59–61.

Streff JW, Wolff BR, Jinks B. Eye tracking and locating skills. Lancaster, Ohio: SA Noel Center, 1985;5.

Winter JD. Clinical oculography. J Am Optom Assoc 1974;45:1308–1313.

Wold RM. Screening tests to be used by the classroom teacher. Novato, Calif.: Academic Therapy Publications, 1970;4–5.

Woodruff ME, Lovasik JV, Spafford MM. Ocular accommodation in juvenile diabetics: A preliminary report. Can J Optom 1987;45:146–149.

6

Vision and School Performance

Leonard J. Press

School is a child's vocation, and the report card the paycheck. The child with excellent grades is considered successful and, as is a wealthy counterpart in adult society, is sought after for sage counsel by peers. Self-esteem mounts and a healthy cycle of self-confidence and performance ensues. Conversely when grades or standardized achievement tests scores are low, self-esteem plummets and parents embark on a search for causative factors.

It has become axiomatic to state that vision is the dominant sense in learning, accounting for 85 percent of the information acquired (Getman, 1984). Since vision is the primary sensory modality used for learning, good vision is a requisite for applying one's intellectual capacity (Woodruff, 1973). Vision should therefore be one of the first areas addressed when school personnel, parents, or allied health care professionals investigate factors associated with adequate school performance. Confusion exists, however, in the semantics of what is meant by good vision. Vision is generally defined as the act or power of seeing with the eye. It is therefore not surprising that the public equates vision with eyesight, but when the professional speaks of vision, a broader definition is implied. To the pediatric optometrist, vision includes a constellation of visual-motor, visual-perceptual, and sensory-motor integrative skills that culminate in the process of visual conceptualization or visual thinking (Furth and Wachs, 1975). The message that vision encompasses more than eyesight must continually be sent to educators as well as allied health care professionals.

Historically one can identify three major areas related to vision that have been identified as integral or supportive to school performance: visual/ocular motor skills, sensory-motor/perceptual integration, and the speech-language-auditory complex. The interplay of these areas is depicted in the interlocking model of circles originally described by Skeffington as cited by Getman (1965) (Figure 6.1). Behavioral, developmental, and functional optometrists consider vision the emergent process in this model. Professionals certified in audiology or speech-language pathology might espouse a similar interlocking model of circles but with language as the emergent process. Vision as the emergent process received much attention in remedial learning programs prior to the 1980s, whereas the 1980s and 1990s witnessed a shift toward the language domain. The distinction

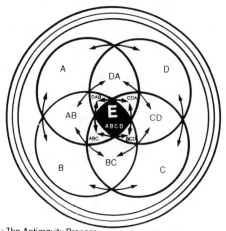

Figure 6.1 The Skeffington interlocking four-circle model of processing with vision as the emergent.

A: The Antigravity Process
B: The Centering Process
C: The Identification Process
D: The Speech-Audition Process
E: The Emergent: Vision

between these two approaches is reflected in the nature of subtypes now recognized in the field of learning disabilities. In addition, the concepts of sequential and simultaneous processing of sensory information as well as the influence of cognitive style on learning demonstrate that there is no satisfactory model of classroom performance that ignores either vision or language.

VISION AND LEARNING DISABILITIES

From a clinical standpoint, concerns associated with children who are not achieving well in school commonly center on learning disabilities (LD). The prevalence of LD in the United States is between 5 percent and 10 percent, somewhat higher among socioeconomically disadvantaged populations and higher among males than among females (NICHD,1987). The most widely adopted definition of LD considers it to be a heterogeneous group of disorders manifested by significant difficulties in the acquisition and use of listening, speaking, reading, writing, reasoning, or mathematical abilities (NICHD, 1987). Visual and perceptual conditions are considered in the same category as are handicapping conditions such as attention deficit disorder (ADD) that may either accompany LD or cause learning problems (Solan & Press, 1989). In some school systems, perceptual impairment (PI) is a distinct classification whereas in others it is included under the umbrella of LD. Visual impairment is equated with partial sight in contrast with more subtle disturbances in visual processing such as ocular-motor or visual-perceptual disorders that are included in the broader categories of PI or LD. Table 6.1 is a sample of conditions listed by a committee on special education and used by that committee in classifying a student's primary handicapping condition.

Table 6.1 Classifications currently used in New York state to specify a student's handicappng condition

Classification	Characteristics of the Handicapping Condition
Autistic	A behavioral disorder that may occur in children of all levels of intelligence. Responses to sensations of light, sound, and feeling may be exaggerated, and delayed speech and language skills may be demonstrated.
Learning disabled	Disability in receiving, organizing, or expressing information. Difficulty in listening, thinking, speaking, reading, writing, or arithmetic results in a significant discrepancy between expected level of achievement and actual school performance.
Perceptually impaired	Disabilities in one or more visual and/or auditory perceptual attributes such as memory, sequencing, or organization.
Visually impaired	Partial sight that may allow residual visual function either through large-print text or low-vision aids. Blind students with no visual resolution will require special braille material.
Hearing impaired	Partial hearing that may allow residual auditory function with or without an aid. May have difficulty following instructions or discriminating sounds, or may have speech and/or language disorders. Deafness requires teaching an alternate means of communication.
Speech impaired	Communication disorder demonstrated by inability to produce sounds, difficulty in understanding or using words in sentences, stuttering, or voice impairment.
Orthopedically impaired	Physical handicap due to conditions such as cerebral palsy, amputation, fractures, or burns that have caused permanent disability.
Health impaired	Limited strength, vitality, or alertness due to problems such as heart condition, asthma, sickle-cell anemia, Tourette syndrome, or epilepsy.
Mentally retarded	Slowed rate of learning due to reduced level of intelligence. Degrees of retardation are subclassified as educable, trainable, severe, and profound.
Emotionally disturbed	Behavior difficulties over a long period of time that interfere with school performance and that are unexplained by intellectual, sensory, or health factors. Students may be generally unhappy or fearful or develop physical symptoms associated with school or personal problems.
Multiply impaired	Students with two or more primary handicaps.

Subtypes of Learning Disabilities

The heterogeneity of LD helps to account for the fact that two clinicians can have success with an LD child using ostensibly different treatment approaches. The younger reading-disabled child with deficits in visual-motor and auditory-visual integration should be differentiated from the older child with deficits in language and formal operations (Satz et al, 1971). This is a useful clinical approach in identifying the two major subtypes of information-processing disorders.

1. Visual-spatial deficits—more heavily weighted on early aspects of reading performance
2. Auditory-linguistic deficits—greater implications in the later elementary school years

One conventional wisdom related to subtyping is the distinction between verbal and performance intelligence quotients (IQ). If verbal IQ is more than 10 points above performance IQ, the visual-spatial domain is suspect. If performance IQ is more than 10 points above verbal IQ, the auditory-linguistic domain is suspect. From a clinical standpoint, the ideal patient to remediate is the child under age nine who is rated as high verbal and low performance. Development of the child's visual-spatial attributes through vision therapy at a young age, as will be reviewed in chapter 16, is expected to have an immediate transfer to classroom performance.

Subtypes of Dyslexia

The subtyping of LD is paralleled in reading disabilities in the consideration of dyslexia (Table 6.2). The child with reading disability reflected in poor auditory-linguistic processing is labeled dysphonetic. This is manifest in poor decoding and phonetic spelling errors with adequate sight vocabulary. In contrast, the dyseidetic child manifests visual-spatial dyslexia with poor sight vocabulary, nonphonetic spelling errors and adequate phonetic spelling ability (Grisham & Simons, 1990). A third category, dysnemkinphonesia, is a combination of the other two forms of dyslexia. The dysnemkinphonetic child has difficulty in developing motor gestalts for written symbols as well as in grapheme-phoneme integration (Griffin & Walton, 1985). The optometrist can administer the Dyslexia Determination Test (DDT) to document the predominant information-processing mode used by the child (Bernell Corp., see Appendix A). The interrelationship between the auditory, visual, and grapheme-phoneme systems is depicted in Figure 6.2.

Table 6.2 Subtypes of dyslexia

Dysphonetic	Dyseidetic	Dysnemkinphonetic
Auditory-linguistic difficulty	Visual-spatial difficulty	Combination of dysphonetic and dyseidetic
Poor decoding	Poor sight vocabulary	Poor grapheme-phoneme integration
Poor phonetic spelling ability	Good phonetic spelling ability	

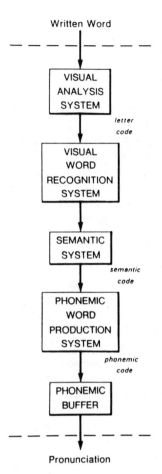

Figure 6.2 A model for the direct visual-recognition comprehension and naming of familiar written words (From Ellis, 1984).

MULTIMODAL PROCESSING

Inherent in the process of subtyping learning and reading disabilities is the differentiation of information-processing modalities. Educators as well as clinicians speak of the relative predominance of one sensory system over another. As was reviewed in Chapter 5, standardized test batteries are administered to the school-aged child to document the child's dominant perceptual modality. Knowing whether the child's strength lies in the visual-spatial domain, the auditory-linguistic domain, or neither helps to structure the remedial approach.

Supramodal Processing and Perceptual Development

Beyond the boundaries of multisensory processing lies the concept of supramodal processing. As was discussed in Chapter 5, the coding of information occurs predominantly in either a successive or a simultaneous processing mode. Furthermore the efficient processing of information shows a strong developmental trend. The verbal child is oriented toward successive processing—the temporal ordering of information serially as when stringing sounds to make a word or stringing words into sentences. This is the predominant mode of processing in efficient readers from kindergarten through second grade. In the middle and upper grades, success in reading and mathematics correlates with a shift toward spatial/simultaneous processing, the ability to perceive the whole picture (Solan, 1987).

Supramodal processing not only shows strong developmental trends but also the relative predominance of simultaneous versus successive processing can vary with the task at hand (Das et al, 1979). For example, accurate copying from the blackboard calls for predominance of simultaneous processing. Conceptualizing entire words, phrases, or units will allow greater speed and precision. This will allow careful inspection of the individual elements involved in the final spatial construct. Consider this:

> While reading this sentence you are using either simultaneous or
> or sequential processing of the printed words.

When reading this sentence aloud, the efficient reader using a visual/spatial or simultaneous processing mode would not detect that the word *or* was repeated. A poor reader who relies on more of a verbal/temporal or successive processing mode would read the word *or* twice exactly as it is written. The efficient reader has the flexibility to switch from simultaneous to successive processing depending on the demand of the task. When reading for general content and comprehension, simultaneous processing is used. When proofreading for print errors, however, successive processing would be used. The inefficient reader is more likely to remain bound to successive processing irrespective of the task demand.

This concept of the maturation of developmental readiness seems to represent the most parsimonious and effective way to describe the behavioral differences that characterize children destined to become the best and poorest readers (Satz et al, 1974); that is, the error patterns observed in all learning disabled children, especially those who are dyslexic, would resemble the behavioral patterns of chronologically younger normal children who have not yet acquired mastery of later developing skills (Satz & von Nostand, 1973).

Supramodal processing is consonant with the Piagetian view of intellectual development (Furth & Wachs, 1974). Intelligence and thinking are not modality-specific and can therefore be considered supramodal forms of processing information. Premature labeling of children as visual, auditory, or haptic learners is therefore undesirable and unproductive; rather the child should be remediated to develop a balance between simultaneous and successive processing strategies. As will be detailed in Chapter 16, this can be done in part through vision therapy.

ORGANIZATION OF SPACE AND TIME

The concept of subtypes in learning and reading disabilities with respect to simultaneous and successive processing is reflected in the relative balance between the child's organization and structuring of space and time.

Structured in Space/Disorganized in Time

The child who is structured in space but disorganized in time is likely to be a fluent reader with poor understanding of content (Kephart, 1971). Spelling is usually inaccurate with frequent reversals, omissions, and additions. Shape recognition, which is a simultaneous and spatial task, is accurate. Shape reproduction, which is a successive and temporal task, is inaccurate. This child can therefore be classified as visual/spatial-simultaneous. In terms of hemispheric lateralization or cerebral dominance, this child's profile is right-brain (parallel) dominant.

Structured in Time/Disorganized in Space

Children who are structured in time but disorganized in space are likely to read laboriously and to subvocalize and creatively substitute their own grammar and syntax. Only when contextual clues are rich do they exhibit good comprehension. These children can therefore be classified as verbal/temporal-successive and left-brain (sequential) dominant.

COGNITIVE STYLE AND ATTENTION DEFICIT
Cognitive Style

Children can be classified as impulsive or reflective in terms of their conceptualization and response style (Kagan, 1966). Impulsive children have limited attention spans, act with little forethought to the consequences of their actions, and respond quickly and inaccurately to questions. Reflective children are quiet, attend to the task at hand, and respond more slowly and accurately.

Impulsivity is a behavioral characteristic associated with a significant number of reading and learning disabled children. Impulsivity enables the child to react to stress or danger but hampers long-term planning, refined discrimination, and covert trial and error. The visual-information processing deficits of these children are part of their generalized cognitive profile (van Meel et al, 1970). Perceptual and vision therapy has a salutary effect on impulsivity (Solan, 1991), thereby transferring directly to observed changes in classroom performance. Lenses and prisms may be used to affect figure-ground and field dependency as well as central and peripheral organization (Kraskin, 1982; Sutton, 1985). Most recently, computerized programs with joystick, keyboard, or mouse controls have facilitated the slowing down of the impulsive child and the speeding up of the reflective child (Groffman & Press, 1989).

Attention Deficit Disorder (ADD)

ADD usually includes hyperactivity, a characteristic of the impulsive child. Some children with ADD, however, are hypoactive to the point of being withdrawn. They may daydream and avoid participating in the classroom. This can be manifest in perseveration and overfixation when tasks are attempted. The child with ADD benefits from individualized or small group instruction with time-related or rhythmically imposed tasks. Auditory-visual and perceptual-motor activities with a metronome are ideal for this population.

AUTOMATICITY OF SKILLS

Many students with learning problems must devote conscious attention to tasks that have become automatic to others. To the optometrist, this is apparent in the investigation of the ocular-motor complex (accommodation, vergence, and motilities) mediated through the frontal motor cortex (Hoffman, 1980). Peachey (1991) recently developed a clinical model of functional automaticity in the developing visual system. When visual skills operate at an automatic level, maximum attention and concentration can be directed toward higher-level cognitive skills such as reading comprehension. The general developmental sequence of vision therapy builds automaticity through (Roberts, 1991):

1. Developing awareness of the process
2. Developing control of the process
3. Improving skill and stamina with conscious control
4. Maintaining skill and stamina with subconscious control

Richman and Cron (1987) demonstrated how vision therapy can be administered to take the child from a control level of performance with intersensory support and feedback to an automatic level of performance with regard to eye movements. At the outset, the child is given unlimited time with few distractions and then set to doing timed tasks with background distractions. When one considers the typical classroom environment with its time structure and distractions, it is no wonder that the child undergoing vision therapy experiences transfer of learned skills to an extent far greater than a traditional ocular-motor examination would portend or than controlled studies of isolated functions can identify.

NEURO-OPHTHALMIC CORRELATES
OF READING DISABILITY

Thus far the principal consideration has been the cognitive aspects of visual development that impact school performance. There are, as well, many traditional optometric functions and others that are in development that lend insight into clinical features of reading-disabled children. These principally involve the neurophysiological pathways and retinocortical functions.

The traditional optometric approach to children who have reading disabilities, but not severe enough ones to be labeled dyslexic, addresses readily quantifiable visual functions. Hyperopia and anisometropia are associated with poor reading performance as compared with myopia (Grisham & Simons, 1986). Certain binocular anomalies such as convergence insufficiency and constricted fusional vergence ranges show a correlation with reading problems (Simons & Grisham, 1987) that has led to a radical treatment approach of occluding one eye as treatment for the visual-spatial subpopulation of reading-disabled children (Stein & Fowler, 1986). The traditional optometric approach to therapy for this population is an appropriate nearpoint spectacle prescription coupled with appropriate vision therapy to normalize the fusional vergence profile. A similar approach should be taken with regard to accommodative, ocular-motor, and visual-perceptual motor skills.

The concept of parallel visual processing has recently received much attention as fertile ground for the basis of certain mechanical reading errors (Williams & Lecluyse, 1990). The concept of dual processing is not new to optometry, having been previously applied in the clinical concept of central versus peripheral visual processing. As reviewed by Flax (1984), this has implications in every facet of visual analysis from Optometric Extension Program (OEP) case-typing to psychophysical processing. The body of research that implicates specific eye movement control and response abnormalities in reading errors stems from the dual processing parallel systems inherent in sustained and transient channels (Breitmeyer & Ganz 1976). Specifically the theory holds that fixation eye movements operate through sustained channels whereas saccadic eye movements operate through transient channels. Fixational eye movements, which last on the order of 250 msecs, have a visible persistence of the image that would trail into the following fixation were it not for the cutoff mechanism that occurs during the 25 msecs of saccadic suppression. The saccadic eye movement therefore not only serves a motor function in moving the eyes from point to point during reading, but acts as a psychophysical barrier to the trailing visible persistence of the preceding fixation. In specific reading disability, experimental evidence has shown that the transient cutoff mechanism of the saccade is defective, allowing words to smear into one another (Lovegrove et al, 1990).

Although applied research in transient versus sustained processing is scant, a connection can be made to the importance of saccadic training in vision therapy and the further importance of integrating saccadic with fixational eye movements. This provides a dual interactive balance between transient and sustained functions that are as essential as the temporal/spatial and accommodative/convergence balance sought from a more traditional therapeutic base. As was noted in the section entitled "Automaticity of Skills," earlier in this chapter, this serves as a further explanation for the reported improvement in reading and classroom performance gleaned through vision therapy that seems removed from the actual therapy techniques (Garzia & Nicholson, 1990).

THE ROLE OF THE OPTOMETRIST

The optometrist should be viewed as one member of the multidisciplinary team that cares for the child. Figure 6.3 depicts a model of care in which vision is an integral part of student evaluation. In 1975, Public Law (PL) 92-142 mandated that public school systems provide a free, appropriate education for all handicapped children. Private and parochial school students are also eligible for special education services from the jurisdiction in which they reside. If there are services identified that will aid in the evaluation or education of the child, these must be identified or provided by the school district. This provision of the law established the formal mechanism whereby an optometrist can become part of the special education process when visual needs are considered. Vision therapy may be considered as a related or supportive service

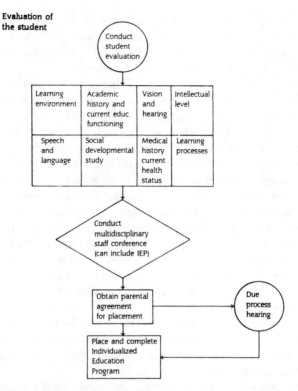

Figure 6.3 Flow diagram of the evaluative process in special education that culminates in the development of an IEP. (MV Pysh, JC Chalfont, Learning disabilities manual: Recommended procedures and practices. Springfield: State Board of Education, Illinois Office of Education, 1978;33. Reprinted with permission.)

required to assist a handicapped child to benefit from special education (Lemer, 1990). Although PL 94-142 is a federal law with specific minimum requirements, it is subject to local interpretation by each state. Special education services and the individual education plan (IEP) process through which optometric evaluation and therapy are identified will be discussed further in Chapter 20.

There are several philosophical and political issues with which the optometrist must be prepared to deal. One revolves around the identification and recognition of visual problems in the school-aged child. Pediatricians and ophthalmologists persistently maintain that there is no interrelationship between vision and learning and that children with learning or reading disabilities have the same prevalence of visual abnormalities as do children without such disabilities. The optometrist must empathize with the confused picture painted to school personnel, who receive negative reinforcement for visual intervention from the ophthalmologic camp and positive reinforcement from the optometric camp. This confusion is reflected in texts in the learning disability field that dismiss the role of vision in learning yet provide extensive support for the role of information processing of the nature discussed in this chapter under the rubric of vision (Smith, 1991). The optometrist must therefore be prepared with scientific documentation, which is abundant (American Optometric Association, 1988; Garzia & Nicholson, 1990).

Another issue revolves around the resources with which localities can budget their special education programs. PL 92-142 guarantees the right of every child to receive special education services and, when the family cannot afford such services, to provide payment for these services. Consequently if extensive optometric evaluation is recommended for the child's IEP, the school system is bound to pay for it. When the parent has the financial means to seek optometric care and therapy or when insurance reimbursement is applicable, the parent can seek direct remediation.

The optometrist is therefore placed in the role of child advocacy. In general, the optometrist acts as an independent vision-care practitioner who educates parents and allied professionals about the interrelationship of vision and learning and about the need for ongoing vision care. In specific instances involving special education services, the optometrist should be prepared to assist the parent and child in a due-process hearing to obtain inclusion of vision therapy services in the IEP, as will be discussed in Chapter 20.

REFERENCES

American Optometric Association. Special Report: The efficacy of optometric vision therapy. J Am Optom Assoc 1988;59:95–105.

Breitmeyer BG, Ganz L. Implications of sustained and transient channels for theories of visual pattern masking, saccadic suppression, and information processing. Psychol Rev 1976;83:1–36.

Das FP, Kirby JR, Jarman RF. Simultaneous and successive processes. New York: Academic Press, 1979.

Ellis AW. Reading, writing and dyslexia: A cognitive analysis. London: Lawrence Erlbaum Associates, 1984.

Flax N. A current look at the OEP B1 and B2 case typings. J Optom Vis Devel 1984;15(1):19–21.

Furth HG, Wachs H. Thinking goes to school: Piaget's theory in practice. New York: Oxford University Press, 1975.

Garzia RP, Nicholson SB. Visual function and reading disability: An optometric viewpoint. J Am Optom Assoc 1990;61:88–97.

Getman GN. The visuomotor complex in the acquisition of learning skills. In Hellmuth J, ed. Learning disorders, vol 1. Seattle: Special Child Publications, 1965, 49–76.

Getman GN. How to develop your child's intelligence. White Plains, Md.: Research Publications 1984.

Griffin JR, Walton HN. Therapy in dyslexia and reading problems including vision, perception and motor skills. Los Angeles: I-Med, 1985.

Grisham D, Simons H. Perspectives on reading disabilities. In Rosenbloom AA, Morgan MW, eds. Principles and practice of pediatric optometry. Philadelphia: JB Lippincott, 1990;518–559.

Grisham JD, Simons HD. Refractive error and the reading process: A literature analysis. J Am Optom Assoc 1986;57:44–55.

Groffman S, Press LJ. Computerized perceptual therapy programs. Optom Extension Prog 1989;61:387–393.

Hoffman LG. Incidence of vision difficulties in children with learning disabilities. J Am Optom Assoc 1980;51:447–451.

Kagan J. Reflection impulsivity: The generality and dynamics of conceptual tempo. J Abnorm Psychol 1966; 71(1):12–24.

Kephart NC. The slow learner in the classroom. 2d ed. Columbus, Ohio: Merrill, 1971.

Kraskin RA. Lens power in action: The visual process. Optom Extension Prog, Curr II 1982(Jun);33–36.

Lemer PS. Education for all handicapped children act, public law 94-142. J Behav Optom 1990, 1(6):150–153.

Lovegrove WJ, Garzia, Nicholson SB. Experimental evidence for a transient system deficit in specific reading disability. J Am Optom Assoc 1990;61:137–146.

NICHD, Office of Research Reporting. Learning Disabilities: A report to the U.S. Congress. Washington, D.C.: Interagency Committee on Learning Disabilities, 1987.

Peachey GT. Minimum attention model for understanding the development of efficient visual function. Behav Optom 1991;3(1):10–19.

Pych MV, Chalfont JC. Learning disabilities manual: Recommended procedures and practices. Springfield: State Board of Education, Illinois Office of Education, 1978; 33.

Richman JE, Cron MT. Guide to vision therapy. South Bend, Ind.: Bernell Corporation, 1987.

Roberts B. The developmental sequence of vision training. Behav Optom 1991;3(1):27–32.

Satz P, Friel J, Rudegair F. Some predictive antecedents of specific reading disability: A two, three and four year follow-up. In Guthrie JT, ed. Aspects of reading acquisition. Baltimore: Johns Hopkins University Press, 1974;111–140.

Satz P, Rardin D, Ross J. An evaluation of a theory of specific developmental dyslexia. Child Devel 1971;42:2009–2021.

Satz P, von Nostand GK. Developmental dyslexia: An evaluation of a theory. In Satz P and Ross J, eds. Disabled learner. Rotterdam: Rotterdam University Press, 1973;121–148.

Simons HD, Grisham JD. Binocular anomalies and reading problems. J Am Optom Assoc 1987;58:578–587.

Smith CR. Learning disabilities: The interaction of learner, task, and setting. 2d ed. Boston: Allyn and Bacon, 1991.

Solan HA. A comparison of the influences of verbal successive and spatial-simultaneous factors on achieving readers in the fourth and fifth grade: A multivariate correlational study. J Learning Disabil 1987;20(4):237–242.

Solan HA. Learning disabilities: The role of the optometrist revisited. Ped Optom Vis Ther 1991;1(2):1–9.

Solan HA, Press LJ. Topical review of the literature: Optometry and learning disabilities. J Optom Vis Devel 1989;20(1):5–21.

Stein J, Fowler S. Occlusion treatment. Optician 1986;11:16–22.

Sutton A. Building a visual space world: The role of lenses and prisms in learning. Optometric Extension Program, Curriculum II, 1985(June):29–36.

van Meel JM, Vlek CAJ, Bruijel RM. Some characteristics of visual information-processing in children with learning difficulties. In Bakker DJ, Satz P, eds. Specific reading disability: Advances in theory and method. Rotterdam: Rotterdam University Press, 1970;97–114.

Williams MC, Lecluyse K. Perceptual consequences of a temporal processing deficit in reading disabled children. J Am Optom Assoc 1990;61:111–121.

Woodfuff ME. The visually "at risk" child. J Am Optom Assoc 1973;44:130–134.

7

Diseases of the Orbit and Anterior Segment

Bruce D. Moore

ORBIT AND WHOLE EYE

Abnormalities affecting the orbit, the globe, and the general appearance of the face will usually be apparent on cursory examination. The dilemma facing the clinician is to make the correct diagnosis from among the possible causes. Once the diagnosis is made, the question of appropriate treatment can be decided.

Proptosis and orbital inflammation will be difficult to detect in their early stages. A careful physical examination and a good history of the child are essential when these disorders are suspected. Diagnostic imaging procedures such as X-ray, computerized tomography (CT) scan, and magnetic resonance imaging (MRI) are invaluable in arriving at the proper diagnosis. Some of these etiologies are of a life-threatening nature and require prompt diagnosis and treatment.

Congenital Orbital Anomalies (Table 7.1)
Size Abnormalities

The size of each orbit and globe is usually about equal. There are a number of conditions in which there are either asymmetries in the size of the eyes and/or orbits or one eye or orbit is larger or smaller than normal. These inequalities of size indicate potentially serious ocular and systemic problems. Some of these are readily apparent, but some are not.

Clinical anophthalmia, the apparent absence of the eye, is a very rare condition that has many possible causes. Patients with anophthalmia almost always have additional major neurological and systemic malformations at birth. It is unlikely that the optometrist will ever see these patients. Anopthalmia is really an extreme form of a much more common condition, microphthalmia.

Microphthalmia occurs in about 1 in 2000 births (Singh et al, 1980). Microphthalmia may present in one or both eyes and can vary from virtually imperceptible to very gross in the case of clinical anophthalmic. It may be an isolated condition or associated with other ocular and systemic conditions such as persistent hyperplastic primary vitreous and congenital cataracts, maternal rubella and toxoplasmosis, trisomy 13, various colobomata, and a number of uncommon systemic anomalies. Isolated cases of microphthalmia without additional systemic or ocular involvement may be unilateral or bilateral and tend to be milder in degree and with better visual potential than are the more complex cases. The orbits and the optic foramina of patients with microphthalmia are usually reduced in size. The growth of the orbit is affected by the size of the orbital contents. Patients with severe microphthalmia or anophthalmia and no visual potential are usually fit with an inert orbital expander after enucleation to increase the size of the orbit during development and improve cosmesis. These expanders need to be enlarged periodically.

An enlarged globe (megalophthalmia) in a patient must be assumed to be due to congenital glaucoma until proven otherwise, but the more likely causes of megalophthalmia are high myopia, Marfan's syndrome, or a hereditary familial pattern. Patients with megalocornea, which must be differentiated from megalophthalmia, may appear to have an enlarged globe, but it is only the cornea and not the entire eye that is enlarged. The appearance of an enlarged globe may also be due to proptosis. This possibility should always be fully investigated as it may be caused by potentially serious medical problems.

Craniofacial Abnormalities

There is obviously a very wide range of normal appearances that children may possess. It is often difficult to determine if a child is simply a variant of normal or if the child is actually dysmorphic. The determination of these abnormalities may be even more difficult in infancy, becoming less so as the child matures and the physical appearance changes. Observing the parents and siblings may prove very helpful in aiding the diagnosis.

Table 7.1   Disorders of the orbit

Congenital orbital anomalies	Acquired orbital disease
Size anomalies	Proptosis
Anophthalmia	Inflammatory
Microphthalmia	Orbital cellulitis
Megalophthalmia	Peri-orbital cellulitis
Craniofacial abnormalities	Cavernous sinus thrombosis
Crouzon's disease	Pseudotumor
Apert's syndrome	Vascular
Plagiocephaly	Capillary hemangioma
Hypertelorism	Lymphangioma
Treacher-Collins syndrome	Orbital dermoid
Goldenhar's syndrome	
Fetal alcohol syndrome	

In general, dysmorphic appearances that are of limited functional or cosmetic significance need little if any intervention. Malformations that are of significant functional or cosmetic concern will require attention. There are a myriad of abnormalities of the facies that may come to the attention of the clinician. The description of these conditions and the determination of the proper treatment if any is required is a very complex area of management for the optometrist and will require the help of other specialties.

One of the more commonly seen groups of craniofacial abnormalities are the craniosynostosis syndromes. These abnormalities are due to a premature closure of one or more cranial sutures, causing a decrease in skull growth perpendicular to the fused suture and an increase in growth parallel to the fused suture. As a result, the skull grows in an abnormal shape. The sutures normally do not completely fuse until around late puberty, allowing for continued growth in the volume of the cranium and the brain. Restricted growth may cause neurologic problems and mental retardation, along with a host of ocular complications. The calvarium is the area of the brain that is most frequently affected in patients with craniosynostosis.

Crouzon's syndrome is a craniosynostosis with marked midface hypoplasia and oxycephaly (*tower skull* or increased height of the skull in relation to its width or length) and brachycephaly (a head with increased width in comparison to its length). There is also a beak-shaped nose, hypertelorism, shallow orbits, maxillary hypoplasia, and an abnormal inferiorly displaced position of the lateral palpebral ligaments that results in an antimongoloid slant to the eyelids.

Patients with Apert's syndrome have a somewhat similar appearance to those with Crouzon's syndrome with the addition of greater oxycephaly, greater incidence of cleft palate, and (of diagnostic importance) syndactyly of the hands and feet and fusion of the digits. Patients with Apert's and Crouzon's syndromes may present with a V-pattern exotropia due to harlequin shaped, shallow orbits. Proptosis from the abnormal shape of the orbits is common, occasionally resulting in corneal exposure and scarring. There is a tendency for high refractive errors, requiring optical correction and attention to amblyopia (Nelson et al, 1981). Fitting spectacles to these patients may occasionally prove difficult or impossible, necessitating the use of contact lenses. The optic nerves may be involved, especially following surgical treatment of the facial abnormalities. Both Crouzon's and Apert's syndrome are autosomal dominantly inherited with variable expressivity, and there appears to be a relatively high rate of new mutations.

Plagiocephaly is a craniofacial abnormality caused by a unilateral fusion of a coronal suture (Shillito & Matson, 1968). Many of these patients possess a form of strabismus that simulates a fourth cranial nerve paresis but is actually due to an underaction of the superior oblique caused by the abnormal configuration of the orbit (Robb & Boger, 1983). These oculomotor abnormalities persist even after craniofacial surgery and may require additional ophthalmic intervention for amblyopia.

Hypertelorism, an increase in separation of the orbits, occurs in a number of conditions. This is due to an increase in the width of the ethmoid resulting in an increased interpupillary distance—sometimes as great as 80mm. There is usually an exotropia due to the increased pupillary distance or to abnormalities in the shape of the orbits similar to that seen in Apert's and Crouzon's syndromes, but occasionally an esotropia may be present. A variant of the Tessier procedure is the treatment of choice when surgical intervention is indicated.

Treacher-Collins syndrome (mandibulofacial dysostosis) is a condition having a number of skeletal and facial abnormalities. The face shows depressed cheekbones, small jaw, beaked nose, abnormally shaped ears, hearing loss, dental abnormalities, and cleft palate. The palpebral fissures slant downward (antimongoloid slant) and give a characteristic facial appearance. There may also be an absence of medial eyelashes, ectropion, and a coloboma of the lower lid. The condition is autosomal dominant with variable penetrance and expressivity.

Goldenhar's syndrome is also called either hemifacial microsomia or the first and second branchial arch syndrome. It is usually unilateral, but a small number of patients may show bilateral deformity. This syndrome results in a hypoplastic facial abnormality affecting the area of the cheek and jaw along with prominent epibulbar dermoids and lipodermoids; small, low-set ears and inferior anomalous auricular tags; and vertebral skeletal anomalies. There may be an associated coloboma of the upper lid and less commonly, strabismus and microphthalmia. The limbal dermoids may cause anisometropic astigmatism and amblyopia in a few patients.

The surgical treatment of choice in patients with craniofacial anomalies is a series of complex and extensive midface procedures named after Paul Tessier (1971), a French surgeon, who first attempted treatment of these conditions. There are potential ocular complications that may result from the extensive surgical shifting of the facial bones (Matthews, 1979). These include residual strabismus (especially exotropia), optic nerve damage, ptosis, corneal exposure, and enophthalmus. The cosmetic improvement for the patient can range from minimal to dramatic, depending on individual factors.

Fetal Alcohol Syndrome and Substance Abuse

This is a multisystem congenital disorder arising from heavy maternal consumption of alcohol (Rosett & Weiner, 1984). The drinking must be heavy, defined as more than 45 drinks per month (1.5 oz liquor, one beer, or one glass of wine is a drink). Binge drinkers are at highest risk. The risk does decrease if drinking is stopped at any time during a pregnancy. The incidence of fetal alcohol syndrome in infants is approximately 30 percent of mothers that are heavy drinkers. There has been some suggestion recently that alcohol in any amount may present risk to the developing fetus, but there as yet is no confirmation of this. Alcohol is the specific teratogenic factor but the actual mechanism is not as yet known. Professional intervention in maternal behavior during pregnancy is the only way of reducing the risk to the infant.

The systemic manifestations include growth retardation; central nervous system (CNS) involvement; developmental delay; mental retardation; and urogenital, cardiopulmonary, and skeletal abnormalities. There is also a facial dysmorphology that includes microcephaly, flat maxilla, thin upper lip, and small palpebral apertures. There is much variability among individuals.

The ocular manifestations are also quite variable. They include ptosis, anterior chamber cleavage syndrome, reduced palpebral aperture, epicanthal folds, telecanthus, strabismus, optic nerve hypoplasia, cataracts, and high myopic and astigmatic refractive errors (Miller et al, 1984).

The recent, dramatic increase in the number of infants born to women that are addicted to crack cocaine has become a major medical and social problem. Many of these pregnant women receive little or no prenatal care, are poorly nourished, and face myriad medical and social problems. The infants have a very high rate of prematurity with all the attendant medical problems. The children appear to have a high incidence of neurological, developmental, and learning problems. There is some evidence that oculomotor and optic-nerve abnormalities may be due to the fetal exposure to crack cocaine, and there is a high incidence of retinopathy of prematurity. The association of all forms of substance abuse to increased risk of neonatal human immunodeficiency virus (HIV) infection has become all too obvious recently.

Acquired Orbital Disorders

Proptosis

Proptosis is an important indicator of orbital disease. It is relatively uncommon in children. When it is present, the differential diagnosis includes hemangioma, lymphangioma, dermoids, orbital cellulitis, hematoma, pseudotumor, craniostenosis, hyperthyroidism, trauma, and neoplasms such as rhabdomyosarcoma. Enophthalmus of the fellow eye may give a false impression of proptosis. Conditions causing either an enlarged anteroposterior diameter of the eye or increased corneal diameter (such as eyes with congenital glaucoma, megalophthalmia, megalocornea, or unilateral high myopia) may also cause a false impression of proptosis in the affected eye. The rate of progression of proptosis is highly variable; it may be stationary or progress slowly or very rapidly. Radiologic and neurologic consults are mandatory in all suspected cases of proptosis in order to arrive at the correct diagnosis. An important consideration in any eye with proptosis, regardless of the cause, is the possibility of corneal exposure leading to keratitis and scarring. Appropriate lubrication of the eye is extremely important to guard against this.

Orbital Inflammation

Most causes of orbital and periorbital inflammation are due to inflammatory processes involving the surrounding tissues. The definitions of orbital and periorbital cellulitis are frequently confused and often used imprecisely (Shapiro et al, 1982). The connective tissue membrane of the orbital septum acts as a somewhat porous barrier between the periorbital and orbital tissues. The periosteum is a connective tissue that is contiguous with the dura and overlies the bones of the orbit. This comprises the major portion of the periorbital tissue. The orbital tissue lies within the periosteum and the periorbital tissues and consists of the globe itself and the areolar tissue and orbital fat surrounding the globe.

Periorbital cellulitis may be a precursor to the more serious orbital cellulitis and occurs much more frequently (Gellady et al, 1978). It may arise from such causes as hordeolum, trauma, and (most commonly) systemic bacterial infections such as from Haemophilus influenza and Streptococcus pneumoniae. Periorbital cellulitis must be treated aggressively with systemic antibiotics to prevent serious and potentially life-threatening sequelae.

Among the causes of acute orbital cellulitis are inflammation of the ethmoid sinus, tooth abcess, dacryocystitis, and periorbital cellulitis. Haemophilus influenza and Streptococcus pneumoniae are the leading bacterial agents in orbital cellulitis. The infected tissues must be drained and intensive antibiotic therapy initiated or there is a major risk of cavernous sinus thrombosis, meningitis, and brain abscess. These cases require hospitalization.

Cavernous sinus thrombosis presents as a severe orbital cellulitis with the development of papilledema, decreased visual acuity, ophthalmoplegia, and various serious neurological signs. This is a life-threatening condition requiring intensive treatment. Pseudotumor is a chronic orbital inflammation of uncertain etiology that often presents as a unilateral proptosis with limitation of extraocular muscle movement. It tends to improve spontaneously over time and is treated with systemic steroids.

Vascular Anomalies of the Orbit

Capillary hemangiomas of the orbit may be associated with similar conditions of the skin and face. They typically are either quite small or are not noted at all at birth, but they develop rapidly during the first few months of life, sometimes to dramatic size. They become a deep red to purplish color that intensifies when the child cries. Orbital capillary hemangiomas may cause a pulsating proptosis. They generally regress spontaneously by age four to seven years but may linger longer in some cases. Management should be conservative, as long as they do not cause amblyopia due to lid involvement (Robb, 1977) or corneal exposure due to proptosis. Surgical intervention should be avoided since there is often direct vascular connection to the carotids and the lesion may bleed profusely if disturbed. Direct injection with steroids is indicated if amblyopia or proptosis develops (Kushner, 1979). This may need to be repeated at frequent intervals but must be monitored very closely because of the possibility of systemic involvement due to growth retardation.

Lympangiomas are similar in many ways to capillary hemangiomas, but they are lymphoid in nature. They may cause unilateral proptosis, strabismus, and amblyopia. They do not tend to regress and may require surgical intervention in extreme cases. Management is usually restricted to preventing amblyopia and the adverse effects of proptosis.

Orbital Dermoids

Orbital dermoid cysts are the most common pediatric orbital tumor. Many orbital dermoids are not noted at birth but become more apparent over the first two to three decades as they grow in size or become inflamed due to various causes. Most orbital dermoids are located superiorly. They may cause proptosis, ptosis, and restriction of ocular motility, requiring surgical excision.

EYELIDS

Many of the conditions affecting the eyelids will be immediately apparent to the parents or the referring optometrist. Congenital conditions are likely to be noted in the newborn nursery. Conditions affecting the maintenance of the tear film may early on cause a red eye and recurrent episodes of inflammation. Many of the less severe eyelid disorders need to be followed closely for signs of ocular inflammation, but most of them will require little if any treatment. Patients with marked ptosis must be monitored for the possibility of amblyopia.

Other conditions that tend to develop in the first few months of infancy (such as eyelid hemangiomas) will be alarming to parents and will generate a quick referral. These cases need to be managed by someone experienced with this disorder. Patients with nevus flammeus need referral to their pediatrician for evaluation for Sturge-Weber disease. Simple observation is most important in making the correct diagnosis for patients with eyelid abnormalities.

Congenital Abnormalities of Size and Shape (Table 7.2)

There are a large number of congenital abnormalities affecting the size or shape of the eyelids. Some are only of cosmetic importance, but others affect the functioning and health of the eye. Many of these abnormalities are associated with other congenital malformations. The appearance of any single abnormality should arouse the suspicion of additional ocular and systemic problems, requiring a thorough internal

Table 7.2   Congenital eyelid abnormalities

Size or shape	
Coloboma	Absence of a portion of the lid
Epiblepharon	Extra skin fold causing entropion
Entropion	Turning inward of the lid
Ectropion	Turning outward of the lid
Blepharophimosis	Small palpebral aperture
Telecanthus	Increased intercanthal distance
Epicanthus	Extra skin fold at inner canthus
Ptosis	Drooping of the upper lid
Vascular tumors	
Hemangioma	Endothelial proliferation
Port wine stain	Associated with Sturge-Weber
Nevus flammeus	Not associated with Sturge-Weber; more benign

and external ocular examination. An important consideration in any patient with eyelid problems is the effect on the maintenance of the tear film and corneal clarity.

Colobomas of the eyelids occur most frequently on the nasal aspect of the upper eyelids and somewhat less commonly on the temporal side of the lower lid. The degree of involvement is quite variable—from a slight indentation of a small portion of one lid to complete absence of one or both lids. Only rarely are there multiple colobomas on the same eyelid. These patients may also have additional colobomas or structural abnormalities of the eyes or face. The preferred treatment of eyelid colobomas is surgical in nature when either the cosmetic appearance of the patient or the proper maintenance of the tear flow over the corneal surface is compromised.

Epiblepharon appears as an extra horizontal fold of tissue across the lower eyelid, which may lead to an entropion or turning inward of the lashes in infants. Johnson (1978) has noted that differentiation between epiblepharon and entropion is important because the treatment is different. The appearance of epiblepharon generally changes over the first years of life as the face and eyelids grow. Surgical treatment is required only if it causes problems with the integrity of the corneal physiology.

Congenital entropion and ectropion rarely occur as isolated findings. When there is true entropion, the condition tends to worsen with age, whereas the opposite tends to be true in patients with epiblepharon. There are often associated problems of the lids or facies in patients with entropion. Ectropion may also be associated with Trisomy 21 and blepharophimosis.

Patients with blepharophimosis show a narrowing of the palpebral aperture and an absence of the transverse fold of the upper lid. The medial canthus is shifted and the nasal bridge is flattened. There may be ptosis, epicanthus, telecanthus, and hypertelorism. Cosmetic surgery may be performed, especially if deprivation amblyopia is threatened or an anomalous head position is required for vision in severely affected patients. Telecanthus appears as an exaggerated intercanthal distance with an essentially normal interpupillary distance. It may be isolated or occur along with epicanthus and blepharophimosis. Cosmetic surgery may be considered.

Epicanthus appears as an extra fold of the eyelid at the medial aspect of the inner canthus at the semilunaris. One fairly common type of epicanthus may be associated with blepharophimosis, but most patients have a simple isolated form. Epicanthus is of considerable clinical importance because it is frequently the cause of pseudoesotropia, one of the more common reasons that parents bring infants to the optometrist's office for examination. The child appears to have an esotropia, especially with the eyes in slight lateral gaze. Examination shows only epicanthal folds paralleling the bridge of the nose. This facial appearance almost always changes by six to eight years of age as the face and especially the bridge of the nose grows. Treatment is not required, but one must be certain that an actual strabismus is not present. Serial exams are useful to completely rule out this possibility.

Congenital Ptosis

Congenital ptosis is a common abnormality affecting the position and function of the upper eyelid. It may be uni- or bilateral and can be isolated or associated with paresis of the superior rectus muscle, the Marcus Gunn jaw-winking syndrome, epicanthus, or blepharophimosis. There may be an autosomal dominant hereditary pattern.

Visual acuity may be impaired in some patients with marked ptosis if the pupillary axis is effectively blocked by the lid, leading to deprivation amblyopia in the affected eye(s). Individuals with marked ptosis may assume a head position with the head thrust back in order to maintain binocularity. Many of these patients become adept at also using the orbicularis muscle to elevate the lids. More commonly the ptosis is less marked and only of cosmetic concern.

The *typical* form of congenital ptosis is due to dysplasia of the levator palpebrae muscle. The skin of the upper eyelid is smooth because it lacks the tarsal fold caused by the presence of the levator. Treatment, when required, is by surgery. A commonly used procedure uses autogenous fascia lata slings of one or both eyes.

The Marcus Gunn jaw-winking syndrome is a type of congenital ptosis that is due to a *miswiring* of the nerves responsible for the muscle actions of the jaw and the eyelids. There is either a retraction or relaxation of the eyelid via the levator muscle when the jaw moves. It is most readily observed when the child is sucking a bottle and tends to become less noticeable over time. The Marcus Gunn jaw-winking syndrome is generally a unilateral condition with considerable variation in appearance among patients.

Vascular Abnormalities of the Eyelids (Table 7.2)
Capillary Lid Hemangioma

These are benign vascular tumors of the eyelids that develop rapidly after birth. They show abnormally rapid turnover of endothelial cells during the early proliferative stages of development of the hemangioma. Most hemangiomas are first noted during the second to fourth weeks of life and are only rarely evident at time of birth. They usually reach maximum size by 1 to 1.5 years of age and then regress over the next 6 to 8 years. Their size varies from a small patch a millimeter or two in diameter on the upper lid to a massively disfiguring growth covering most of one side of the face. There is a predilection for the upper lid. They are most common in females and rarest in blacks. They become a darker red or blue color when the child cries due to an increase in blood volume within the abnormal capillary bed. They are of significant ophthalmic concern because of the possible development of amblyopia by occlusion of the pupillary axis (causing deprivation amblyopia) or because of the effect of the tumor mass pressing against the globe and inducing an astigmatic anisometropia with the axis of astigmatism perpendicular to the eyelid tumor mass (Robb, 1977). Either type of amblyopia is difficult to treat effectively. When anisometropia does develop, it must be corrected optically and occlusion therapy must be instituted as quickly as possible. The refractive error caused by the growth and presence of the hemangioma in the early years is not generally reduced later as the hemangioma mass regresses.

Treatment is required if the tumor mass causes amblyopia. The current best method of treatment is direct steroid injection into the hemangioma (Kushner, 1979). This may need to be repeated a number of times if the mass does not show sufficient resolution. In some cases, the results of steroid injection can be dramatic; in others, it may be relatively ineffective. There is always the potential of systemic steroid side effects such as adrenal suppression and growth retardation along with Cushingoid effects. There have also been reports of eyelid necrosis following injection (Sutula & Glover, 1987). The capillary hemangioma is very fragile and has a propensity to show vascular breakdown and spontaneous massive bleeding. Surgery is very risky for this reason. Most patients with lid hemangioma will have a nearly complete resolution by age seven to ten, with the only significant ocular sequelae being amblyopia of varying degree. Very careful and aggressive amblyopia treatment may minimize this problem. There may be some redundancy of the skin overlying the region of the old tumor mass that is of continued cosmetic concern to the parents and the child.

Port Wine Stains and Nevus Flammeus

These two terms have been used interchangeably, but are now considered by some authorities to be two different types of vascular malformations. The *port wine stain* is a vascular lesion of the upper eyelid and adjacent facial areas that is often associated with Sturge-Weber disease (Mulliken & Murray, 1982). They are composed of masses of dilated capillaries within the skin, differing from hemangiomas in not having any abnormal endothelial proliferation. It is a flat lesion (in contrast to lid hemangiomas, which are elevated) that is purple in color and follows a pattern over the distribution of the trigeminal nerve, not usually extending beyond the midline. Port wine stains tend to darken when the child cries. These lesions are of ocular importance because of their association with choroidal hemangiomas and glaucoma and with the systemic effects of Sturge-Weber disease. Recent treatment includes the use of the Argon laser to improve cosmesis. Surgery is not indicated for the skin lesions. All patients with port wine stains must be monitored closely for the development of glaucoma and choroidal hemangiomas, which can cause hyperopic anisometropia and amblyopia.

Nevus flammeus is a term that should probably be restricted to a much more benign type of skin lesion that is very common in infants. These occur most often on the face and neck and do not necessarily follow the distribution of the trigeminal nerve. They often fade in the first few years of life but may remain into the adult years. Treatment is generally not indicated.

Acquired Eyelid Disorders

Acquired Ptosis

Acquired ptosis can be due to several primary causes—myogenic (senile, progressive external ophthalmoplegia, myasthenia gravis, congenital fibrosis), neurogenic (third nerve due to various specific causes), and mechanical (lid tumors and inflammations, microphthalmia and vertical strabismus). Accurate diagnosis is critical to rule out potentially serious neurological problems. Old photos may be of great help. Ptosis derived from third nerve involvement tends to be severe with only minimal residual levator function remaining. Depending on the specific location of the lesion, effects may be noted in the superior rectus muscle only (the superior branch of the third cranial nerve) or in each of the extraocular muscles and pupillary fibers innervated by the third cranial nerve. Ptosis secondary to Horner's syndrome is less severe since only the sympathetic innervation to Muller's muscle is affected, and there remains normal levator function. Patients with Horner's syndrome have in addition to the partial ptosis a concomitant miosis and anhydrosis on the affected side. Birth trauma from forceps delivery may damage the third nerve causing an aberrant regeneration of the nerve and abnormal movement of the ptotic lid. Surgical intervention for the various types of ptosis can aid cosmetic appearance, but results are dependent on the etiology and can be very unpredictable. The specific surgical procedure is selected depending on the cause of the ptosis. A ptosis crutch of dental wire inserted into an ophthalmic frame may also aid cosmesis.

Infection
These conditions are described in more detail in the section on infectious eye disease in Chapter 9. The most common inflammatory disorders of the eyelids in children are the same as for adults and include hordeolum, chalazion, and blepharitis. Several additional causes seen more often in children than in adults include molluscum contagiosum, primary herpes simplex blepharitis, impetigo, vaccinia, and pediculosis.

Trauma
Trauma to the periorbital areas during sports or careless play among children may easily result in damage to the eyelids. Lacerations, contusions, and burns occur often. These injuries may affect the functioning of the lids adversely and compromise the tear film and corneal clarity. Trauma may also directly cause ptosis.

LACRIMAL APPARATUS

Dry eyes of the type commonly seen in adults are exceedingly rare in young children. Overly wet eyes usually indicate a nasolacrimal duct obstruction. Conservative treatment is generally preferred for these patients.

Alacrima and Dry Eyes

Alacrima is a very uncommon absence or severe reduction of tear production. Many neonates show a delay in the onset of normal tearing for several weeks (Sjogren, 1955) after birth but should exhibit at least some tear production by one month of age. Tearing in response to crying may take several months after birth to develop fully. Alacrima may be due to a true absence or hypoplasia of the lacrimal gland, to neurological abnormalities, or to a blockage of tear flow into the eye. It is usually bilateral but may be unilateral.

The eyes of these patients will probably look dry and are likely to show a reduced corneal light reflex. Schirmer or Jones testing (instillation of fluorescein into the conjunctival sac and a cotton swab in the nose to catch the dye after it has traversed the nasolacrimal duct) will confirm a lack of tear production or drainage. Rose Bengal staining may be evident. Patients with truly deficient tearing will present with photophobia, corneal staining and scarring, and bulbar and palpebral conjunctival injection.

Treatment is difficult and is directed at conserving whatever limited tear output is available. A variety of artificial tears should be tried until the particular brand that works best is found. Ointments should be used at night and at other times if they can be tolerated. Punctal occlusion, therapeutic and collagen contact lenses, swim goggles and other moisture barriers, and tarsorrhaphy may also be tried when lubricants fail to prevent further corneal scarring and photophobia.

The Riley-Day syndrome is a multisystem autosomal recessive disease, having alacrima as the prominent ocular complication. Patients with this syndrome have a reduced, but still present, tear production and a greatly diminished corneal sensitivity. This often results in corneal scarring, ulceration, or perforation (Liebman, 1956). Patients may have a tonic pupil. Systemic manifestations include lability of blood pressure, skin blotching when behaviorally upset, and greatly reduced sensation to pain in general. Children often exhibit unusual behavior and hyperactivity. The basic defect is unknown, but the decreased tearing seems due to abnormal parasympathetic innervation of the lacrimal gland. Ocular treatment can be very difficult due to the child's behavior and is directed at keeping the corneas moist and preventing corneal injury.

The form of keratitis sicca commonly found in adults is very rare in otherwise healthy children. Tear production, particularly of the aqueous component, tends to be high in most children. A few systemic and ocular conditions can cause changes in the constituency of the tear film, occasionally leading to corneal problems. Blepharitis and other external ocular inflammations can produce toxic effects on the cornea. Patients with cystic fibrosis may have an abnormal mucoid secretion in their tears. This can cause heavy coating of contact lenses.

Patients that have been treated with radiation for leukemia and other neoplastic diseases frequently exhibit signs and symptoms of ocular dryness. This is due to direct damage to the structures that produce the components of the tear film and to effects on the corneal epithelium. These patients often develop cataracts as a result of the radiation treatment, requiring the subsequent use of aphakic contact lenses. The ability to wear the contact lenses successfully may be affected adversely by the decreased tear production and compromised corneal epithelium. Supplemental ocular lubrication may be required.

Nasolacrimal Duct Obstruction

This is a common, unilateral or bilateral blockage of the lacrimal drainage system, usually at the nasal end of the duct. Patients present with an epiphora over one or both cheeks, a *wet* appearance to the eye, and a tendency toward recurrent conjunctivitis. The blockage is usually complete, but some patients may have a partial, somewhat intermittent obstruction. The Jones test will show an absence or significant decrease of tear outflow to the nose. Parents tend to be very sensitive to the presence of nasolacrimal duct obstruction, wanting something done immediately. The best treatment, however, is to delay a probing procedure until at least six to eight months of age (Petersen & Robb, 1978). The nasolacrimal duct obstruction often opens spontaneously after parents are instructed to massage the duct between the lower punctum and the nose daily. Episodic use of antibiotic ointments to control purulent conjunctivitis may be necessary. When it is required, probing is usually performed under anesthesia to prevent the child from struggling and to minimize trauma to the area, but some surgeons feel comfortable performing the procedure in a sedated child in the office setting. Probing is successful 90 percent of the time (Robb, 1986), and if it is not successful initially, it may be repeated as needed.

Dacryocystitis may be a complication of chronic nasolacrimal duct obstruction. There will be a fullness and tenderness to the area inferior and nasal to the lower punctum. Antibiotics and drainage may be required.

CORNEA AND CONJUNCTIVA

Infections of the cornea and conjunctiva are discussed in the section on infectious eye disease in Chapter 9. Limbal dermoids are usually easy to diagnose because of their characteristic appearance and size. Abnormalities of corneal size are usually apparent if the condition is unilateral, but bilateral patients with mild size inequalities may be much less obvious. These patients must have a full ocular evaluation to rule out other potentially serious problems such as glaucoma and cataracts.

Among the most difficult of all pediatric eye disorders to diagnose accurately are corneal opacities, both congenital and acquired. Careful biomicroscopy will be helpful but may be difficult in a young child although a hand-held slit lamp may prove very useful. Since most causes of corneal opacities are uncommon, referral to a corneal specialist will probably be necessary. Keratoconus can be readily managed by the optometrist with contact lenses.

Dermoid Cysts (Figure 7.1)

Dermoid cysts are histologically classified as *choristomas*, normal tissue that is abnormally located. Dermoids are composed primarily of connective tissue that may contain hair follicles and sebaceous glands, and they have a keratinized epithelial surface. There may also be a varying presence of lipid or bony materials. Dermoids may be found in various locations in and around the eyes or eyelids including the orbit, or they may be epibulbar (cornea, conjunctiva, and limbus). The size is variable but can be quite large. The color is usually light. Dermoids are a common tumor in young children.

Conjunctival dermoid cysts are most often located at the temporal aspect of the limbus and may extend onto the cornea several millimeters. Dermoids may be very deep, in some cases arising from the bones of the orbit. They may either be congenital or become clinically apparent only sometime later. The mass of the dermoid can cause deformation of the globe, inducing astigmatism and amblyopia, requiring early treatment of the refractive error and occlusion therapy.

Limbal dermoids may be associated with either Goldenhar's syndrome (auricular abnormalities, epibulbar dermoids, and vertebral malformations) (Feingold & Gellis, 1968) or microphthalmia. Most dermoids are sporadic in nature, but there is evidence of infrequent autosomal recessive inheritance. Dermoids that are not of

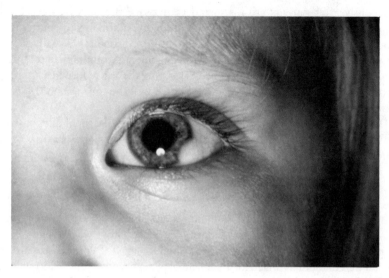

Figure 7.1 Typical limbal dermoid extending onto the cornea. There is often a significant degree of irregular astigmatism associated with this type of dermoid.

functional or cosmetic concern are generally left alone, but they may be surgically removed if desired. Care must be taken to prevent rupture of the cyst, which can cause a serious inflammatory response. Since dermoids sometimes extend very deeply into the surrounding ocular tissue, surgical complications may occur during excision.

Corneal Size Anomalies

The normal horizontal corneal diameter in a neonate is 9.5 to 10mm. This reaches the typical adult diameter of 11.5 to 12mm by three to four years of age. The change in corneal diameter is simultaneous with a change in the corneal vault, or corneal sagitta. The central corneal curvature is relatively steep at birth, but because of the minimal corneal vault, the corneal plane is very similar to that of the sclera. By six months of age however, the cornea rises out of the plane of the sclera, assuming an adultlike configuration by three to four years of age. The central corneal curvature also flattens rapidly during this same period (Moore, 1987). There are simultaneous growth changes in the structure of the entire anterior segment as well.

Megalocornea is indicated when the corneal diameter is greater than 11.5 to 12mm in an infant or greater than 13mm in a fully grown eye. Other ocular parameters are normal. There are several possible etiologies to be considered in these neonates. The most important consideration is the possibility of congenital glaucoma, which may be unilateral or bilateral. The initial presentation is a steamy cornea, prominent photophobia and tearing along with increased corneal diameter, which should not be confused with true megalocornea. Infants with this anomaly likely will not have normal visual behavior. Megalocornea is a bilateral condition (rarely unilateral) with a variable hereditary pattern, perhaps most commonly X-linked recessive (XR). In the form known as anterior megalophthalmus, there may be a number of associated ocular abnormalities, including high refractive errors, iridodonesis, iris atrophy, cataracts, and ectopia lentis. Megalocornea is usually nonprogressive and by itself is visually non-threatening. Patients with typical megalocornea possess a normal corneal endothelial cell density in contrast to patients with congenital glaucoma who have a reduced endothelial cell density (Skuta et al, 1983). Megalocornea is also commonly seen in patients with Marfan's syndrome. Along with enlarged corneal diameter goes the possibility of ectopia lentis, myopia to extreme degrees, and retinal detachments. All patients with large corneas should have a thorough eye examination to check for corneal clouding, increased intraocular pressure, myopia, lens changes, and retinal problems.

Microcornea is indicated by corneal diameter of less than 9mm at birth or asymmetric corneal diameters at a later age with one or both corneal diameters being smaller than normal size. Microcornea may occur as an isolated finding in otherwise normal eyes. There may be an autosomal dominant (AD) or recessive (AR) inheritance pattern. It is most frequently seen, however, in patients with persistent hyperplastic primary vitreous and/or congenital cataracts. These patients possess additional abnormalities of the eyes beyond the microcorneas. Microcorneas may also occur in the anterior chamber cleavage syndromes, often along with a central corneal leukoma in the variant known as Peters anomaly.

Corneal Opacities (Table 7.3)

The conditions that cause corneal opacification in children are both numerous in type and individually quite rare. Only the more commonly encountered conditions that cause these opacities in children will be discussed here.

Neonatal Corneal Opacities

Sclerocornea is a nonspecific description of a congenital corneal opacification with vascularization that is essentially continuous with the sclera. Most patients with sclerocornea show bilateral and nonprogressive opacifications. The limbus is usually not readily definable, but the central cornea may be somewhat clearer than the

Table 7.3   Corneal opacities

Causes of neonatal corneal opacities	Causes of acquired corneal opacities
Sclerocornea	Anterior
Birth trauma	Meesmann's dystrophy
Glaucoma	Reis-Buckler dystrophy
Congenital hereditary endothelial dystrophy	Stocker and Holt dystrophy
Congenital hereditary stromal dystrophy	Grayson and Wilbrandt dystrophy
Posterior polymorphous dystrophy	Stromal
Infection	Macular dystrophy
Mucopolysaccharidosis	Granular dystrophy
Mucolipidosis	Lattice dystrophy
Fabry's disease	Band keratopathy

periphery. The major defect is in the stroma, with a disruption of the typical lamellar structure and an appearance quite similar to that of the sclera. There may also be disorganization of other corneal layers, especially of the endothelium and Descemet's layer. Variations of sclerocornea include eyes that are otherwise relatively normal and retain at least a modest degree of vision; eyes with small, very flat corneas and anterior segments; microphthalmic eyes; eyes with the anterior chamber cleavage syndrome; and eyes with completely white, opaque corneas and an absence of vision. This undoubtedly encompasses a large number of separate conditions that are not as yet adequately described. The visual prognosis obviously depends on the degree of opacification. Penetrating keratoplasties can be attempted on those eyes having some potential for visual rehabilitation, especially if the condition is bilateral and asymmetric where the "poorer" eye may be operated on to give the infant at least a chance of vision. These cases are very difficult to treat because of deprivation amblyopia and the irregular corneal surfaces resulting from the surgery. Early intervention is critical. The use of rigid contact lenses in the subsequent optical correction provides the most regular corneal surface possible. Because of the poor optical character of these operated eyes, arriving at the correct refractive correction may be extremely difficult.

Tears or opacification of Descemet's layer and the endothelium can be caused by birth trauma and by congenital glaucoma. Injuries from birth trauma may be caused by the use of forceps to aid in the delivery of the infant (Angell et al, 1981). They will be unilateral and typically appear as vertical striae in Descemet's layer. Decreased visual acuity is caused by both the opacities themselves and the astigmatism and amblyopia they cause early in the infant's life. If it is identified early enough, amblyopia treatment may be considered. Congenital glaucoma tends to cause horizontal striae in Descemet's along with megalocornea. It must be pointed out that, although the direction of the striae due to glaucoma and trauma often follows the orientations described, this is by no means a certainty.

Only a few corneal dystrophies are seen at birth. Congenital hereditary endothelial dystrophy (CHED) is thought to be an AR inherited condition presenting as variable, bilateral corneal clouding, and sensory nystagmus if the opacities are dense enough to impair vision severely. There is minimal photophobia, blepharospasm, or tearing and normal corneal diameters in contrast to congenital glaucoma. There is a less common, dominantly inherited form that is more progressive and symptomatic than is the recessive form (Judisch & Maumenee, 1978). Penetrating keratoplasty should be considered if vision is severely compromised.

Congenital hereditary stromal dystrophy (CHSD) is encountered less frequently than CHED is. It is an AD inherited condition appearing as a dense, central stromal opacification and somewhat clearer periphery. Vision may not be as adversely affected as it is in CHED due to the possibility of some degree of vision through the relatively clearer peripheral cornea.

Posterior polymorphous dystrophy is a unilateral or asymmetric bilateral dystrophy affecting the corneal endothelium (Cibis et al, 1977). It is quite commonly noted in patients at later ages. Most patients are completely asymptomatic. Only rarely is the dystrophy severe enough to cause some visual loss. The endothelium and Descemet's layer appear to have horizontal bands of vesicles that are usually translucent or transparent. Severe cases may show stromal clouding. Progression is rare. Treatment is not required. Patients with posterior polymorphous dystrophy that eventually desire contact lenses should be fitted only with lenses of very high oxygen permeability because of the possibility of somewhat reduced corneal endothelial functioning.

There are a number of other conditions that rarely cause corneal opacities in the neonate, but do occur more often somewhat later in life. Corneal infection by Herpes simplex is a major cause of corneal opacity but is seen only rarely in neonates, mainly as a sequela of disseminated congenital herpes disease. Several common and usually mild systemic diseases of later life can have devastating effects when there is congenital infection. Examples of this are cytomegalovirus and rubella. Certain of the mucopolysaccharidoses, the mucolipidoses, and the tyrosinosis—all of them very rare—may manifest corneal opacities at birth. Fabry's disease may initially present in patients with an unusual, whorl-like corneal opacity (Sher et al, 1979). There may be a similar whorl-like or propellerlike opacification of the lens as well. The differentiation of these conditions is very complex.

Acquired Corneal Opacities
Corneal Dystrophies
There are a large number of acquired corneal dystrophies that cause corneal opacification and decreased visual acuity during childhood. They all are bilateral, often asymmetric in appearance, hereditary in nature, more central than peripheral, nonvascularized, and without inflammation. These tend to become manifest at some point during childhood and may progress throughout life. The conditions discussed in this section are only the most common corneal dystrophies of childhood. They are often classified according to location in the cornea.

The anterior corneal dystrophies are located in the epithelium or in Bowman's layer. The hereditary juvenile epithelial dystrophy of Meesmann is dominantly inherited and seen in early childhood. It may cause visual acuity loss to about the 20/50 to 20/60 level. The degree of corneal opacification is usually only mild. On retroillumination, the opacities appear as cysts within the epithelium. The condition is not progressive. Penetrating keratoplasty is generally not indicated. Reis-Buckler dystrophy is a dominantly inherited condition seen in early childhood that may cause significant visual loss to 20/200 or less. The opacities are gray and splotchy within the deep epithelium and Bowman's layer, gradually increasing in size and density and involving the stroma. Corneal sensitivity eventually decreases, often leading to recurrent corneal erosions, inflammation, and neovascularization at the limbus. Bandage contact lenses may be useful for acute phases, and penetrating keratoplasty is indicated if acuity becomes poor. The hereditary epithelial dystrophy of Stocker and Holt and the hereditary anterior membrane dystrophy of Grayson and Wilbrandt are only rarely encountered.

The stromal dystrophies are not seen in early childhood. Their first appearance is not usually until the second decade of life. The earliest to become apparent and the least common is the macular corneal dystrophy. This shows a recessive hereditary pattern. The opacities are grayish, indistinct in shape, and may be quite dense. Penetrating keratoplasty is usually required because of significant visual loss, but the graft may later develop the identical type of opacities. Granular dystrophy causes only mild visual impairment. There is an autosomal dominant inheritance pattern. The opacities are well defined and scattered with much clear cornea remaining. The epithelium remains unaffected, and treatment is generally not required. Lattice dystrophy is also dominantly inherited. There is a slow progression of linear stromal opacification, primarily centrally. These opacities may appear similar to prominent corneal nerves, but they are thicker and there may be a haze around them. Later in life, the epithelium may become involved, leading to recurrent corneal erosions and inflammation. Vision is often compromised enough to require corneal transplantation.

Keratoconus

Keratoconus is a common corneal degeneration (Krachmer et al, 1984) that may first be noted during the teenage years. Only rarely will it become manifest in the first decade of life, and when it happens, patients invariably develop a severe form of degeneration. A small percentage of cases have a familial incidence, but most appear to have no hereditary predisposition. There has been a strong association between keratoconus and habitual eye rubbing. Many patients have a concomitant history of allergy, eczema, or blepharitis. It was previously thought that individuals with Down syndrome manifested keratoconus as part of the condition, but studies have indicated that those patients with Down syndrome that do develop keratoconus are often noted to be habitual eye rubbers (Pierse & Eustace, 1971). The amount of force that can be applied to the eye by rubbing with a finger or knuckle is sufficient to cause a mechanical thinning of the cornea. Poorly fitting hard contact lenses may cause a form of apical corneal distortion that appears very similar to keratoconus. There has also been a long-standing suggestion that contact lenses may actually cause keratoconus. Some cases of keratoconus undoubtedly are due to this.

The earliest sign of keratoconus is a variable and increasing degree of astigmatism. A typical scenario is for a patient reporting previous visits to one or more eye doctors for refractions and spectacles that were effective for only a limited period of time. Subsequent refractions by each eye doctor found significant differences from the previous ones, and there was an implication that perhaps the previous eye doctor prescribed inaccurately. Finally enough corneal distortion and irregular astigmatism becomes manifest to make the correct diagnosis. This scenario has been experienced by virtually every optometrist.

The irregular, dark, scissors reflex that is seen on retinoscopy is the most apparent and universal sign of keratoconus. It is due to the central area of the cornea bulging out of its normal plane and creating a highly irregular refracting surface. Other early signs include an increased visibility of the peripheral corneal nerves, a series of vertical Vogt striae in the stroma of the central area of the cornea, the brownish-red circular or semicircular Fleischer's ring at the base of the cone, and central corneal thinning. Later signs include corneal clouding and scarring, corneal hydrops and breaks in Descemet's layer, and occasionally corneal neovascularization, which may in some cases be the sequelae of poorly fitting keratoconic rigid contact lenses.

The current best method of treatment for keratoconic patients is with rigid gas-permeable contact lenses. Experienced contact lens practitioners consider the fitting of lenses to keratoconic eyes to be among the most difficult of eyes to fit with lenses. There is usually a trial and error period, during which a number of lens designs will be tried until a reasonably good fit is achieved. This depends on the degree of the keratoconus, the shape of the cone, and the tolerance of the patient to the lenses. Most patients can eventually be fitted with lenses. These patients must be educated to the fact that their visual acuity will not be as good under most circumstances as it was before the condition developed. Current fitting techniques generally attempt to distribute the weight of the lens onto the healthy peripheral corneal areas in the so-called three-point touch technique. The degree of central corneal touch is minimized in order to reduce pressure on the corneal apex, the least healthy area of the cornea. Some of the older fitting techniques that attempted excessive central touch gave excellent vision but may have caused a more rapid progression of the disease and in some cases probably led directly to central corneal hydrops. The current techniques are in a sense a compromise between good fit and vision and good ocular health.

The problem of progression is a real one for the patient and the practitioner. Just when the lens appears to fit well, the corneal configuration changes, causing a previously well-fitting lens to fit less well, adversely affecting the comfort and the vision. Fitting lenses to these patients is definitely an ongoing process, requiring frequent follow-up. Better techniques and better lens materials in the future promise some improvement in this process. A small percentage of patients either will prove lens intolerant or will develop enough corneal scarring to prevent a level of visual acuity sufficient for the patient's life style and will therefore require a penetrating keratoplasty. These patients need to understand that this surgical procedure is no panacea as their vision will in most cases still be less than that they desire, particularly for the first year or so. Most will still require contact lens correction in order to mask the inevitable corneal irregularities resulting from the surgery. It is important to pursue contact lenses for as long as is reasonable because of the less than perfect results from penetrating keratoplasty.

Band Keratopathy
Band keratopathy is a calcific degeneration of the cornea following chronic anterior uveitis or the sequela of an alkaline burn to the cornea. It appears as a grayish to milky white opacification at about Bowman's layer and initially is concentrated at the nasal and temporal limbus. There is usually a lucid interval at the limbus due to the absence of Bowman's layer there. It eventually may extend centrally but is almost always less dense centrally than peripherally and is clearer superiorly and inferiorly. It occurs most commonly secondary to chronic anterior uveitis due to juvenile rheumatoid arthritis. Band keratopathy may cause reduced visual acuity when the opacification becomes centrally located. Treatment is by chelation with EDTA, which can dramatically clear the cornea. Patients with uncontrolled long-term anterior uveitis may require repeated treatments by chelation.

IRIS AND CILIARY BODY

Many of the congenital abnormalities of the iris are apparent by observation alone although the specific diagnosis may require more extensive evaluation. There has been considerable confusion, in both the literature and clinical practice, about the various etiologies comprising the anterior chamber cleavage syndrome. The most important factor in arriving at the correct diagnosis is a very careful evaluation of the anterior segment and consideration of exactly which structures are affected and the ways in which they are affected. The diagnosis will follow from these observations.

Aniridia, colobomas, and pupillary anomalies will generally be quite obvious as will oculocutaneous albinism, but ocular albinism may be difficult to determine. Albinos usually have early onset sensory nystagmus, reduced visual acuity, and a lack of a foveal reflex. These characteristics may be difficult to observe in a young child, however, and there are other conditions that may have a similar appearance. It may require multiple examinations over a period of time to confirm the diagnosis.

Uveitis in adults is very difficult to diagnose specifically. This is true for children as well. A single, mild, unilateral episode of uveitis may not require extensive evaluation, but multiple episodes of bilateral uveitis that do not respond to treatment must be fully worked up both in the eye and systemically. A full battery of laboratory tests should be performed in these patients. The standard treatment for uveitis is with topical and systemic steroids and cycloplegic agents. These should always be used very cautiously due to the potential systemic and ocular adverse effects.

Congenital Abnormalities (Table 7.4)
Anterior Chamber Cleavage Syndrome
The anterior chamber cleavage syndrome comprises a diverse group of congenital mesodermal abnormalities of the anterior segment of the eye. The structures involved include the cornea, the iris, and the anterior angle. There may also be various systemic abnormalities associated with the anterior chamber cleavage syndrome. Waring and colleagues (1975), in a now classic paper, devised a stepladder classification scheme for these conditions that has proved particularly useful in their

Table 7.4 Uvea

Congenital abnormalities	Causes of uveitis
Anterior chamber cleavage syndrome	Kawasaki's disease
Aniridia	JRA
Coloboma	Lyme disease
Pupillary anomalies	Systemic lupus erythematosus
Albinism	Crohn's disease
Choroidal hemangioma	Sarcoid
Choroideremia	Pars planitis
	Fuchs' heterochromic iridocyclitisis
	Reiter's syndrome
	Ankylosing spondylitis
	Behcet's disease
	Vogt-Koyanagi-Harada
	Sympathetic ophthalmia
	Infection
	Trauma

categorization. Prior to the publication of this paper, considerable confusion in the diagnosis and classification of those conditions now considered included within the anterior chamber cleavage syndrome existed.

Specific abnormalities are separated into two main groupings—central and peripheral defects—with a third grouping made up of a combination of the first two. The peripheral abnormalities are the easiest to classify and describe because they are the easiest to view during examination. Certain of the central abnormalities may not be apparent during examination because their view is obscured by the central corneal opacities. The ocular abnormalities may be unilateral but are more frequently bilateral and asymmetric. The cause of these defects is presently unclear but probably is related either to intrauterine inflammation or a developmental abnormality. There may be an AD inheritance pattern in several of the conditions.

The simplest of the peripheral defects is a prominent Schwalbe's line (posterior embryotoxon). It appears as a whitish ring within the cornea just inside the limbus and is separated by a lucid interval from the limbus. The ring may be incomplete with the most likely visible location temporal. The posterior embryotoxon is very common and usually not associated with the anterior chamber cleavage syndrome. There are generally no significant ocular problems that result from isolated posterior embryotoxons.

A prominent Schwalbe's line coupled with fine iris attachments that insert from the iris is called Axenfeld's anomaly. The appearance of these iris strands is quite variable, ranging from small numbers of intermittent, fine fibers, to a thick, almost continuous membrane extending around the entire angle. Many patients with Axenfeld's anomaly will develop glaucoma, resulting in the entity known as Axenfeld's syndrome (Henkind et al, 1965). The glaucoma may develop either at a very young age precluding early diagnosis and treatment and resulting in significant visual loss or as late as the second decade of life (Figure 7.2).

Reiger's anomaly has in addition to Axenfeld's anomaly a hypoplasia of the anterior iris stroma. The iris appears stringy and without the normal architecture of the collarette and remaining iris, and there is often a variable correctopia. Glaucoma is common, appearing anytime from early childhood to middle age. Reiger's anomaly is usually inherited in an autosomal dominant pattern with high penetrance and variable expressivity. When facial and dental abnormalities are associated, the condition is called *Reiger's syndrome* (Feingold et al, 1969). There may also be neurological, cardiologic, and skeletal abnormalities as well. A variant of Reiger's syndrome is iridogoniodysgenesis, which appears similar except for an absence of the prominent Schwalbe's line, and a greater tendency for megalocornea.

The central defect of the anterior chamber cleavage syndrome is a corneal opacity caused by an absence or hypoplasia of the central corneal endothelium and Descemet's membrane. The peripheral cornea often looks normal. The appearance of this corneal opacity may change considerably after birth, either clearing somewhat or becoming denser and vascularized. There is a wide spectrum of central abnormalities that may be encountered with the effect on visual acuity being also quite variable.

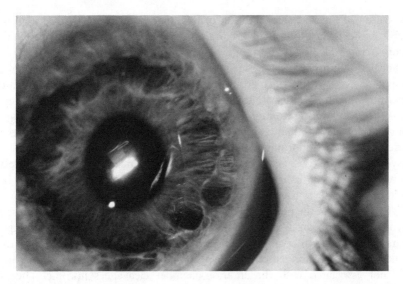

Figure 7.2 This patient exhibits a prominent anteriorly displaced Schwalbe's line with fibers extending to the iris along with hypoplasia of the anterior iris stroma. The risk of later onset glaucoma is greatly increased in these patients with the anterior chamber cleavage syndrome.

Posterior keratoconus appears as a central posterior corneal depression with an area of hazy corneal stroma anteriorly to the posterior defect. This is very different from the typical anterior corneal keratoconus that is a degeneration of the anterior cornea. It may be unilateral, and vision is often only mildly affected.

Peter's anomaly is a central corneal leukoma with iris strands arising from the iris collarette and attaching to the posterior surface of the leukoma. The density and configuration of the iris strands are variable as is the size and density of the leukoma. The anatomy of the anterior angle is often abnormal, and there is a high incidence of glaucoma. Cataracts, which are due to an anteriorly displaced lens being in contact with the cornea, may be seen. There may be microphthalmia or microcornea. Anterior synechiae are common. There may also be a number of systemic abnormalities. Vision is likely to be severely compromised.

The major ocular complications from the variants of the anterior chamber cleavage syndrome are visual loss secondary to the central corneal leukoma and the likelihood of the development of glaucoma. All patients, even those with only the minor characteristics of the condition, must be closely monitored for glaucoma, particularly during the early years. Examination under anesthesia should be performed as early as possible after the diagnosis is made with particular attention to measurement of the intraocular pressure, clarity of the media and the configuration of the anterior angle. Patients with bilateral dense corneal leukomas must be evaluated shortly after birth for consideration of corneal transplantation in order to salvage some level of visual acuity. These patients are difficult to operate on and to manage, but prompt intervention may be the only way to forestall the development of bilateral deprivation amblyopia and blindness.

Aniridia

The term *aniridia* is a misnomer that implies an absence of an iris. Actually patients with aniridia always retain at least a small residual iris root that may not be visible behind the corneal-scleral junction (Figure 7.3). There are a host of other ocular abnormalities that may be associated with aniridia, including foveal and macular hypoplasia, keratopathy, optic nerve hypoplasia, anterior polar cataracts and ectopia lentis, persistent pupillary membrane, sensory nystagmus, and photophobia. Patients are invariably legally blind. There are also abnormalities of the aqueous drainage and the anterior angle resulting in a high incidence of developmental glaucoma sometimes with onset as late as adulthood. This may be due to trabeculodysgenesis or occlusion of the trabeculum from hyperplasia of the iris stroma. It is very difficult to treat. The corneal dystrophy develops in the anterior layers of the cornea at the limbus along with a slowly advancing pannus. The central cornea is usually relatively clear even late in the course of the disorder.

Familial aniridia is inherited in an autosomal dominant pattern with high penetrance and variable expressivity. The sporadic form, present in about 20 to 35 percent of infants with aniridia, has an important association with Wilm's tumor of the kidneys. Most of these patients are found to have a deletion of the short arm of chromosome 11 (Riccardi et al, 1978). Since this tumor can develop at any time in childhood, especially in the first three to four years of life, all infants and

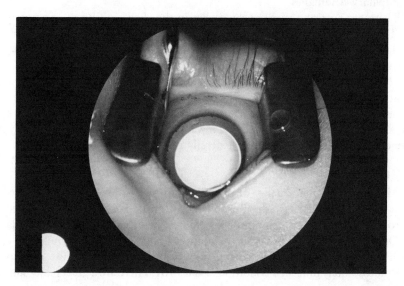

Figure 7.3 Although often thought of as the absence of the iris, there is always at least some evidence of hypoplastic iris tissue in patients with aniridia. The thin rim of iris tissue is easily visible in this patient.

children with aniridia must be closely monitored by a pediatrician for any potential development of this tumor. There is a school of thought that maintains that all infants with aniridia should have a chromosome analysis to help in the early diagnosis of this condition. Infants with the sporadic form of aniridia may also be at risk for a host of systemic abnormalities, including mental retardation, craniofacial abnormalities, microcephaly, and genitourinary disorders.

There have been attempts at fitting darkly tinted contact lenses to patients with aniridia as early as possible to help in the development of visual acuity. The hypothesis is that excessive light to the retina is a prime cause of the decreased acuity, but there is no confirming evidence that this improves the potential for vision. It is likely that much of the reduced acuity is due to foveal and macular hypoplasia and not to photophobia.

Iris Coloboma
Colobomas of the iris are relatively common and may be associated with other ocular colobomas of the choroid, ciliary body, lens, retina, and optic nerve. There may be an autosomal dominant hereditary pattern. The typical position of an iris coloboma is inferonasally, which corresponds to the last area of closure of the fetal fissure, but they may occur in other positions. Visual acuity is usually relatively unaffected unless there is an associated coloboma of the posterior segment of the eye that includes the macula or the optic nerve head. Colobomas may be of cosmetic concern in some patients and, if they are large enough, can be a source of photophobia. Cosmetic tinted contact lenses may be helpful for these patients.

Pupillary Anomalies
There are a great variety of anomalies in the shape, position, and size of the pupil. These pupillary abnormalities may be congenital or acquired and due to trauma or infection of the eye. The congenital iris anomalies are often sporadic in nature but may in some cases be hereditary. Partial forms of aniridia can cause multiple aberrant pupils (polycoria) due to iris aplasia. There is also a wide spectrum of persistent pupillary fibers, ranging from a few fine iris fibers across the pupil to thick fibers that cause an anomalous pupil shape (correctopia) and under rare circumstances can effectively block the visual axis, resulting in varying degrees of deprivation amblyopia. Treatment of pupillary anomalies is generally not indicated.

Albinism
Albinism is an abnormality of pigmentation that is due to an inborn error of metabolism. The uvea is often the most obviously affected ocular structure. There are two broad classifications of albinism—generalized or oculocutaneous and ocular.

Oculocutaneous albinism is fairly common, occurring in 1 of 20,000 people, but is much more common in certain isolated populations and ethnic groups. It is thought to be an autosomally inherited condition, usually AR. There are a great many subtypes of oculocutaneous albinism that depend on genotypic and phenotypic characteristics, but a classification system based on the presence or absence of tyrosinase in the hair bulbs is the one most commonly used today. The tyrosinase-negative group of patients lack the enzyme *tyrosinase*. When their hair bulbs are incubated in tyrosinase, they are unable to produce melanin. The tyrosinase-positive group is able to produce melanin in the presence of tyrosinase. Other subtypes have been identified that have variations of these tyrosinase findings, including the yellow mutant variant found in the Amish. In general, the tyrosinase-negative patients have a greater deficit of pigmentation and greater degree of ocular problems than do the tyrosinase-positive patients. The tyrosinase-positive patients usually retain some degree of pigmentation and have less severe visual loss.

Ocular albinism is thought to be primarily an X-linked condition, but some subtypes exhibit an AR pattern of inheritance. There is usually normal or near normal skin pigmentation, but a disturbance of melanosome production (O'Donnell et al, 1976) has been noted in the skin, indicating that this is actually a more systemic disorder than was previously assumed. Certain patients may possess enough ocular pigmentation that they do not exhibit iris transillumination and may have brown iris coloration.

There are a number of abnormalities that occur in the eye as a result of albinism. There is usually some degree of transillumination of the iris, especially in oculocutaneous albinos. A bright light shined through the sclera is visible through the iris and the sclera in a completely darkened room. The eye shows a bright red reflex whereas a normally pigmented eye will not. The color of the iris will usually be blue or very lightly pigmented. It will be lighter in color (less pigmented) in tyrosinase-negative individuals than it is in those with some residual degree of pigmentation. There may be a pupillary hippus. There is also some degree of foveal hypoplasia, which is the major cause of visual acuity loss and a major contributor to the nystagmus that is almost always present (Figure 7.4). The foveal hypoplasia appears as an absence of normal macular pigmentation and an absence of the foveal light reflex. The cones in the region where the fovea normally would be present resemble more closely the cones that would normally be in parafoveal areas (Fulton et al, 1978). There is usually no identifiable foveal depression due to an abnormal layer of ganglion cells where they should not be present normally.

There is a tendency toward moderately high hyperopic and astigmatic refractive errors, which also contribute to the nystagmus, strabismus, and visual acuity loss that is often present (Taylor, 1978). Strabismus is common and due in large measure to the nondecussation of nerve fibers at the chiasm (Creel et al, 1974). Corrective strabismus surgery is relatively unsuccessful because of this anatomic fact; there is not a simple misalignment of the eyes that can be mechanically corrected. Photophobia is present to some degree because of the lack of normal pigmentation but is often much less than one might assume. It was previously felt that this was the main cause of the visual loss, but it is now understood to be due much more to foveal hypoplasia than it is to photophobia. Color vision is often relatively normal, as is the ERG (electroretinogram) response. Some patients may have surprisingly good visual acuity (there are patients with ocular albinism with visual acuity of 20/25 or better), an absence of nystagmus and strabismus, and a partial foveal light reflex. These patients are sometimes classified as albinoid as opposed to albinotic.

There is little that can be done to correct the visual problems caused by albinism in its many forms. Because of the high incidence of significant refractive error, it is important to correct any refractive error carefully. Since most albinos have nystagmus,

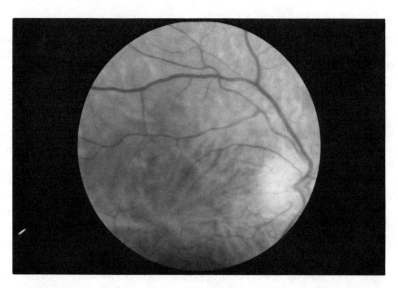

Figure 7.4 This patient retains a considerable degree of fundus pigmentation but has foveal hypoplasia, a hallmark of the disorder. Patients with partial albinism may maintain a surprisingly good level of visual acuity.

spectacles do not provide the optimal mode of correction. Contact lenses move with the eye during the nystagmoid eye movements, allowing the pupillary axis of the eye to coincide with the optic center of the lens and minimize the prismatic effects caused by off-axis viewing through spectacles. The lenses can also be tinted to decrease the intensity of ambient light, reducing to some degree the photophobia and its adverse effects on visual acuity. Strabismus surgery, as previously mentioned, is of little value, except for cosmesis. All oculocutaneous albinotic patients should use effective skin protection against ultraviolet (UV) light exposure to prevent severe sunburn and the possibility of various types of skin cancers. They are at significantly high risk for these problems.

Uveitis

Uveitis is the inflammation of the uveal tract of the eye. It causes a number of pathologic changes to the vasculature of the uvea. These changes include leakage of protein and inflammatory cells into the aqueous and vitreous, which appears as flare and keratic precipitates (KPs). The degree of flare and KPs is somewhat proportional to the degree and type of inflammation of the tissue. KPs are often classified as *fine* or *mutton-fat*, depending on their size and appearance. The uveal tissue may also become swollen and thickened. The combination of exudate and swelling can cause adhesions between the iris and cornea (anterior synechia) and the iris and lens (posterior synechia), which can be temporary or permanent. Under certain conditions, a posterior synechia can impair the drainage of aqueous, causing acute glaucoma. Chronic uveitis can lead to the formation of membranes of inflammatory debris that can block the pupillary axis and lead to a reduction in visual acuity. This can also occur at the ciliary body, creating a *snowbank* of inflammatory cells inferiorly and may lead to detachment of the choroid or pars plana. A similar process in the choroid can lead to necrosis of both the choroid and adjacent retina, causing visible scarring and visual field loss.

The general symptoms of uveitis include pain, tearing, photophobia, and decreased visual acuity. Pain may be surprisingly absent in young patients with severe uveitis, particularly in peripheral or intermediate uveitis (pars planitis), so it is not as good an indicator of uveitis as it tends to be in adults. Photophobia may be a more significant symptom in children, even in cases of mild uveitis. It is important to keep in mind, however, that uveitis in children is sometimes completely symptom free. This is especially true in uveitis that occurs secondary to juvenile rheumatoid arthritis. Young children with chronic uveitis may have decreased visual acuity due to inflammatory material in the ocular media and to lens and corneal opacification. Amblyopia and strabismus can result from this inflammation, particularly if the uveitis is unilateral.

The signs of uveitis include flare, cells, and KPs in the aqueous and vitreous and anterior and posterior synechiae, chorioretinal lesions of various types, and band keratopathy in chronic (especially from juvenile rheumatoid arthritis) uveitis. Cataracts can form in response to chronic or severe acute uveitis as can vitreous membranes. Intraocular pressure is usually quite low in juvenile uveitis except for those with iris bombe or massive anterior chamber membranes that may block the drainage of the aqueous.

The general treatment of uveitis includes the use of topical steroids and cycloplegic agents. Acute uveitis may require frequent instillation of one percent prednisolone acetate drops or dexamethasone ointment as often as hourly, but usually the dosage is four or five times per day, along with cycloplegic agents such as cyclogyl, atropine, or scopolamine. The steroids should be tapered when the uveitis begins to resolve. Care must be taken to minimize the total amount of steroids, because of the potential for cataract formation and the development of glaucoma and the concern over adrenal suppression and growth retardation. In most patients, these complications occur only when the topical steroids must be maintained for extended periods of time, but of course, steroid responders will develop problems much earlier. Occasionally systemic steroids may be required, especially in cases of posterior and peripheral uveitis.

Anterior Uveitis
Kawasaki Disease
Kawasaki disease (mucocutaneous lymph node syndrome) is a somewhat mysterious disease that has only recently been recognized by pediatricians. Its cause is unknown, but it has certain characteristics that imply an infectious etiology. Kawasaki disease is more frequently diagnosed in Japan where there have been recent epidemics that have affected thousands of people, but it is now being increasingly diagnosed in the United States as well.

It often begins as an acute febrile episode in toddlers lasting about one week. Children often present with reddened lips and tongue (*strawberry tongue*), reddening of the extremities and skin rash, and cervical lymphadenopathy. The ocular signs are a bilateral conjunctivitis and an acute anterior uveitis. Serious cardiovascular disease may ensue, and there is significant mortality. Optometrists should be aware of the association of conjunctivitis, uveitis, fever, and rash and should refer these patients to an appropriate source.

Juvenile Rheumatoid Arthritis

Juvenile rheumatoid arthritis (JRA) is a common inflammatory disease of the joints that can have serious ocular manifestations in children. There are estimates of about 200,000 children with JRA in the United States (Baum, 1977). Onset of the disease can occur in infancy when diagnosis may prove very difficult. The first presentation may be as a skin rash and fever of undetermined origin. Joint disease may not be evident in some patients during the pediatric examination for the rash and fever. The joint disease may first be noted when the child shows difficulty with movement or in a few cases when the child refuses or is unable to move at all. The degree of joint swelling ranges from minimal to severe. Histocompatibility antigens and antinuclear antibody (ANA) testing may help in the diagnosis, but a thorough pediatric physical examination should allow for clinical diagnosis. The condition is more common in females by around a 3:1 ratio. The etiology is presently uncertain, but is thought to have an autoimmune component.

Clinically JRA is divided into three groups based on the number of joints that are involved: Pauciarticular has five or less joints involved with the smallest incidence of serious systemic manifestations. Polyarticular has more than five but less than most joints involved. Systemic has almost all joints involved along with more frequent systemic manifestations in addition to the joint disease (Spiera, 1982). Ocular involvement is much more common in the pauciarticular form for reasons that are not yet understood with the very highest incidence of ocular involvement in young girls with pauciarticular JRA and positive ANA titers.

The ocular involvement does not follow a similar time course as does the systemic involvement. For example, a systemic flare-up may occur with no ocular inflammation evident while there may be no systemic problems for years prior to an acute inflammation in the eye. The ocular inflammation can be unilateral or bilateral although not necessarily at the same time. Ocular symptoms are usually surprisingly absent. Only rarely do patients with acute inflammation present with any complaints. The ocular inflammation may, in some cases, precede the onset of joint or systemic disease by years. Anterior uveitis is the predominant eye problem initially with the chronic sequela of the uveitis becoming more important later (Wolfe et al, 1987). The uveitis tends to show more flare than cells, but this is not pathognomonic. Posterior synechiae can occur quickly in the course of the uveitis and may even occur in the absence of significant cells and flare. There is a tendency toward the formation of cataracts from the chronic inflammation or from the treatment with steroids. These cataracts require surgical removal when the visual acuity drops below functionally useful levels. There may be a vitreous haze evident in some patients. There may also be a pupillary membrane that arises from the inflammatory cells in the anterior chamber that can have a similar effect on vision as secondary membranes from cataract extraction have. Band keratopathy is a frequent result of the uncontrolled, long-term uveitis that these patients manifest. In unilateral or asymmetric bilateral cases, the threat of amblyopia must always be considered in young children.

There is invariably great difficulty in controlling the uveitis with topical agents. It is routine to require steroids for years to minimize the inflammation to a *tolerable* level since complete remission of the uveitis is uncommon through the childhood years. Many patients will be unable to taper the steroids completely because severe uveitis returns. Steroid-induced glaucoma must always be considered during treatment. The goal of the treatment is to taper the dosage to the minimal degree possible without encountering a flare-up of the inflammation. Concomitant use of cycloplegic agents is usually required. The refractive effects of the long-term use of these cycloplegic agents must also be kept in mind; near adds should be considered when appropriate. Constant attention to amblyopia must always be kept in mind.

Systemic treatment is initially by the use of high doses of aspirin, which controls the disease well in most patients. For those developing gastrointestinal problems from the aspirin, a number of nonsteroidal anti-inflammatory drugs are used. In a small number of patients, gold therapy and Plaquenil are used. Plaquenil is a drug that has significant toxicity to the retina; patients must be closely followed for color vision and Amsler grid changes along with pigmentary changes to the retina, cornea, and lens.

All patients with the pauciarticular form of JRA must be followed for ocular involvement at four- to six-month intervals to guard against a silent flare-up of ocular disease. Patients with the other forms of JRA should still be seen about every six to nine months for routine slit lamp evaluations.

Lyme Disease

No current discussion of JRA would be complete without mention of Lyme disease, caused by a spirochete and spread by ticks. It was first described in 1975 in Lyme, Connecticut, but appears to now be widely distributed around the United States and Europe. Lyme disease is a multisystem disorder that includes a bull's-eye appearing skin rash, flulike symptoms, arthralgia, and, late in its course, cardiac and neurologic disease. There are also a number of eye findings, including conjunctivitis, anterior and posterior uveitis, retinal vasculitis, pseudotumor and optic neuritis, and keratitis (Aaberg, 1989). The ocular complications are quite variable, except for the conjunctivitis, which is a common sign of the disease. Any patient with acute arthritic symptoms should be evaluated for Lyme disease.

Crohn's Disease and Ulcerative Colitis

These are inflammatory diseases of the lower gastrointestinal tract that occasionally have the ocular manifestations of acute anterior uveitis. There may also be an association to juvenile rheumatoid arthritis. Episcleritis, corneal ulcers, and scleritis have also been reported (Petrelli et al, 1982). These patients often require long-term use of systemic steroids to control their gastrointestinal (GI) disease. They need to be followed about every six to nine months for the potential ocular sequelae of the steroid treatment and the possibility of occult uveitis.

Sarcoid

Sarcoid is a multisystem disease of unknown etiology that in the United States occurs primarily in young and middle-aged black females living along the Atlantic and Gulf coastal plains. It is relatively uncommon in children but is seen occasionally. Many organs of the body are affected—including the skin, lungs, liver, spleen, nervous system, and kidneys—along with the eyes. The primary features are noncaseating granulomas and vasculitis.

The ocular manifestations include a granulomatous uveitis with large, mutton-fat KPs, granulomatous nodules of the iris and conjunctiva, vitritis, and retinal vasculitis. The chronic uveitis may lead to band keratopathy. This retinal vasculitis may appear as *candlewax drippings* that are white exudates surrounding retinal arteries. Similarly appearing exudates may be seen at the optic disc, and their size may be quite extensive and can obscure the disc completely. Anterior synechiae secondary to the granulomatous uveitis can lead to glaucoma.

The course of the disease is highly variable as is the severity. Treatment is with systemic and topical steroids. The dosage is titrated to the minimal level that reduces the ocular and systemic disease to a level that allows the patient to function reasonably well. It is often impossible to completely eliminate the uveitis. The condition may resolve on its own as the patient reaches middle age.

Other Causes of Anterior Uveitis

There are a number of less common causes of anterior uveitis in children that must be considered in the differential diagnosis. Fuchs' heterochromic iridocyclitis is more commonly seen in older patients, but has been reported in children occasionally. The most apparent sign is a difference in the color and texture of the irides with the affected eye being lighter in color. Cells but not flare may be seen, and there will not be synechiae. Cataracts and glaucoma may cause decreased vision. There is some suggestion that toxoplasmosis and trauma may be associated with this condition.

Reiter's syndrome is seen mostly in young males and is associated with HLA-B27. There is urethritis, pauciarticular arthritis, conjunctivitis, and anterior uveitis. Chlamydial and gonococcal venereal diseases have been implicated in the etiology.

Ankylosing spondylitis causes arthritis in the sacroiliac joints and occasionally in the peripheral joints of young males. There is a strong association with HLA-B27. Anterior uveitis is often a feature of the disease. This uveitis may follow a course much like the uveitis of JRA. Behcet's disease and Vogt-Koyanagi-Harada disease are both rarely seen in the United States but are considerably more common in Japan. Among the many signs of these conditions are anterior and posterior uveitis. Sympathetic ophthalmia can produce a granulomatous anterior uveitis. This condition is precipitated by trauma, particularly penetrating trauma to one eye with the inflammation occurring in the fellow eye even after the eye is enucleated. Various types of intraocular surgical procedures have also precipitated sympathetic ophthalmia. Fortunately this condition is much rarer today than it was in the past.

Perhaps the most common category of uveitis in children is *cause unknown*. This is the same as for adults, where the cause of uveitis is not adequately diagnosed, at least on the first acute episode. If there are subsequent episodes, there is greater likelihood that a specific diagnosis can be arrived at. If the first episode resolves without significant ophthalmic sequelae, extensive testing is probably not indicated. Even with a full ophthalmic and pediatric work-up, a specific diagnosis is not likely to be found. This is certainly true in clinical populations.

Finally by far the most common identifiable cause of anterior uveitis in children is due to trauma. This may be through accident or, increasingly, through violence from child abuse. Most eyes that have received mild to moderate degrees of concussive force will develop a low-grade and self-limited anterior uveitis. These eyes will improve rapidly with or without treatment by topical steroids and cycloplegics. Care must be exercised to be certain that there is no further ocular damage that is unapparent on initial examination.

CONGENITAL GLAUCOMA

The detection of congenital and early onset glaucoma is usually easy, but the treatment is difficult to carry out successfully. Once the diagnosis of congenital glaucoma is made, these patients are best managed by a specialist in pediatric glaucoma.

Signs and Symptoms of Congenital Glaucoma

Open-angle glaucoma in adults, the most common type of glaucoma in that age group, usually requires extensive examination to detect. This is not the case with glaucoma in infants. Most infants with congenital glaucoma have an obvious ocular problem. There is usually little question that something is wrong.

There are a number of cardinal signs and symptoms of infantile glaucoma. The cornea exhibits a number of abnormalities as a result of congenital glaucoma. Most apparent is increased corneal diameter. Megalocornea in young children can be caused by other factors, including primary hereditary megalocornea and Marfan's syndrome, but any enlarged corneal diameter in the infant should immediately arouse suspicion of congenital glaucoma. The increased corneal diameter usually indicates an enlargement of the eye itself. Most patients with congenital glaucoma and megalocornea will be myopic as well (Robin et al, 1979). In unilateral or asymmetric bilateral cases, this may lead to anisometropia and amblyopia even in patients with early controlled glaucoma.

Corneal clouding is another abnormality noted in infants with congenital glaucoma and may be the most common sign of the disease in newborns (Figure 7.5). There are many other conditions that will cause corneal clouding, but the combination of enlarged and cloudy corneas is highly suggestive of congenital glaucoma. Both of these signs can be rapidly progressive and quite dramatic in appearance if only one eye is affected. Horizontal breaks in Descemet's layer, called Haab striae, may be seen. This is accompanied by a flow of aqueous into the cornea through the corneal endothelium. These breaks in Descemet's layer occur only with onset of glaucoma in the first year or two of life and are a valuable diagnostic indicator in later years of the presence of congenital glaucoma. The ruptures in Descemet's tend to greatly exacerbate the degree of symptoms in these patients.

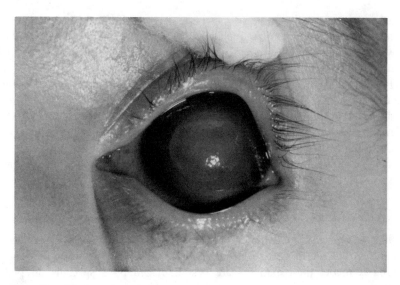

Figure 7.5 The cloudy, enlarged cornea in this patient is typical of infants with congenital glaucoma.

Patients with congenital glaucoma almost invariably have certain distinct behavioral patterns that aid in the diagnosis. Photophobia tends to be extreme. It is very typical on the initial examination to have the mother bring the child in to the examination room with the child's head buried in the mother's shoulder, trying to block out any light. This is accompanied by intense blepharospasm and epiphora, making attempts at examination very difficult especially when the lights are turned on in the room. Eye rubbing may also be seen. This behavior tends to worsen before treatment is instituted and the pressure brought under control. It is often this reclusive behavior, more than any physical signs, that brings the parent and child in for examination.

Other, less apparent signs of congenital glaucoma that may be visible only during an examination under anesthesia include a deep anterior chamber and surprisingly extensive glaucomatous optic disc cupping. The optic nerve head of infants is much less able to resist the effects of increased intraocular pressure than adults, and cupping develops very rapidly and extensively. This cupping can regress if the pressure is brought under control before optic atrophy ensues (Quigley, 1977). This change may occur in only a matter of days. Increased intraocular pressure is another important finding in congenital glaucoma, but the degree of elevated pressure may be much less than is generally found in open-angle glaucoma in adults.

Etiology of Congenital Glaucoma

The basic etiology of congenital glaucoma lies in abnormalities of the filtering angle of the eye. In general, it is the outflow of aqueous that is abnormal, not the inflow. Several theories have been advanced as to the specific defect. One concept is that there is some sort of film or membrane (Barkan's membrane) that covers the trabecular meshwork, impairing the drainage of aqueous. Another pertains to an absence or maldevelopment of Schlemm's canal. Other patients with primary congenital glaucoma are found to have a type of trabeculodysgenesis. This may take several forms with either an anomalous, anteriorly displaced insertion of the iris into the trabecular meshwork at the scleral spur as opposed to its normal insertion posterior to the scleral spur, or an anomalous configuration of the iris itself at the point of insertion into the trabeculum (Wright et al, 1983). The iris may show additional abnormalities of the anterior stroma and iris vessels. It is likely that each of these mechanisms, along with additional ones, is responsible for cases of congenital glaucoma.

Examination of Infants with Congenital Glaucoma

A comprehensive examination of every infant with presumed congenital glaucoma is the first step in diagnosis. A complete history, including family history, pregnancy and delivery, and general medical history must be obtained. While eliciting this information, the infant's behavior should be closely observed. Visual acuity testing by an objective technique, such as preferential looking or visual evoked potential, should be obtained, looking particularly for any asymmetry in acuities between eyes. If this is not possible, assessing fixation behavior will suffice at this point. Then an external ocular examination, including pupils, lids, cornea, anterior chamber, and tearing should be performed. If possible, a hand-held slit lamp should be used. Depending on the intensity of photophobia, this may be difficult or impossible. Retinoscopy and direct ophthalmoscopy, in part to evaluate the presence and appearance of a red reflex, should be done. A measurement of intraocular pressure with a hand-held applanation tonometer should be obtained. With the help of the mother or an assistant, reasonably accurate pressures can usually be obtained. Schiotz tonometry is less useful than applanation tonometry because of the likelihood of abrading the cornea with the metal footplate, and because of differences in the scleral rigidity factor between infants and adults (the sclera is very much softer and more pliable in infants, giving a different rigidity function) leading to potential inaccuracy of the results. Koeppe gonioscopy should be attempted to evaluate the anterior angle if the cornea is relatively clear and the child is adequately restrained.

The next major step will be to schedule an examination while the child is under anesthesia. This will allow a more thorough and less traumatic examination to be performed than may be possible in an office setting. A good look at the anterior segment of the eye with the aid of a slit lamp or operating microscope is invaluable. Measurement of intraocular pressure while under anesthesia may differ from that obtained in the office because of the effects of the anesthesia medication itself (Quigley, 1982). The pressure can be much lower while under anesthesia, with readings that would be considered normal in the office indicating high pressures under anesthesia. Thorough examination of the anterior angle and the fundus with gonioscopy and the indirect ophthalmoscope should follow.

The last step in the examination of infants with congenital glaucoma is to send the patient back to the pediatrician for a thorough physical examination to check for the presence of systemic disease that may be associated with the glaucoma. After all this has been done, a proper diagnosis can be made and a treatment plan developed. While awaiting completion of the evaluation, initial medical treatment can be instituted.

Conditions Causing Congenital Glaucoma
Primary Congenital Open-Angle Glaucoma

The major cause of congenital glaucoma is primary congenital open-angle glaucoma. This is a usually a sporadic, primary ocular condition without systemic manifestations although a small percentage of cases appear to be hereditary in nature. About 10 percent of patients have an autosomal recessive hereditary pattern. Seventy-five percent of cases are bilateral, and congenital glaucoma is somewhat more prevalent in males (about 65 percent of cases). The estimated incidence of the disease is approximately 1 in 10,000 births (Miller, 1962). The presenting signs and symptoms are primarily enlarged and cloudy cornea, photophobia, epiphora, and optic disc cupping that is usually present in the first year of life. The etiology of primary congenital glaucoma is related to structural and functional abnormalities of the drainage angle as has been described already.

Treatment of congenital glaucoma is eventually surgical in nature, as the antiglaucoma drugs that are typically used in adults are of only limited usefulness. Diamox, however, may have some effectiveness on an interim basis in selected patients. Many patients with congenital glaucoma will require multiple surgical procedures before the intraocular pressure is brought under reasonable control. It is important to understand that congenital glaucoma is a very difficult disease to treat, and many patients will never achieve adequate control of the increased intraocular pressure, eventually going on to significant visual loss. This is a disease that is best treated by an experienced pediatric glaucoma specialist, not a general practitioner.

Other Causes of Congenital Glaucoma

There are many other ocular and systemic conditions that may have congenital glaucoma as a manifestation. Patients with aniridia have, in addition to iris hypoplasia, about a 50 percent incidence of congenital or early onset glaucoma. This is due to either a physical blockage of the traebeculum by the remnant of the iris, or trabeculodysgenesis that is typically seen in primary congenital open-angle glaucoma. Glaucoma secondary to aniridia is a particularly difficult type of congenital glaucoma to treat (Walton, 1986). Goniotomy surgery and medical therapy are the current best treatments. Aniridia patients without early onset glaucoma must still be closely followed throughout life because of the high risk of developing glaucoma later.

Patients with many of the subtypes of the anterior chamber cleavage syndrome are susceptible to congenital or early onset glaucoma. There are a number of abnormalities of the anterior angle, including an anteriorly displaced Schwalbe's line, adhesions between the iris and Schwalbe's line, and iris hypoplasia. Glaucoma may be present in approximately 50 percent of these patients (Waring et al, 1975). All patients with the anterior chamber cleavage syndrome must be followed throughout life for possible late development of glaucoma. Treatment is initially by medication with surgery indicated later if the medical therapy is ineffective.

Two of the phakomatoses, Sturge-Weber disease and neurofibromatosis (Von Recklinghausen's disease), have a significant incidence of congenital and early onset glaucoma. Sturge-Weber disease causes glaucoma in 30 to 50 percent of patients, most commonly in those having the typical port wine stain on one side of the face with its distribution following the course of the fifth (trigeminal) cranial nerve. Often this is found in association with a hemangioma of the leptomeninges of the affected side (Phelps, 1978). This is the most commonly seen systemic disease that causes congenital glaucoma. The angle is affected by what is thought to be a membranous film over the traebeculum. There are usually additional abnormalities of the uveal vasculature, which may limit the ability of the traebeculum to pass aqueous, but the mechanism of the glaucoma is not yet known for certain. This is also a difficult type of glaucoma to treat.

Glaucoma from neurofibromatosis is most often associated with plexiform neuromas of the eyelids on the affected side. The cornea may become greatly enlarged in congenital cases. The etiology of the glaucoma is quite variable but may include trabeculodysgenesis, synechiae, or a membranous covering over the traebeculum.

There are a number of less common causes of congenital glaucoma. Patients with Marfan's syndrome and homocysteinuria may develop congenital glaucoma from pupillary block of a dislocated lens or as a result of abnormalities of the drainage angle. Patients with Lowe's syndrome, Hurler's syndrome, Weill-Marchesani syndrome, and Pierre Robin syndrome also have a significant risk of the development of congenital glaucoma.

ACQUIRED GLAUCOMA IN CHILDREN

Each of the conditions discussed above that cause congenital glaucoma may not become manifest until some time after birth, thus technically falling into the category of acquired glaucoma. This is true especially of the phakomatoses. The detection and diagnosis of these secondary glaucomas is not very different than detection of the congenital types. It is easier to examine these older patients than the neonates, and it is likely that examination under anesthesia will not be required to the same degree as it is in younger patients.

Trauma is the leading cause of all glaucomas in children with hyphema being the single most important predisposing event. Several specific factors increase the risk of development of secondary glaucoma: the size of the hyphema, the occurrence of rebleeds, and the presence of significant angle recession. Treatment includes paracentesis of the anterior chamber and trabeculectomy along with medical treatment. Angle recession without hyphema may cause glaucoma soon after the injury or many years later. The greater circumference of angle that is recessed, the greater the risk of glaucoma. If three-quarters of the angle is involved, glaucoma at some point in the future is almost assured.

Glaucoma secondary to chronic or acute uveitis is also an important cause of acquired glaucoma in children. This can occur as a result of blockage of the trabeculum by inflammatory cells and debris or by neovascularization of the angle. Iris bombe and angle closure due to inflammation may also cause secondary glaucoma. JRA is a relatively frequent cause of this type of glaucoma (Kanski, 1988). It must be pointed out that the primary treatment for most forms of uveitis is topical or systemic steroids, which itself can cause glaucoma, making it somewhat unclear if it is the uveitis, the treatment, or, more likely, a combination of both that precipitates the glaucoma. Regardless of the cause, the treatment consists initially of medical therapy followed when needed by surgical intervention.

Additional causes of secondary glaucoma in children include those resulting from cataract extraction even many years after surgery, retinopathy of prematurity, congenital systemic infections with ocular sequelae, and ocular neoplasms.

LENS AND CATARACTS (TABLE 7.5)

Ectopia lentis, or dislocated lens, is not an uncommon finding in children. It is important to arrive at the correct diagnosis in these patients, because of the potentially serious systemic manifestations found in many of its causes. For example, early diagnosis of aortic aneurysms in patients with Marfan's syndrome may prevent premature death.

Many cases of congenital and early onset cataracts in young children are impossible to categorize as to their etiology. There are a large number of uncommon systemic disorders that cause cataracts that can be diagnosed by careful evaluation. Early detection and treatment of these cataracts greatly facilitates a favorable outcome while late treatment virtually guarantees failure. These patients should be referred to an appropriate facility for treatment as expeditiously as possible.

Table 7.5   Lens

Causes of ectopia lentis	Causes of cataracts
Marfan's syndrome	Unknown etiology
Homocystinuria	Autosomal dominant
Ehlers-Danlos syndrome	Galactosemia
Weill-Marchesani syndrome	Fabry's disease
Hyperlysinemia	Refsum's disease
Sulfite-oxidase deficiency	Hypoglycemia
Trauma	Hypocalcemia
	Hallerman-Streiff syndrome
	Conradi's syndrome
	Stickler's syndrome
	Zellweger's syndrome
	Lowe's syndrome
	Rubella and other infections
	Persistent hyperplastic primary vitreous
	Diabetic
	Uveitis, especially JRA
	Steroids and other drugs
	Atopic disease
	Radiation

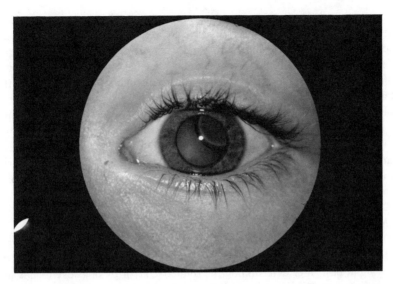

Figure 7.6 Lens dislocation in a superotemporal direction is most common in patients with Marfan's syndrome.

Ectopia Lentis

Ectopia lentis, or dislocation of the anatomic lens, occurs as a result of trauma, as part of a systemic disease syndrome, or as an isolated ocular event (Nelson & Maumenee, 1982). The lens is normally held in position by the zonules, fine, elastic fibers that connect the ciliary body muscle to the vicinity of the equator of the lens. There are several types of zonular fibers that originate in different geographic areas of the ciliary body and terminate either exactly at the equator or just anterior or posterior to the equator of the lens. Weakness, trauma, or absence of any or all groups of these zonules determines the direction and the magnitude of the lens dislocation (Figure 7.6).

Of major concern to patients with ectopia lentis is the irregular refractive error resulting from the malpositioned anatomic lens. This is caused by a tilting of the lens from its approximately normal position or a displacement of the lens out of its normal position. This results in light rays either falling on the lens in a nonparaxial orientation or the light rays falling on a noncentral or peripheral region of the lens. This induces an irregular form of astigmatism and myopia that cannot be corrected properly with spectacles or contact lenses. Patients with ectopia lentis are among the most difficult to perform retinoscopy on because of the aberrant retinoscopic reflexes caused by the malpositioned lens. These patients often cannot be corrected to a reasonably good level of visual acuity. Patients with early onset of ectopia lentis will in addition be subject to refractive amblyopia. There is also a strong likelihood that the refractive error will change as the lens continues to change position. Occasionally the lens may be dislocated to such a great extent that the eye is in effect aphakic. These patients can then be corrected with a standard aphakic refractive correction, often obtaining a higher level of visual acuity than that previously reached when the eye was functionally phakic.

There are several other important ocular sequelae of ectopia lentis. Uveitis is a not infrequent complication. Usually this is due to direct contact of the lens to the iris or ciliary body (Nirankari & Chaddah, 1967). Rarely, a ruptured lens may cause a phacolytic uveitis. Glaucoma is a frequent complication of ectopia lentis. This may result from pupillary block, secondary to uveitis, or displacement into the anterior chamber. Displacement of the lens into the anterior chamber can cause damage to the corneal endothelium and lead to an opacified cornea. Retinal detachment occurs with many of the underlying causes of ectopia lentis. Iridodonesis is also found in patients with ectopia lentis regardless of the etiology.

Management

The goal of the management of patients with ectopia lentis is generally to provide the best refractive correction possible. As was mentioned before, this is challenging at best since determining the refractive error by objective means such as retinoscopy is very difficult and requires great skill and patience. There is often high to extreme degrees of myopia and irregular astigmatism. Unilateral or asymmetric bilateral ectopia lentis will produce anisometropia and amblyopia, particularly in young children. Careful attention to this possibility must always be considered, and appropriate treatment applied. Frequent refractions should be performed because the refractive error may be quite unstable.

All patients with ectopia lentis need frequent, thorough evaluations of their retinas by dilation and binocular indirect ophthalmoscopy because of the increased risk of retinal detachment. These patients are one of the few groups where the use of miotic drops after examination to reverse dilation and to reduce the risk of anterior lens displacement is acceptable. The possibility of glaucoma must also be considered.

Lens removal has in the past been a controversial treatment modality for patients with ectopia lentis. At this time, most experts feel that lensectomy should be performed only when there is a specific indication, such as recurrent anterior chamber displacement, cataract, and phacolytic uveitis. Lensectomy performed on these patients carries a greater than normal risk of retinal detachment, glaucoma, and cystoid macular edema.

Anteriorly Displaced Ectopia Lentis

Although it is a rare event, a lens can become dislocated into the anterior chamber (Figure 7.7). These patients may present without any symptoms or may complain of blurred vision or pain in the eye. The cornea may be mildly to severely hazy, depending on the length of time and degree of touch of the lens to the corneal endothelium. It may on initial examination appear remarkably like an anterior chamber intraocular lens. The pupil will probably be mid-dilated and fixed.

It is essential that an attempt at repositioning the lens into the posterior chamber be made as soon as possible in order to limit the potential damage to the corneal

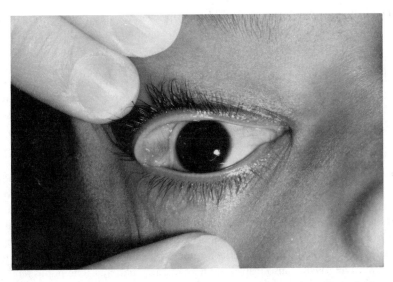

Figure 7.7 This patient presented with a complaint of decreased vision in both eyes and bilateral anteriorly displaced lenses. Medical evaluation confirmed a diagnosis of homocystinuria. After repeat episodes of anterior lens dislocation and in spite of the recommended use of miotic agents, clear lens extraction was performed on both eyes.

endothelium and reduce the risk of glaucoma. If the pupil is not already dilated, a short acting mydriatic agent such as Mydriacyl (Tropicamide) should be instilled as the patient lies quietly on her back. The lens may then fall back into the posterior chamber spontaneously if the pupil is sufficiently dilated. If the lens does retract, the pupil should then be constricted with pilocarpine to keep it in the posterior chamber. The intraocular pressure should be checked and the angle evaluated by gonioscopy. A decision then needs to be made whether to keep the patient on a miotic agent to prevent recurrence of the anterior lens displacement or to remove the lens surgically. If there is any indication that the anterior lens displacement is recurrent, as evidenced by history or the appearance of corneal endothelial damage, lens removal is indicated. Since this condition is more likely to occur in homocystinuria and Weill-Marchesani syndrome, a thorough work-up for systemic disease is indicated.

Causes of Ectopia Lentis
Marfan's Syndrome
Probably the single most common systemic cause of ectopia lentis is Marfan's syndrome. The prevalence is estimated at about 5 cases per 100,000 population (Pyeritz & McKusick, 1979). Marfan's syndrome is an AD inherited disease with a high degree of penetrance and variable expressivity that systemically affects connective tissue. Some patients appear to have new, spontaneous mutations.

The systemic manifestations include tall and slender stature, very long extremities, kyphosis, scoliosis, hyperextensibility of the joints, and cardiovascular abnormalities. Of major concern are the cardiovascular problems, which include abnormalities of the aortic valves and a high incidence of aortic aneurysms that tends to dissect suddenly, causing death. One study has indicated that greater than 95 percent of all premature deaths in Marfan's syndrome are due to cardiovascular causes (Murdoch et al, 1972). All patients diagnosed with this syndrome must have a complete cardiovascular work-up to determine the presence of these anomalies. Prophylactic surgery is now being performed to correct these defects before catastrophe occurs.

The ocular manifestations include congenital megalocornea, microspherophakia, enormous degrees of myopia (up to −30D) and astigmatism, blue sclera, retinal detachment, iridodonesis, and dislocated lenses. Vision may be severely reduced, but amblyopia may be improved with proper refractive correction and occlusion therapy. The high myopia found in some patients may be caused by the marked optical blur present from a very early age causing an increase in axial length. The iris often appears abnormal with a marked decrease in the number and consistency of iris crypts, ridges, and furrows. The iris may also transilluminate in a few patients. The pupils tend to be small and are frequently difficult to dilate. The anterior angle may show various abnormalities as well. Ectopia lentis is present in a majority of patients. It is usually bilateral and somewhat symmetrical. There is some tendency for the lenses to dislocate superotemporally, but this should not be considered diagnostic. Surgery to remove a clear lens should only be considered if the lens subluxates into the anterior chamber, which can lead to compromise of the corneal endothelium and iris bombe glaucoma. There is significant risk of retinal detachment in Marfan's patients who are left phakic throughout life, but this risk is increased tremendously if lens extraction is performed.

Homocystinuria

Homocystinuria is a metabolic disease with an AR hereditary pattern. There is a deficiency of an enzyme, cystathionine-β-synthase, which leads to excess levels of homocystine excreted in the urine. Many patients are mentally retarded. Many of the other systemic manifestations of patients with homocystinuria appear to be quite similar to patients with Marfan's syndrome. In fact, the two conditions have in the past been frequently confused and sometimes lumped together. The major difference other than the biochemistry is the frequent presence of mental retardation in those patients with homocystinuria. The major cause of premature death in patients with homocystinuria is thrombotic vascular occlusions.

The ocular effects are also quite similar to patients with Marfan's syndrome, although there is a tendency for the ectopia lentis to be inferiorly displaced in homocystinuria. There is also a greater likelihood of lens displacement into the anterior chamber in patients with homocystinuria than from the other causes of ectopia lentis.

Other Causes of Ectopia Lentis

A few other uncommon conditions can also cause ectopia lentis, including Ehlers-Danlos syndrome, Weill-Marchesani syndrome, hyperlysinemia, and sulfite-oxidase deficiency. Patients with aniridia have a very high incidence of dislocated lens.

The other major cause of ectopia lentis, in addition to Marfan's, is undoubtedly due to trauma to the eye (Jarrett, 1967).

CATARACTS
Congenital Cataracts

Congenital cataracts are estimated to occur in approximately 1 in 10,000 live births in the United States (Edmonds & James, 1985)—somewhere around 400 to 500 babies per year. There are perhaps an additional 400 to 500 cases per year that develop in the first year or so of life. This is not a very high incidence compared to many other eye problems, but congenital cataracts are one of the leading causes of serious visual impairment in young children. Research by Hubel and Wiesel in the 1960s and 1970s showed that the absence of form vision (caused by eyelid suturing or media opacity) in young animals caused a deep form of amblyopia, termed *deprivation amblyopia*, to occur (Weisel & Hubel, 1963). They also determined that, if this deprivation of form vision is maintained throughout the so-called *critical period* of visual development, permanent and severe visual loss occurred (Hubel & Weisel, 1970). If the eyelids of animals were sutured only after this critical period, relatively little visual loss occurred.

It has been determined that in human infants there does not appear to be an abrupt end to the critical period as there is in other animals but rather a more gradual change over the first four to eight months of age. For example, an infant born with a congenital cataract that is surgically removed, optically corrected, and patched for amblyopia prior to two to three months of age stands a far better chance of obtaining good visual acuity than an infant that does not have treatment initiated until sometime later. There are a great many factors that bear upon the success of treatment, but in general, the earlier the diagnosis is made and the treatment initiated, the better the chance of good visual acuity at the end of the treatment years later. The issue of critical period as it relates to amblyopia will be discussed further in Chapter 11.

Patients with unilateral congenital cataracts will almost always develop amblyopia in the affected eye. The noncataractous eye will generally develop a relatively normal level of visual acuity unless the degree of patching is so intensive that it develops a degree of deprivation amblyopia. Great care must be exercised during the period of treatment to prevent this possibility from occurring. The best means of prevention is by frequent monitoring of visual acuity by an objective method such as by preferential looking techniques (Mayer et al, 1989).

Causes

Congenital cataracts can be due to a great many different causes. The specific etiology, however, is often impossible to identify in patients, particularly in those with unilateral congenital cataracts. The causes of congenital cataracts can be roughly divided into several groups.

A large group of patients with bilateral cataracts have a hereditary form with no other ocular or systemic manifestations. These patients typically show an AD inheritance pattern with mixed penetrance and variable expressivity. It may appear in every generation, or it may miss one or more generations. It is almost always bilateral. The cataracts are usually quite dense, are present at birth, and may cause a sensory nystagmus from a very early age. Early treatment often results in good visual acuity.

Cataracts due to maternal infection during the pregnancy no longer account for as many cases as before, in large measure because of the development of vaccination for rubella. In the 1960s before the widespread use of rubella vaccination, there were a great many patients born with the congenital rubella syndrome (cataracts, chorioretinitis, mental retardation, deafness, and heart disease). Recently with a decrease in the percentage of children being vaccinated due to a number of factors, there are again some patients with the congenital rubella syndrome. Certain other infectious agents, including herpes simplex, cytomegalovirus, and syphilis, may also cause congenital cataracts as part of a disseminated congenital disease pattern.

Cataracts due to prematurity are on the rise. They are the result of the improving ability of neonatologists to keep very small birth weight babies alive. These infants are also at risk for retinopathy of prematurity. Some infants with unilateral congenital cataracts will also have persistent hyperplastic primary vitreous. This is a condition in which the embryonic hyaloid artery extending from the disk to the lens does not resorb during fetal development, leaving a glial and sometimes vascular mass retrolentally, along with an opacified lens. This is usually seen only in unilateral congenital cataracts. Many of these eyes are microphthalmic. Formerly it was felt that the presence of persistent hyperplastic primary vitreous made any attempt at treatment impossible, but it is now apparent that this is not necessarily true (Karr & Scott, 1986). The surgery is more involved than it is with simple cataract extraction, but in experienced hands, it is often successful.

There are a large number of rare metabolic diseases that have cataracts as a manifestation. Galactosemia is important to consider because the cataract, if it is promptly diagnosed, may be reversed and treated with a change in diet (Figure 7.8). Others include Fabry's and Refsum's diseases, hypoglycemia, and hypocalcemia. There are also a number of nonmetabolic inherited diseases that have cataracts as a manifestation, most of which are very rare. Included among these are Hallerman-Streiff, Conradi's Stickler's, Zellweger's, and Lowe's syndromes. All patients with congenital cataracts should have a complete physical examination to screen for metabolic and systemic abnormalities.

The majority of congenital cataracts, particularly in patients with unilateral congenital cataracts, are of unknown etiology. There is no evidence of any previous family history; there is no evidence of any systemic disorder; and the child appears otherwise completely normal. In some ways, these patients may present more problems for the parents than does a child with an identifiable cause. The mother in particular may carry a significant degree of guilt over her belief that the cataract resulted from something she did during her pregnancy. This may lead to difficulties in her relationship with both the child and her husband unless this problem can be worked out. It is important to try to allay these concerns in discussions with the parents during the earliest stages of the treatment.

Acquired Cataracts
Acquired cataracts are generally considered less difficult to treat than are congenital cataracts because deprivation amblyopia does not develop to as great an

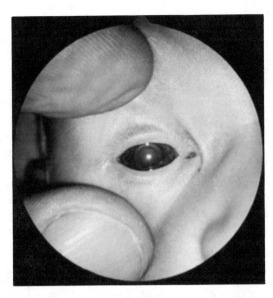

Figure 7.8 The *oil droplet* appearance centrally is due to a difference in refractive index between the nucleus and the cortex of the lens. Early dietary elimination of galactose can lead to a regression of the lens opacity.

extent as it does in truly congenital cataracts. These are still difficult and complicated conditions to treat, however. By far the most common cause of acquired cataracts in children is trauma. Penetrating and concussive trauma to the eye occurs frequently in young children (Nelson et al, 1989). This may be due to toy (especially broken toy), or sports injuries, violence, or accidents. Any patient with a penetrating eye injury also runs the risk of intraocular infection. There is great variability in the appearance of a traumatic cataract, but sometimes it may show a snowflakelike characteristic, and there may be a Vossius ring of pupillary pigment on the anterior lens surface. Severe trauma may also lead to rupture of the capsule and release of lens material into the aqueous or vitreous causing severe inflammation.

Diabetic cataracts are seen in adolescents with insulin-dependent diabetes, especially those under poor medical control. There is a higher incidence of this among adolescent female diabetic patients. These cataracts may require removal somewhat earlier than other types of cataracts because of the importance of a clear view of the retina to spot diabetic retinal disease. Other causes of acquired metabolic cataracts include hypocalcemia, galactokinase deficiency, and hypoglycemia.

Chronic uveitis is a frequent cause of acquired cataracts. In particular, the long-term smoldering uveitis associated with pauciarticular juvenile rheumatoid arthritis often leads to cataracts. In addition, the treatment for anterior uveitis, topical steroids, is a significant cause of cataracts. Approximately half the patients that have used eight bottles of topical steroids per eye, even over a long period of time, will develop posterior subcapsular cataracts. It is often impossible to know if the cataracts found in a patient with juvenile rheumatoid arthritis were caused by the steroids, the inflammation, or a combination of the two. There are also many systemic diseases that require long-term treatment with high dosages of systemic steroids (Figure 7.9), including asthma, arthritis, lupus, leukemia, and Crohn's disease. These patients need to be examined about every six months or so to evaluate the possibility of cataracts or glaucoma secondary to the use of the steroids. Atopic diseases may also cause cataracts. There have been recent, dramatic improvements in survival rates of children with leukemia and rhabdomyosarcoma (as well as other cancers) as a result of advances in chemotherapy, directed and whole-body radiation, and bone marrow transplantation. This has led to an increase in radiation-induced cataracts (Figure 7.13). Cumulative exposure of 800 rads to the lens is sufficient to cause cataracts. Optical correction after cataract extraction is often complicated by permanent damage to the lacrimal gland and the corneal epithelium, leading to problems wearing contact lenses.

Morphology of Cataracts

There is wide variability in the shape, position, density, and appearance of cataracts. In general, those cataracts that are densest and closest to the posterior nodal point of the eye have the greatest adverse effect on vision. It is necessary to evaluate the effect on visual acuity before deciding on the efficacy of cataract removal. Many types of cataracts have little, if any, adverse effect on vision and visual development, particularly those involving only a portion of the anterior lens capsule, which is

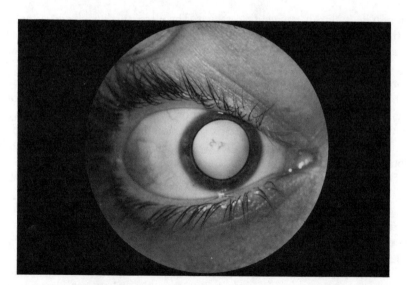

Figure 7.9 The long-term use of systemic steroids results in the development of posterior subcapsular cataracts. This patient had a renal transplant and will require the continued use of steroids to prevent rejection although continued use will lead to a visually disabling cataract that will require extraction. In other patients when it is medically advisable, discontinuation of steroids at this stage of lens opacification can sometimes allow partial regression of the cataract.

furthest from the nodal point of the eye. In patients with bilateral congenital cataracts, the presence of early onset nystagmus is an indication of dense and visually significant cataracts, whereas an absence of early nystagmus may be an indication that vision is much less affected. There may be a surprising difference in the examiner's estimate of the density of the cataracts by appearance and the cataracts' effect on vision. The objective measurement of visual acuity by preferential looking procedures or by visual evoked potential is the only accurate method of assessing vision and should be done routinely in every young patient with cataracts.

Anterior polar cataracts are the most anteriorly positioned cataracts (Figure 7.10). They appear as small white opacities in the pupillary aperture. On slit lamp exam it is evident that they are protruding from the anterior capsule, only rarely extending into the cortex. They are usually unilateral or bilateral and asymmetric and generally do not progress. There may be a positive family history, and there may also be an association with aniridia, microphthalmus, and pupillary membranes. Because they lie furthest from the nodal point of the eye, they have the least effect on vision if their size is not greater than that of the pupil. Treatment is not indicated unless they are very large or adversely affect vision, but there is a tendency for progression in some patients (Jaffar & Robb, 1984). Posterior polar cataracts may appear similar to the anterior polar type. Their effect on vision may be greater because of their proximity to the nodal point of the eye. Vision must be closely monitored in these patients, and surgical removal should be considered if vision is significantly affected.

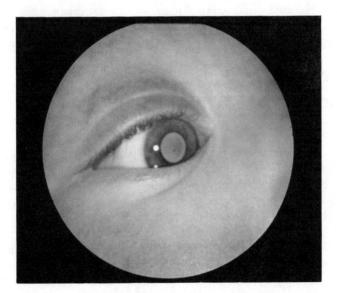

Figure 7.10 The small central opacity protrudes forward from the anterior lens capsule. Anterior polar lens opacities often produce minimal visual compromise because they are the furthest cataracts from the nodal point of the eye.

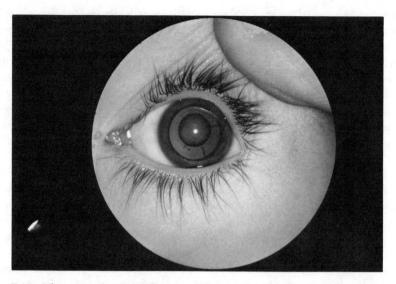

Figure 7.11   This patient has a sharply demarcated zonular cataract. Cursory observation may confuse this cataract with the *oil droplet* galactosemia cataract.

Sutural cataracts occur at the anterior and posterior Y sutures of the fetal nucleus of the lens. They are common, have a variable hereditary pattern, and only rarely cause decreased visual acuity. Zonular or lamellar cataracts are very common morphological types of congenital cataracts. They may be hereditary in origin, or due to pre- or postnatal insult to the developing lens. There is a clear zone of lens cortex that surrounds the more central lamellar area of opacification (Figure 7.11). The opacification often becomes denser over time. Patients with zonular cataracts may be quite photophobic. The effect on visual acuity is quite variable, depending on the size, density, and position of the opacity.

Nuclear cataracts are one of the more common visually significant congenital cataracts. They are often bilateral and asymmetric in density, and they may be progressive. The progression is sometimes initially very slow but with a sudden opacification later. Cortical cataracts of many types are also often progressive. They may cause little or no visual problems if they are primarily peripheral but can be visually significant if they are central.

Posterior lenticonus cataracts may have surprisingly little effect on visual acuity (Figure 7.12). They are outpouchings from the surface of the posterior capsule almost appearing like keratoconus. They are often unilateral. Posterior lenticonus cataracts have a tendency to progress and often require removal during childhood. It is very important to follow these patients closely with frequent visual acuity testing and to patch as needed to minimize the development of amblyopia prior to surgical removal.

Posterior subcapsular cataracts are frequently due to chronic uveitis and/or to the use of steroids (see Figure 7.9). The degree of visual disturbance is very great because of the proximity to the nodal point of the eye. Visual acuity may be subjectively more compromised than that found by objective testing. For this reason, these cataracts often need removal sooner than do other acquired cataracts.

The Treatment of Pediatric Cataracts

The treatment of congenital cataracts has progressed tremendously in the past ten years. It was formerly felt by most experts that unilateral congenital cataracts were not worth attempts at treatment because of difficulties in surgery and long-term treatment of the aphakia and amblyopia (Costenbader & Albert, 1957). More recent studies have shown that, with persistence, the results can be quite good (Beller et al, 1981; Robb et al, 1987).

There are enormous differences between the treatment of young children with cataracts and that of adults. Adults have had many years of normal vision before cataracts forms. The development of amblyopia as a result of the cataract is of no concern at all in these older patients. Amblyopia, however, is *the* problem in young children. If the cataract is congenital or of early onset, the visual system has not as yet had an opportunity of development. If the visual system is not properly stimulated by the end of the critical period of visual development, there is essentially no possibility of attaining any reasonable degree of visual acuity. The exact upper age limit of this critical period in humans is not currently known for certain, but it is thought to be more gradual in development than it is in lower animals. It is known that dense congenital cataracts left untreated at nine months of age are almost impossible to

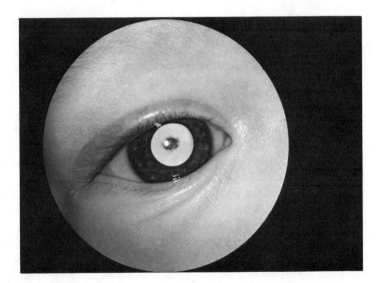

Figure 7.12   The lens is usually clear at birth but later develops an outpouching of the posterior lens capsule. This opacifies, resulting in reduced vision. Because relatively normal vision occurred during the critical period of visual developement, the visual prognosis is often much better in patients with posterior lenticonus than it is in true dense congenital cataracts.

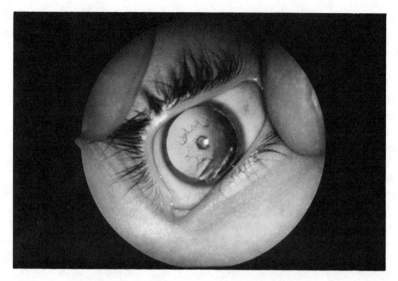

Figure 7.13 A common sequela to radiation therapy to the head when the total exposure to the lens is greater than 800 rads. Subsequent fitting with an aphakic contact lens is complicated by a combination of decreased aqueous tear production and superficial punctate keratitis, which are both common adverse affects of the radiotherapy.

treat. There is still some possibility of a good result up to about six months of age, and the rate of success is still better at three months of age. In general then, it is best to begin treatment as early as possible.

Older children with acquired cataracts often are able to achieve better levels of vision than are children with congenital cataracts. It is also clinically apparent that the shorter the period of time these patients with acquired cataracts have their vision obscured by the cataract, the better the prognosis of regaining good vision. Cataracts that are very dense have a more adverse effect on vision than do cataracts that only partially obscure the retinal image. In general, the greater the density of the opacity and the longer it obscures a clear retinal image, the greater the depth of amblyopia and the more difficult it is to rehabilitate.

Once it is understood that timing is of such importance in the treatment of pediatric cataracts, the necessity of rapid treatment becomes apparent. Surgical removal of the cataract must be completed as soon as it is determined that it is impairing visual acuity. Within the past ten years, improvements in the surgical techniques of cataract extraction by aspiration methods and a decrease in the risk of complications from anesthesia and surgery have allowed routine surgery in the first months of life for congenital cataracts. One ongoing problem has been the early detection of the cataracts. Pediatricians should be the first to see the congenital cataract when they are looking for a red reflex during the newborn physical examination that takes place at the time of discharge from the hospital, but this is not always the case. Some infants with congenital opacities are unfortunately not detected for months when the onset of strabismus may be the first obvious clinical sign of a serious ocular problem.

After the surgery has been performed, the next step, once the eye is healed sufficiently, is to provide an optical correction for the aphakia. In theory, there are several ways of accomplishing this. Spectacles work well in bilateral aphakes, but they usually work less well in unilateral aphakes. This is due to the enormous difference in the prescription between the lenses, which causes difficulty in getting the spectacles to fit properly on the child's face, causes magnification effects in the aphakic lens in comparison to the nonaphakic lens, and affects the peripheral vision. They may be useful, though, on a temporary basis for children who have lost their contact lens or when a child's behavior over the issue of contact lens wear becomes too difficult for the parents to deal with. A few patients with unilateral cataracts were unsuccessful with contact lenses but did very well with spectacles. An occasional break from contact lens wear may alter the child's behavior in a more favorable direction. The most important point to make here is to use whatever means of correction that works and to not be overly concerned with theory.

Intraocular lens implants (IOLs) have been used in the eyes of young children by a handful of ophthalmologists in the United States (Hiles, 1984), but there is a greater risk of serious complications, including uveitis, improper refractive correction, corneal problems, and glaucoma. There seems to be little reason to use IOLs in young children. Epikeratophakia has lately been advocated by some ophthalmologists as an alternative to contact lenses, especially in those patients intolerant of contacts. These ophthalmologists have found that it is more difficult to obtain a proper refractive correction in infants than it is in older children (Arffa et al, 1986), and they advocate the use of epikeratophakia only for those patients who have had acquired cataracts or for those who have failed with contacts. This is an evolving technology that may become a better alternative in the future. It is important to remember that the refractive error of young children changes greatly in the first decade of life and that IOLs and epikeratophakia do not allow for changes in power as do contact lenses or spectacles.

The best optical correction at present is with the use of contact lenses. In general, aphakic neonates can be easily fitted with contact lenses that are especially designed for this purpose in the office (Moore, 1985; 1990). Lenses are chosen based on the age of the patient and the size of the eye (Moore, 1987; 1989). A lens of approximately the correct size, shape, and optical correction is placed on the eye, and retinoscopy is performed over the contact lens in order to minimize the possibility of error by off-axis retinoscopy. Both the fit and the power of the lens is then adjusted until the examiner is satisfied that the parameters are correct. The lens may then be either ordered in the correct parameters or, if it is in stock, dispensed at this time. Lens power is often in excess of $+35D$.

Lenses only on a daily wear basis are highly recommended when possible, in part because of the issue of infection and safety but more importantly because it is much easier for the parent and the child to adapt to daily handling of the lens when the child is very young. This becomes much more difficult when the child is a year or two old. Although it does take time and effort to instruct parents properly in the care and handling of the lenses on a daily wear basis, virtually all parents are able to learn the appropriate techniques without too much difficulty. In this way, the parents become much more skilled daily observers of their child's eyes, and are able to spot problems immediately. Parents of extended wear patients are usually less able to manage the frequent minor lens-related problems that invariably occur.

The most difficult aspect of the treatment of children with early onset unilateral cataracts involves patching for amblyopia. In general, most children with unilateral cataracts will require some degree of amblyopia therapy until about age eight years, plus or minus a year or two. Consistency of patching is the single most critical part of the process of visual rehabilitation. It is easy to ask parents to keep a patch on their child's eye every day but quite another thing actually to accomplish it. Patch the normal eye for approximately three-quarters of waking time in the beginning of treatment, then titrate this regimen by measuring on each follow-up visit the visual acuity of each eye by the preferential looking technique. As the children reach about a year of age, patching typically becomes more difficult with adhesive eye patches, so shift to a black occlusive soft contact lens in those patients that become intolerant to the patching (Moore, 1991). This will often work well. It seems that many children object more to the feel of the patch on their face than they do to the effect on their vision that the patching causes. Also encourage the parents in the strongest way possible to maintain the patching schedule even if their child is rebelling strongly. If their third birthday can be reached with reasonably good patching compliance, regaining a significant degree of visual acuity is usually possible. Robb's and colleagues (1987) study on a large group of patients with unilateral congenital cataracts shows that about one-third of patients end up with acuity worse than 20/200, another third with acuity between 20/80 and 20/200, and the remaining third with acuity better than 20/80. Many of this last group attain acuity in the 20/30 range. Lenses need to be changed often in order to keep up with the changes in refractive error and the size and shape of the eyes as they grow. In some patients, this may be about every three to four months through the first year or two of treatment.

Bilateral aphakic patients often do not have significant amblyopia and therefore do not require any patching. Many of these patients are able to obtain virtually normal levels of visual acuity although some will have nystagmus. Use both contact lenses and spectacles for this group of patients, letting the parents decide which they and their children prefer to use. The parents usually report that the children have more improved gross motor abilities when they wear contacts than when they wear glasses. Almost every aphakic child has some problems with photophobia. Hats with long visors and sunglasses work acceptably, but tinted contact lenses may be a better option. At this point, such lenses are not readily available in the preferred soft lens materials. Overcorrect the refractive error by about +2.50D in young children to allow for focusing at near. When the children enter kindergarten, provide bifocal spectacles in polycarbonate material with an astigmatic correction included if necessary.

There are a number of possible complications that may arise as a result of the treatment of cataracts in young children. The first and most obvious is the inability to obtain good visual acuity. As was already mentioned if the parents are able to effect good patching for a consistent, long period of time, the results are usually quite good.

If the patching is not consistent, the results suffer. If there is no patching in unilateral patients, the results will be as expected, which is very poor (less than 20/200). Most of these unilateral patients will develop a strabismus, usually an esotropia. This can be easily dealt with by surgery later, if it is a cosmetic issue. Stereopsis is generally not possible in these patients because of the intensity of the patching. Other problems that may affect bilateral patients also include the possibility of a nystagmus, glaucoma, and retinal detachments due to the surgery and the 20–30 percent chance of the development of a secondary membrane due to opacification of the posterior lens capsule, which is usually left in place during cataract removal. If this occurs, either a second surgical procedure or the YAG laser is required to cut through the membrane.

REFERENCES

Aaberg TM. The expanding ophthalmologic spectrum of Lyme disease. Am J Ophthalmol 1989;107:77–80.

Angell LK, Robb RM, Berson FG. Visual prognosis in patients with ruptures in Descemet's membrane due to forceps injuries. Arch Ophthalmol 1981;99:2137–2139.

Arffa RC, Marvelli TL, Morgan KS. Long-term follow-up of refractive and keratometric results of pediatric epikeratophakia. Arch Ophthalmol 1986;104:668–670.

Baum J. Epidemiology of juvenile rheumatoid arthritis. Arthritis Rheum 1977; 20:158–160.

Beller R, Hoyt CS, Marg E, et al. Good visual function after neonatal surgery for congenital monocular cataracts. Am J Ophthalmol 1981;91:559–565.

Cibis GW, Krachmer JA, Phelps CD, et al. The clinical spectrum of posterior polymorphous dystrophy. Arch Ophthalmol 1977;95:1529–1537.

Costenbader FD, Albert DG. Conservatism in the management of congenital cataract. Arch Ophthalmol 1957;58:426–430.

Creel D, Witkop CJ, King RA. Asymmetric visually evoked potentials in human albinos: Evidence for visual system anomalies. Invest Ophthalmol 1974;13:430–440.

Edmonds LD, James LM. Temporal trends in the incidence of malformation in the United States, selected years, 1970–71, 1982–83. MMWR: CDC Surv Sum 1985; 34:1SS-3SS.

Feingold M, Gellis SS. Ocular abnormalities associated with first and second arch syndromes. Survey Ophthalmol 1968;14:30–42.

Feingold M, Shiere F, Fogels HR, et al. Reiger's syndrome. Pediatrics 1969;44:564–569.

Fulton AB, Albert DM, Craft JL. Human albinism: Light and electron microscopy study. Arch Ophthalmol 1978;96:305–310.

Gellady AM, Shulman ST, Ayoub EM. Periorbital and orbital cellulitis in children. Pediatrics 1978;61:272–277.

Henkind P, Siegel IM, Carr RE. Mesodermal dysgenesis of the anterior segment: Rieger's anomaly. Arch Ophthalmol 1965;73:810–817.

Hiles DA. Intraocular lens implantation in children with monocular cataracts 1974–1983. Ophthalmol 1984;91:1231–1237.

Hubel DH, Weisel TN. The period of susceptibility to the physiologic effects of unilateral eye closure in kittens. J Physiol 1970;206:419–436.

Jaffar MS, Robb RM. Congenital anterior polar cataracts: A review of 63 cases. Ophthalmology 1984;91:249–252.

Jarrett WH. Dislocation of the lens: A study of 166 hospitalized cases. Arch Ophthalmol 1967;78:289–296.

Johnson CC. Epicanthus and epiblepharon. Arch Ophthalmol 1978;96:1030–1033.

Judisch GF, Maumenee IH. Clinical differentiation of recessive congenital hereditary endothelial dystrophy and dominant hereditary endothelial dystrophy. Am J Ophthalmol 1978;85:606–612.

Kanski JJ. Uveitis in juvenile chronic arthritis: Incidence, clinical features and prognosis. Eye 1988;2:641–645.

Karr DJ, Scott WE. Visual acuity results following treatment of persistent hyperplastic primary vitreous. Arch Ophthalmol 1986;104:662–667.

Krachmer JA, Feder RS, Belin MW. Keratoconus and related noninflammatory corneal thinning disorders. Survey Ophthalmol 1984;28:293–322.

Kushner BJ. Local steroid therapy in adnexal hemangioma. Ann Ophthalmol 1979;11:1005–1009.

Liebman SD. Ocular manifestations of Riley-Day syndrome. Arch Ophthalmol 1956;56:719–725.

Matthews DN. Ophthalmic complications of craniofacial surgery. J Royal Soc Med 1979;72:19–20.

Mayer DL, Moore BD, Robb RM. Assessment of vision and amblyopia by preferential looking tests after early surgery for unilateral congenital cataracts. J Pediatr Ophthalmol Strab 1989;26:61–68.

Miller MT, Epstein RV, Sugar J, et al. Anterior segment anomalies associated with the fetal alcohol syndrome. J Ped Ophthalmol and Strabismus 1984;21:8–18.

Miller SJH. Genetic aspects of glaucoma. Trans Ophthalmol Soc UK 1962;81:425–434.

Moore BD. Contact lens therapy for amblyopia: In Rutstein R, ed. Problems in optometry: Amblyopia. Philadelphia: Lippincott, 1991;3:355–368.

Moore BD. Contact lens problems and management in infants, toddlers, and preschool children. In Scheiman M, ed. Problems in optometry: Pediatric optometry. Philadelphia: Lippincott, 1990;2:365–393.

Moore BD. Changes in the aphakic refraction of children with unilateral congenital cataracts. J Ped Ophthalmol Strab 1989;26:290–295.

Moore BD. Mensuration data in infant eyes with unilateral congenital cataracts. Am J Optom & Physiol Optics 1987;64:204–210.

Moore BD. The fitting of contact lenses in aphakic infants. J Am Optom Assoc 1985;56:180–183.

Mulliken JB, Murray JE. Natural history of vascular birthmarks. In Williams HB. Symposium on vascular malformations and melanotic lesions. vol 22. St. Louis: CV Mosby, 1982.

Murdoch JL, Walker BA, Halpern BL, et al. Life expectancy and causes of death in the Marfan's syndrome. N Engl J Med 1972;286:804–808.

Nelson LB, Ingoglia S, Breinin GM. Sensorimotor disturbances in craniostenosis. J Ped Ophthalmol Strabismus 1981;18:32–41.

Nelson LB, Maumenee IH. Ectopia lentis. Survey Ophthalmol 1982;27:143–160.

Nelson LB, Wilson TW, Jeffers JB. Eye injuries in childhood: Demography, etiology, and prevention. Pediatrics 1989;84:438–441.

Nirankari MS, Chaddah MR. Displaced lens. Am J Ophthalmol 1967;63:1719–1723.

O'Donnell FE, Hambrick GW, Green WR, et al. X-linked ocular albinism: An oculocutaneous macromelanosomal disorder. Arch Ophthalmol 1976;94:1883–1892.

Petersen RA, Robb RM. The natural course of congenital obstruction of the nasolacrimal duct. J Ped Ophthalmol Strab 1978;15:246–250.

Petrelli EA, McKinley M, Troncale FJ. Ocular manifestations of inflammatory bowel disease. Annals Ophthalmol 1982;14:356–360.

Phelps CD. The pathogenesis of glaucoma in Sturge-Weber syndrome. Ophthalmol 1978;85:276–286.

Pierse D, Eustace P. Acute keratoconus in mongols. Br J Ophthalmol 1971;55:50–54.

Pyeritz RE, McKusick VA. The Marfan syndrome: diagnosis and management. New Engl J Med 1979;300:772–777.

Quigley HA. Childhood glaucoma: Results with trabeculotomy and study of reversible cupping. Ophthalmology 1982;89:219–225.

Quigley HA. The pathogenesis of reversible cupping in congenital glaucoma. Am J Ophthalmol 1977;84:358–370.

Riccardi VM, Sujansky E, Smith AC, et al. Chromosomal imbalance in the aniridia-Wilm's tumor association: 11p interstitial deletion. Pediatrics 1978;61:604–610.

Robb RM. Probing and irrigation for congenital nasolacrimal duct obstruction. Arch Ophthalmol 1986;104:378–379.

Robb RM. Refractive errors associated with hemangiomas of the eyelids and orbit in infancy. Am J Ophthalmol 1977;83:52–58.

Robb RM, Boger WP. Vertical strabismus associated with plagiocephaly. J Pediatr Ophthalmol Strab 1983;20:58–62.

Robb RM, Mayer DL, Moore BM: Results of early treatment of unilateral congenital cataracts. J Pediatr Ophthalmol Strab 1987;24:178–181.

Robin AL, Quigley HA, Pollack IP, et al. An analysis of visual acuity, visual fields, and disc cupping in childhood glaucoma. Am J Ophthalmol 1979;88:847–858.

Rosett HL, Weiner L. Alcohol and the fetus: A clinical perspective. New York: Oxford University Press, 1984.

Shapiro ED, Wald ER, Brozanski BS. Periorbital cellulitis and paranasal sinusitis: A reappraisal. Ped Infect Dis 1982;1:91–94.

Sher NA, Letson RD, Desnick RJ. The ocular manifestations in Fabry's disease. Arch Ophthalmol 1979;97:671–676.

Shillito J, Matson DD. Craniosynostosis: A review of 519 surgical patients. Pediatrics 1968;41:829–853.

Singh YP, Gupta SL, Jain IS. Congenital ocular abnormalities of the newborn. J Pediatr Ophthalmol Strab 1980;17:162–165.

Sjögren H. The lacrimal secretion in newborn premature and fully developed children. Acta Ophthalmol (Copenh) 1955;33:557–560.

Skuta GL, Sugar J, Ericson ES. Corneal endothelial cell measurement in megalocornea. Arch Ophthalmol 1983;101:51–53.

Spiera H. Rheumatic diseases in children. J Pediatr Ophthalmol Strab 1982;19:103–107.

Sutula FC, Glover AT. Eyelid necrosis following intralesional corticosteroid injection for capillary hemangioma. Ophthalmic Surg 1987;18:103–105.

Taylor WOG. Visual disabilities of oculocutaneous albinism and their alleviation. Eldridge-Green Lecture 1978. Trans Ophthalmol Soc UK 1978;98:423–445.

Tessier P. Relationship of craniostenosis to craniofacial dysostoses, and to faciostenosis. Plast Reconstr Surg 1971;48:224–237.

Walton DS. Aniridic glaucoma—the results of goniosurgery to prevent and treat this problem. Trans Am Ophthalmol Soc 1986;84:59–68.

Waring GO, Rodrigues MM, Laibson PR. Anterior chamber cleavage syndrome. A stepladder classification. Survey Ophthalmol 1975;20:3–27.

Weisel TN, Hubel DH. Effects of visual deprivation on morphology and physiology of cells in the cat's lateral geniculate body. J Neurophysiol 1963;26:978–993.

Wolfe MD, Lichter PR, Ragsdale CG. Prognostic factors in the uveitis of juvenile rheumatoid arthritis. Ophthalmol 1987;94:1242–1248.

Wright JD, Robb RM, Deuker DK, et al. Congenital glaucoma unresponsive to conventional therapy: A clinicopathological case presentation. J Pediatr Ophthalmol Strab 1983;20:172–179.

8

Diseases of the Posterior Segment and Neuro-ophthalmic Disorders

Bruce D. Moore

CHOROID

Disorders of the choroid are usually not readily apparent unless they grossly affect visual acuity, leading either to severe bilateral visual loss and nystagmus or visual inattentiveness or, if they are unilateral, to strabismus. A thorough examination of the fundus is required to ascertain the etiology and extent of the disorder.

Although it may be technically incorrect to consider "congenital" toxoplasmosis and cytomegalovirus and herpes infections as congenital since they are probably (in many cases at least) acquired during transit of the birth canal, they are clinically different than the "acquired" forms of the disorders. For this reason, these disorders are placed in the congenital uveitis section of this chapter.

Congenital Abnormalities of the Choroid

Colobomas

Choroidal colobomas tend to occur at the inferonasal margin of the optic disc. The size of the coloboma varies greatly from minimal and of little visual consequence to massive and causing blindness. Eyes that are seriously affected may present as a congenital or early onset strabismus. There is an increased possibility of retinal detachments in patients with choroidal colobomas.

A number of chromosomal abnormalities have been associated with ocular colobomas, including Trisomy 13 and 18, incomplete deletions of chromosomes 13 and 18, and Turner's and Klinefelter's syndromes. Other syndromes associated with ocular colobomas include Aicardi's, CHARGE (an acronym for the following signs: coloboma, heart disease, choanal atresia, retarded growth and development, genital hypoplasia, and ear abnormalities), basal cell nevus, and Goldenhar's syndromes. CHARGE is an increasingly frequently made diagnosis that involves ocular colobomata (Pagon et al, 1981). The colobomata vary from minimal to severe with visual functioning consistent with the size of the coloboma.

Choroidal Hemangioma

There are two general categories of choroidal hemangiomas—localized and diffuse. Both are usually present at birth but may not become apparent until later. The diffuse type is most commonly associated with Sturge-Weber disease and rarely with the Klippel-Trenaunay-Weber syndrome. It appears as a large, red lesion that is usually located temporal to or underlying the macular area of one eye. It may be stationary or very slowly growing. The lesion is almost impossible to visualize with the direct ophthalmoscope since the border is quite indistinct. A dilated fundus examination with binocular indirect ophthalmoscopy is required for diagnosis. These patients have a high risk of glaucoma. An additional complication is the possibility of the lesion causing a hyperoptic shift in refractive error due to displacement of the macula forward. This can lead to anisometropic amblyopia. Isolated cases of choroidal hemangioma are seen infrequently, but the presence of this lesion should always arouse a strong suspicion of Sturge-Weber disease.

The localized form of choroidal hemangioma often appears as an oval, raised, yellowish-red mass usually in the posterior pole of the eye. There may be a pigmented rim. The overlying retina may have cystic characteristics that may make the lesion more apparent. Due to the risk of retinal detachment and cystoid macular degeneration, these patients should be closely followed.

Choroideremia

Choroideremia is an uncommon, bilateral, progressive atrophy of the choroid and the retinal pigment epithelium. There is an X-linked recessive (XR) inheritance pattern with full expression in males and incomplete expression in female carriers. Nyctalopia and visual field loss develops during childhood in males along with a strikingly white fundus appearance due to a loss of pigmentation. Female carriers may show only a mild pigmentary change in the macular area.

Posterior Uveitis

Congenital Posterior Uveitis

True congenital or very early onset uveitis is rare, but when it does occur, it is usually associated with disseminated congenital infections that are of a serious nature. The signs, symptoms, and nature of these congenital infections are much more severe than are the acquired infections of these same agents later in life, and the consequences to the child are much graver. Most patients with disseminated congenital infections will be detected at birth and followed in major teaching hospital settings, but a few less severely affected babies may eventually be seen by the optometrist in the office setting. These diseases are fortunately relatively rare for these are sick infants with generally poor outlooks.

Congenital toxoplasmosis is first acquired by the mother during pregnancy by eating contaminated, poorly cooked meat or during the cleaning of a cat litter box containing cat feces that is contaminated with the Toxoplasma gondii organism. The earlier the transmission of the organism to the fetus during fetal development, the greater the severity of infection, but the incidence of transmission is greater with maternal infection during later pregnancy (Desmonts & Couvreur, 1974). Most infected infants have no manifest disease. In its most severe form, the infant may have a number of severe neurologic manifestations, including mental retardation, microcephaly, intracranial calcifications, seizure disorder, strabismus, and nystagmus. The child may also be premature and have failure to thrive. The chorioretinal lesions are similar to the typical form, and there may be severe or mild anterior uveitis.

Congenital cytomegalovirus (CMV) infection is among the more common intrauterine infections (Hanshaw, 1971). The neonate with congenital CMV infection may be born prematurely and with low birth weight, jaundice, hepatitis, hepatosplenomegaly, thrombocytopenic purpura, and pneumonia. There may be severe neurologic manifestations, including mental retardation, microcephaly, hydrocephalus, seizure disorders, and strabismus. The chorioretinal lesions may appear very similar to toxoplasmosis, but are more likely to appear as small, discrete white foci with overlying vitreous haze that leads to small pigmented chorioretinal scars. The infection may be passed through the fetal circulation from the mother or may be acquired during transit through the birth canal. The drugs Foscarnet and gancyclovir have recently proven useful in treating the retinopathy resulting from CMV infection.

Herpes simplex type II can also be transmitted to the neonate during passage through the birth canal. There may be systemic manifestations that are very similar to that of CMV in addition to encephalitis. In the eye, there is sometimes a hazy media with patches of grayish white chorioretinal focal lesions and areas of retinal hemorrhage. These lesions cause pigmented scarring of the retina. Treatment currently includes acyclovir with other experimental drugs being actively investigated.

Acquired Posterior Uveitis

Systemic Lupus Erythematosus (SLE)

SLE is a relatively common multisystem disease that primarily affects females. Like juvenile rheumatoid arthritis (JRA), the specific etiology of SLE is uncertain but is also thought to be an autoimmune disease. Almost all patients will exhibit the presence of antinuclear antibodies. The major systemic affects include joint inflammation; various skin problems; and necrosis of the heart and peripheral vasculature, kidneys, and brain. Death may result from these causes. The ocular manifestations include retinal vascular disease, cotton wool spots, papilledema, retinal detachment (Figure 8.1), and less commonly, chronic anterior uveitis. Systemic treatment is similar to that of JRA patients with the frequent addition of antimalarial agents such as Plaquenil and steroids. These patients should be followed at least yearly even in the absence of eye disease, particularly if they are on steroids or Plaquenil.

Pars Planitis

Pars planitis, also called peripheral or intermediate uveitis, is a uveitis affecting the region of the pars plana and the ciliary body. It is a disease most prevalent in young boys four to five years of age. Its onset is insidious and may not become apparent until it is picked up on a school vision screening as badly decreased visual acuity or by a pediatrician unable to find a red reflex on ophthalmoscopy. It is almost always

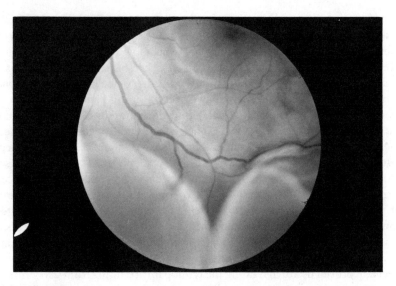

Figure 8.1 This patient has an extensive retinal detachment due to massive subretinal exudation secondary to SLE.

bilateral. There is usually an absence of symptoms such as photophobia or pain and signs of conjunctival or limbal injection. Posterior synechiae almost never occur. There may be a dense postlenticular cyclitic membrane composed of inflammatory cells and a fibrotic response within the vitreous that is the prime cause of the decreased vision. A "snowbank" of white inflammatory debris and collagen is located in the area of inflammation at the inferior pars plana. There is a definite three-dimensional quality to this mass. Additionally there may be retinal edema of the nerve fiber layer and the macular that can affect vision. The disease tends to be chronic with periods of quiescence and flare during which the density of the postlenticular cyclitic membrane varies along with the effect on vision. Cataracts may occur from the chronic inflammation. There is an increased risk of late retinal detachments and retinoschesis. There is a tendency for the disease to lessen in intensity by around 10 to 15 years of age. There may be only minimal residual vision loss due to the membrane and the cataracts. Amblyopia caused by the opacified membrane at earlier ages must be considered particularly if there is asymmetry in the density of the membranes. Treatment is with the use of the minimal dosage of topical and systemic steroids that decreases the inflammation to a reasonable level. It is usually impossible to rid the eye of all signs of inflammation completely, and one must keep in mind the effects on the patient of long-term use of steroids.

Toxoplasmosis

Toxoplasmosis is the most common cause of posterior uveitis in the United States. Toxoplasmosis chorioretinitis is caused by the parasitic organism Toxoplasma gondii. It is thought to be transmitted to the fetus through the placenta as a result of acute infection during the mother's pregnancy. The characteristic hyperpigmented chorioretinal lesions are due to recurrent episodes after the initial primary infection occurs (Figure 8.2). Encysted organisms are released by spontaneous rupture of the cyst, causing a fresh foci of inflammation adjacent to old lesion. The exact mechanism of this recurrence is not well understood at this time. The fresh lesions are surrounded by intense inflammation in the retina, choroid, and vitreous, often completely obscuring the lesion itself. Several antibody tests are used to look for an increasing titer of antibody to the organism in order to confirm the diagnosis.

Treatment is usually undertaken only when the recurrent lesions threaten the macula or optic disc areas of the retina. Peripheral, nonvision-threatening lesions are generally not treated. A combination of oral drugs is used in the treatment of toxoplasmosis, including pyrimethamine, sulphonamides, steroids, and Clindamycin. These drugs have significant toxicity and must be monitored closely. One can expect recurrences of toxoplasmosis, and at least yearly follow-up exams are recommended. Patients should be taught to check monocular visual acuity daily for signs of uveitis indicated by decreased acuity.

Toxocara

Ocular toxocara infection occurs by ingestion of the ova of the toxocara canis or catis parasite by young children often as a result of playing in a sandbox contaminated by cat or dog feces that harbor the organism. The larvae hatch in the child's digestive tract, pass into the bloodstream, and migrate to the choroid, where they can penetrate into the retina or even into the vitreous. They may cause a white mass on

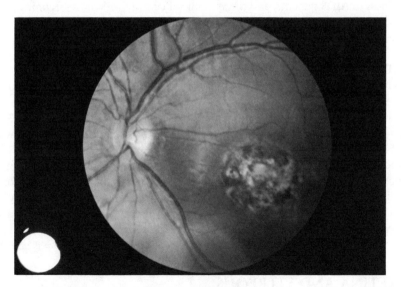

Figure 8.2 This patient exhibits the typical hyperpigmented macular scar resulting from toxoplasmosis chorioretinitis.

the retina often in the vicinity of the macula, and there is usually a severe inflammatory reaction that may completely obscure any view of the fundus. The inflammation can be so severe that it may appear as a totally white pupil (leukokoria), forcing one to consider the possibility of retinoblastoma. Vision is usually completely lost because of the massive inflammation. Cataracts and optic atrophy may ensue. There is no effective treatment, but steroids have been used to quiet the inflammation and various antiparasitic drugs are used to try to control the systemic effects of the parasite. Fortunately it is almost always unilateral.

Cytomegalovirus (CMV) and Acquired Immunodeficiency Syndrome (AIDS)

The severe congenital form of CMV disease has already been discussed. The acquired form of CMV ocular disease has until recently been seen only rarely. It appears as discrete, usually white chorioretinal lesions that may be pigmented and that are smaller than those of toxoplasmosis. These are areas of necrosis of all layers of the retina. There may be considerable vitreous haze adjacent to the chorioretinal lesions. CMV disease was formerly seen primarily in immunosuppressed patients. Recently however, this disease has been seen commonly in conjunction with AIDS. The appearance of CMV retinopathy in these patients, both young children and adults, is much more severe (Levin et al, 1989). Instead of the relatively discrete lesions that were formerly seen, the eyes of some pediatric AIDS patients have been described as looking like "pizza" with enormous amounts of exudates and hemorrhage covering large areas of the fundus. Other patients, at least initially, show a milder form of eye disease with smaller areas of retinal thickening, cotton wool spots, and hemorrhage and vitritis (Dennehy et al, 1989). CMV ocular disease has now become a major cause of blindness in AIDS patients, and the systemic effects of CMV have become a major cause of death in these patients. Very recently, the drugs Foscarnet and gancyclovir have been used as a treatment for ocular CMV with considerable success.

Histoplasmosis

Histoplasmosis is a mycotic organism that is endemic to certain areas of the United States, in particular the Ohio River valley. It is thought to be a major cause of uveitis in those areas. Eye doctors in other areas of the United States rarely see the disease in the native population. For example, the disease is virtually unknown in native New Englanders and is seen only in transplanted patients from the *histo belt* of the Midwest. The organism has not actually been histologically proven, but the evidence is strong enough that experts call the clinical disease presumed histoplasmosis disease. The lesions appear as large numbers of small, discrete, lightly pigmented lesions over the posterior pole of the eye. If the lesions affect the macula, vision can be seriously affected. There are also a host of significant systemic effects, and it is a cause of considerable morbidity in the geographic areas where it is endemic.

RETINA AND VITREOUS

The diagnosis and treatment of retinal disease in children is very complex. The first step is the detection of the disorder, which may turn out to be the most difficult

Table 8.1   Retinal disorders

Congenital	*Juvenile macular degenerations*
Stickler's syndrome	X-linked retinoschisis
Choroidal coloboma	Best's vitelliform degeneration
Medullated nerve fibers	Fundus flavimaculatus
Retinal dysplasia	Cone degeneration
Persistent hyperplastic primary vitreous	
Achromatopsia	*Exudative retinopathies*
	Familial exudative vitreoretinopathy
Tapetoretinal degenerations	Coat's disease
Leber's congenital amaurosis	
Retinitis pigmentosa	*Retinal vascular disease*
Usher's syndrome	Hemoglobinopathies
Laurence-Moon-Bardet-Biedl syndrome	Retinopathy of prematurity
Metabolic tapetoretinal degenerations	

part of all. Signs of poor vision are generally all that can be noted by the parents or pediatrician. Adequate examination of the young child's fundus is not easy, but with persistence, it can be accomplished with the use of the indirect ophthalmoscope. Electrophysiologic testing is essential in arriving at many diagnoses. Fundus photography is also very useful. The examiner should perform the evaluation in a systematic manner, and should not be satisfied with a less than complete view of the fundus before making a tentative diagnosis (see Table 8.1).

Congenital Abnormalities
Stickler's Syndrome

Stickler's syndrome includes a variety of ophthalmic and skeletal anomalies. There is an autosomal dominant (AD) hereditary pattern. The most prominent ocular features are high myopia and progressive retinal detachments along with cataracts and retinal pigmentary changes. Stickler's syndrome is one of the most common systemic disorders associated with high myopia (Opitz, 1972). Associated systemic findings include flattened facies, skeletal dysplasia, cleft palate, and mental retardation. Prophylactic treatment of retinal breaks is recommended. Cataract surgery and the subsequent management of the aphakia in these patients is greatly complicated by the association of retinal detachments. Close follow-up is required throughout life.

Chororetinal Colobomas

Choroidal colobomas have already been discussed, but an important issue to be considered in patients with choroidal coloboma is the increased likelihood of retinal detachment in areas adjacent to or overlying the choroidal coloboma. The abnormally thin retinal tissue is poorly attached to the underlying scleral tissue. These detachments may be particularly difficult to visualize because of the absence of the typical color patterns and contrasts that one associates with retinal detachments and holes. The presence of posterior staphylomas may also reduce the visibility of these retinal problems. There are several ocular conditions that are associated with choroidal colobomas, including Goldenhar's and Aicardi's syndromes, Trisomy 13, and the CHARGE association (Pagon, 1981). Isolated choroidal colobomas may also be sporadic in nature.

High Myopia

Perhaps the most common retinal problems that are seen in patients are those caused by high (sometimes called *pathological*) myopia. The epidemiology and progression of myopia will be discussed in Chapter 17, but a very brief discussion of the fundus changes is appropriate here. These changes affect the vitreous, the disc and peripapillary regions, the macula and fovea and the retinal periphery as well as those that are more widely disseminated throughout the retina.

Vitreous opacities and detachments are a very common feature of adult high myopes but are infrequently seen in children. The complaint of vitreous opacities or floaters is rare in young children. Vitreous detachment may be seen during careful examination of older children, particularly those high myopes engaged in contact sports.

There are a number of ophthalmoscopic changes that are seen at the disc in children with high myopia. The myopic or scleral crescent or ring is probably the single most common easily visible finding in any patient with moderate to high myopia. The disc may be tilted if the nerve exits eccentrically or if there is a posterior staphyloma (Figure 8.3). High myopes are more succeptible to the effects of elevated intraocular pressure (or even to normal pressures) because of structural compromises to the nerve head. This type of glaucoma, however, is encountered only infrequently in children.

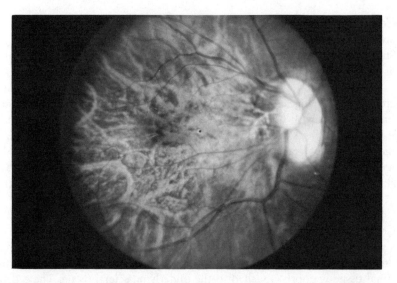

Figure 8.3 This patient with myopic retinal degeneration has conus formation, peripapillary atrophy, tilted disc, posterior staphyloma, macular changes, and choroidal thinning. The best corrected vision is 20/100.

Choroidal thinning is evident in most patients with high myopia (see Figure 8.3). The thinning may be severe enough to lead to breaks in Bruch's membrane. Posterior staphyloma, which is an ectasia or outpouching of the eye, is due to weakness in the structure of the eye from excessive stretching. This tends to be progressive and can lead to extreme degrees of myopia. These eyes are at very high risk of retinal detachment. The most common cataclysmic event occurring in the eyes of high myopes is that of retinal detachment. All high myopes and their families must be clearly warned of the signs and symptoms of retinal detachments and should be strongly cautioned to avoid activities that increase the risk.

Changes at the macula lead directly to decreased vision. Breaks in Bruch's membrane at the macula cause a Fuch's spot. Pigmentary abnormalities resulting from high myopia are often visible in the macula of older children, but may go undetected ophthalmoscopically in younger children. There is more often a decreased visibility of the foveal reflex in these patients that may be confused with other retinal abnormalities. The retinal stretching can affect the density and orientation of the photoreceptors and cause a variable degree of visual loss.

Peripheral retinal degenerations are not often seen in young children, in part because of the difficulty of complete examination. They are certainly seen, however, in older high myopes.

Medullated (Myelinated) Nerve Fibers

This common anomaly of the retinal nerve fiber layer is due to a continuation of the myelination of the ganglion cells beyond its normal termination at the lamina cribrosa. This is typically seen adjacent to the optic disc, but it is not unusual to see patches of myelination in discontinuous areas of the retina. It may be bilateral but is more commonly seen as a unilateral incidental finding on routine examination. There is a feathery edge to the starkly whitish patches of myelinated fibers (Figure 8.4). An absolute visual field defect corresponds to the area of myelination. It is uncommon to have any significant central visual loss caused by isolated cases of myelinated nerve fibers. There is a subgroup of patients that have unilateral high myopia, extensive patches of myelinated nerve fibers off the disc sometimes extending to the fovea, and dense amblyopia. Some of these patients respond to amblyopia treatment, but others show absolutely no improvement. This leads to the assumption that the amblyopia is of organic origin that is related to the myelination (Straatsma et al, 1979).

Retinal Dysplasia

Retinal dysplasia is an abnormal development of the retina causing a series of folds, gliosis, and generalized disorganization of the retina. It may be unilateral or bilateral and associated with a host of systemic abnormalities, or it may be an isolated finding (Fulton et al, 1978). The hallmark of retinal dysplasia is the histopathologic finding of dysplastic retinal rosettes. These rosettes are categorized into several types depending on their degree of organization (Lahav et al, 1973). This can vary from a relatively normal retina that is only partially folded over itself to completely folded retinal tissue containing only a few layers of retinal cells. Some of these eyes may

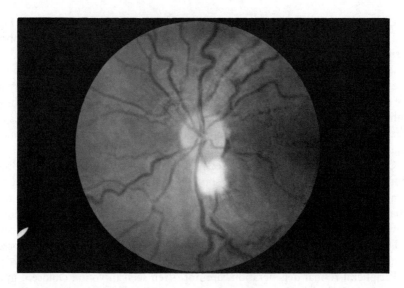

Figure 8.4 The feathered edge of the patch of medulated nerve fibers is starkly visible against the normal fundus coloration.

appear to be normal on examination, but more typically the eyes will be micro-ophthalmic, have a white pupil due to massive gliosis in the posterior segment, and be blind. Patients with severe bilateral retinal dysplasia will have a congenital searching nystagmus. Retinal detachments are common in the more severe forms. There is no treatment. Systemic disorders with ocular manifestations of retinal dysplasia include Trisomy 13-15, Norrie's disease, and Meckle's syndrome. Possible prenatal causes include radiation, toxic chemical exposure, trauma, and viral infection.

Persistent Hyperplastic Primary Vitreous (PHPV)

PHPV is due to failure of embryologic development of the vitreous beyond the earliest primary stage. This results in the continued presence of the fetal hyaloid vasculature to a variable degree and of its attendant glial elements within the retrolental space. There are a number of ocular features that may be present, depending on the severity and location of the condition.

The mildest form of PHPV is Bergmeister's papillae, which appears as a vessel, often corkscrew in configuration, arising perpendicularly out of the optic disc. The size of this vessel is variable, but generally it causes no visual problems unless there is attachment to the posterior surface of the lens. There are isolated reports of this vasculature bleeding because of severe trauma. Mittendorf's dot is the remnant of the fetal vasculature at its point of attachment on the posterior surface of the lens. It is of no visual importance.

Pruett (1975) has described three clinical forms of PHPV—anterior, interme-diate, posterior—and has shown characteristics of each. The anterior variety manifests microphthalmia, a whitish glial mass in the retrolental area that is usually vascularized, vascular traction of the ciliary body, and persistent hyaloid artery. The posterior form shows microcornea, vitreous membranes, retinal folds, and the presence of hyaloid artery remnants. The intermediate type may have a combination of anomalies found in each of the other categories. No matter which form is present, patients often have a shallow anterior chamber and cataracts and may also develop glaucoma, retinal detachments, and vitreous hemorrhages. The most common presenting sign of patients with PHPV is leukocoria although milder forms may present only with strabismus. PHPV is usually unilateral, but bilateral cases exist.

These patients have been considered very difficult to treat. With recent advances in the treatment of congenital cataracts and in neonatal retinal surgery, however, attempts at treating these patients have been more successful. Early removal of the lens and the retrolental tissue by combined aspiration and vitrectomy along with aggressive optical and amblyopia treatment has proven successful in some patients with less severe cases of PHPV (Karr and Scott, 1986).

Achromatopsia (Rod Monochromatism)

The normal color vision system is composed of three types of cones, each with visual pigments that absorb light preferentially at different wavelengths. Color vision defects are caused either by an absence of one or more types of cones or by a shift in the absorption spectrum in one or more of the cone types. The vast majority of patients with color vision anomalies are only mildly affected visually.

Achromatopsia is the most extreme form of color vision defect. It is either the absence of all cones or a deficiency in the functioning of the cone system (O'Connor et al, 1982). The rod system is generally intact. The result is a complete absence of color vision, markedly reduced visual acuity, nystagmus, and severe photophobia. Patients often have high refractive errors, particularly hyperopic astigmatism. There may be a reduced foveal reflex, but otherwise ophthalmoscopically the fundus appears relatively normal. The electroretinogram (ERG) shows a very reduced or absent photopic response with a normal scotopic function. The flicker fusion frequency is also markedly reduced. An autosomal recessive (AR) hereditary pattern is more frequently noted than an XR form, which may show a less severe effect on visual functioning. Achromatopsia is a fairly rare condition with an incidence of about 3 per 10,000 births (Krill, 1977). These patients may be helped by darkly tinted contact lenses for correction of the refractive error and reduction in retinal illumination. There have been dramatic improvements in visual behavior with contact lenses of this type.

Tapetoretinal Degenerations

Leber's Congenital Amaurosis

Leber's congenital amaurosis is a frequent cause of congenital blindness. It usually has an AR inheritance pattern. Leber's is a tapetoretinal degeneration consisting of dystrophic and degenerative changes in the ganglion cells, pigment epithelium, and photoreceptor outer segments of the retina (Mizuno et al, 1977).

At birth, patients are usually completely blind or at least severely visually impaired and have sensory nystagmus. Pupillary reactions are very sluggish or absent, and there may be marked photophobia. Optic atrophy, pigmentary retinopathy, and attenuation of retinal vessels develop by a later age although the fundus appearance of the infant may be normal. High hyperopic refractive errors are common (Foxman et al, 1985). Keratoconus secondary to habitual eye rubbing and cataracts also may occur later in the course of the disorder. Mental retardation and a wide range of neurological problems are frequently associated with a subgroup of Leber's patients, but many of them show relatively normal intelligence levels (Nickel & Hoty, 1982). The diagnosis is confirmed by absence of, or severe decrease in, the ERG response, which should be obtained in any infant with connatal blindness. There is no treatment. Many of these children have been institutionalized.

Retinitis Pigmentosa

Retinitis pigmentosa is a very heterogeneous group of conditions that have a dystrophy of the retinal pigment epithelium as a common finding. Most patients with retinitis pigmentosa have a genetically inherited disease with all types of hereditary patterns noted, but sporadic and presumably noninherited patients are known.

The pigmentary changes are usually present in the first decade of life, but there is much variability as to the time of onset with some patients becoming evident in the first year of life, others in the second and third decades. The earliest retinal signs are fine spots of pigmentation and depigmentation (the classic *salt and pepper fundus*), and the later typical ophthalmoscopic appearance is a *bone spicule* pigmentary retinopathy with small areas of dark pigment in stellate patterns interspersed with whitish areas of depigmentation in the midperipheral areas of the retina (Figure 8.5). This geographic retinopathy spreads gradually anteriorly and posteriorly, resulting in a widening ring scotoma visual field defect. Choroidal sclerosis develops later. There are in addition many atypical forms of retinitis pigmentosa that may show widely variable ophthalmoscopic changes even within the same families (Krill et al, 1970; Yee et al, 1976). It is important to keep in mind that the specific appearance of the fundus is not diagnostic for the specific etiology or classification of the disease.

Histologically the rods are first affected by the dystrophy of the pigment epithelium, leading to sclerosis of the retinal vasculature. The nerve fiber and ganglion cell layers are unaffected even late in the course of the disease process.

The ERG is a major tool in diagnosing retinitis pigmentosa. There is an absent or subnormal ERG response in affected patients, and many female carriers of the XR variety may also show a subnormal B-wave. These changes in the ERG generally precede visual function and ophthalmoscopic changes.

There are a great many conditions that are related to retinitis pigmentosa and that also have a retinal pigment epithelial dystrophy as part of the condition. Usher's syndrome includes a pigmentary dystrophy along with hearing loss. Usher's patients show an AR inheritance. Laurence-Moon-Bardet-Biedl syndrome patients have an atypically appearing pigmentary dystrophy along with mental retardation, hypogenitalism, polydactyly, and obesity (Lahav et al, 1976). Young retinitis pigmentosa

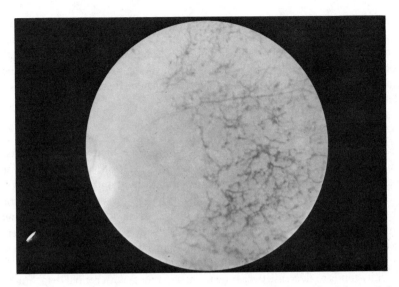

Figure 8.5 The typical bone spicule pigmentary clumping in the midperiphery of the retina and the attenuation of retinal vessels are typical of retinitis pigmentosa.

patients have occasionally been confused with patients incorrectly diagnosed as having Leber's congenital amaurosis. This is particularly true of young children that develop the earliest onset forms of retinitis pigmentosa but that do not present at an early age with the severely reduced visual acuity and nystagmus so typical of classic Leber's patients.

Metabolic Tapetoretinal Degenerations

There are a large number of rare metabolic diseases that have as an ocular manifestation a pigmentary retinopathy. Francois (1982) has divided these conditions into three primary classifications based on the general biochemical abnormalities of lipid, carbohydrate, and protein metabolism. These disorders usually show an AR inheritance pattern although several appear to be XR. The only common denominator is the presence of pigmentary retinopathy at some point in the course of the disease. These conditions are briefly discussed in Chapter 10.

Juvenile Macular Degenerations

The diagnosis and classification of the juvenile macular degenerations has been the source of considerable confusion over the years. The original macular disease described by Stargardt (1909) consisted of an atrophic macular lesion and visual loss in several young patients in two families. This became known as Stargardt's disease. Several additional unrelated diseases with somewhat similar appearances were subsequently included within the category of Stargardt's disease. Another condition, known as *fundus flavimaculatus*, that was thought to be a completely separate disease has a very different initial appearance, consisting of a variable number of white flecks that are visible in the fundus. Krill and Deutman (1972) eventually differentiated the juvenile macular degenerations into a coherent scheme based on anatomical and electrophysiologic correlates. Krill's classification of the juvenile macular degenerations include X-linked retinoschisis, vitelliform macular degeneration, fundus flavimaculatus, and cone degeneration.

X-Linked Retinoschisis

X-linked retinoschisis is an XR hereditary disease of males that results in a splitting of the nerve fiber layer of the retina (Yanoff et al, 1968). Ophthalmoscopically it is seen most frequently in the inferotemporal periphery and at the macula. There is a spokelike pattern of cystoid macular changes that is very characteristic, but its appearance may be difficult to visualize early in the course of the disease. Peripherally, there is a visible splitting of the retina, with vessels present on the outer layer, and retinal holes on the inner layer. Retinal detachments and vitreous hemorrhages may be seen. The ERG shows a reduction in the B-wave with a normal A-wave remaining. Visual acuity tends to decrease over time in most patients with retinal detachments up to, but not including, the ora serata common in later stages. Progression may be quite slow with good vision remaining in some patients even during the late adult years.

Best's Vitelliform Degeneration

This is an AD inherited disease with mixed expressivity and penetrance. The ophthalmoscopic appearance is a macular lesion that appears like a sunny-side up egg yolk in the early stages. The lesion is sharply defined and cystic in appearance with a yellow to orange color, which eventually "scrambles," leaving a pigmented macular lesion. It is only rarely unilateral. It is usually first noted between 3 and 15 years of age, often on routine examination, and there may be a complete absence of any symptoms or perhaps only a mild metamorphopsia on examination. The vision is normal or only slightly reduced until the yolk begins to "scramble" when the acuity may decrease to the 20/200 level, but it is not unusual to maintain good visual acuity throughout life whether the yolk "scrambles" or not. Color vision may be affected even before acuity is seriously compromised with a tritan defect being most commonly noted. ERG, peripheral visual fields, and dark adaptation are normal, but the electro-oculogram is abnormal even for phenotypically normal carriers. The EOG (electro-oculogram) is the key diagnostic tool in this disease. There may be a diffuse abnormality of the pigment epithelium in these patients. Treatment is supportive, and genetic counselling should be performed.

Fundus Flavimaculatus

This condition includes the original disease described by Stargardt. There are actually two forms that have distinctly different appearances in the earlier stages of the disease. These two forms have been considered separate disease entities by some authors but are here treated as one. There is marked variability of the appearance of this disorder, and many authors differentiate the forms based solely on the ophthalmoscopic appearance (Bither & Berns, 1988).

Fundus flavimaculatus is an AR inherited disease. The characteristic retinal lesions are large numbers of yellowish-white flecks of variable shape, size, and density (Figure 8.6). The lesions may become confluent over time, becoming less distinct in color and border. New lesions continue to appear as old ones fade. They tend to be located mainly in the posterior pole and the equator.

Stargardt's disease is the second and more commonly seen lesion of fundus flavimaculatus. It appears between ages 8 and 14 as an atrophic macular degeneration—first with a decreased foveal reflex, then with a round pigmented macular degeneration. It is progressive and usually lowers visual acuity to the 20/200 level. Histologically there is a loss of photoreceptors and pigment epithelium in the perimacular area.

Many patients have both forms of retinal lesions during the course of their disease. Patients with only the retinal flecks may be spared significant visual loss unless a fleck directly affects the fovea. A few of these patients will in addition have a diffuse cone degeneration that appears similar to that of primary cone degeneration patients. This group of patients will show a reduced photopic and flicker ERG as expected. Scotopic function is not impaired. Patients without the cone degeneration have normal or only slightly abnormal ERG responses. The EOG is abnormal, and dark adaptation is slower than normal. Peripheral fields are generally intact. It is now thought that a massive accumulation of an abnormal lipofuscin material within the pigment epithelium is the metabolic cause of the disease (Eagle et al, 1980).

Cone Degeneration

This is an uncommon juvenile macular degeneration with an AD hereditary pattern. The appearance of the macular lesion is usually that of a bull's-eye with a

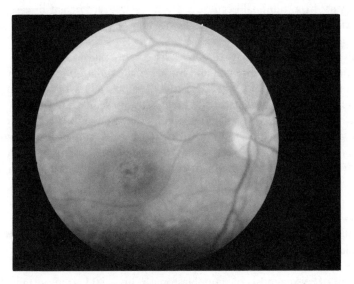

Figure 8.6 Both yellowish-white retinal flecks and pigmentary macular degeneration are visible in this patient with fundus flavimaculatus.

central, dark red area surrounded by a sharply defined ring of depigmentation. It appears similar to chloroquine retinopathy. Rarely the lesion will show only pigment clumping and a diffuse atrophic macula instead of the bull's-eye. Attenuation of the retinal vessels and a peripheral pigmentary retinopathy and optic atrophy may be noted later.

Visual acuity deficits range from mild to severe (20/25 to 20/200), and there is usually some degree of progression. Photophobia and nystagmus are frequently noted. The level of vision loss is related to the degree of destruction of the photoreceptors. There are two patterns of photoreceptor involvement: one affecting only the cones, the other affecting both the rods and cones. Cone outer segment and pigment epithelial destruction may begin at a young age with rod involvement, if any, beginning later in most cases. Peripheral fields tend to remain normal unless there is extensive rod involvement. Color vision is affected when visual acuity is still only mildly decreased. There seems to be an early propensity toward protan/deutan color defects in contrast to many other macular diseases that show a tritan defect, but these patients often progress to severe tritan defects as well. There is an abnormality of the photopic ERG in all cone degeneration patients with scotopic abnormalities in patients having simultaneous rod involvement. Dark adaptation, even in those with rod involvement, remains unaffected.

Exudative Retinopathies

Familial Exudative Vitreoretinopathy

This is a rare AD inherited disease that has clinical features that resemble aspects of retinopathy of prematurity, Coat's exudative retinopathy, and peripheral uveitis (Criswick & Schepens, 1969). Individual patients and probands may have clinical signs that vary from minimal occult disease to very severe ocular disease, the latter causing major visual loss. Although the disease may be progressive, many patients are asymptomatic and have minimal disease.

Fully manifested familial exudative vitreoretinopathy may present as dense vitreous membranes and subretinal and intraretinal exudation particularly temporal to the ora serrata. A fold of retinal detachment temporally, which may appear very similar to retinopathy of prematurity, is generally present when there is significant exudative retinopathy. Neovascular retinopathy may be found in this region beyond the age noted in retinopathy of prematurity. Retinal detachment may occur at later stages of progressive disease. Three stages of the familial exudative vitreoretinopathy disease have been described. Treatment consists of laser photocoagulation and cryotherapy for proliferative retinopathy and retinal detachment.

Coat's Disease

Coat's disease is a type of retinal telangiectasia that is found most typically in young males (Figure 8.7). It is usually unilateral and may present at a very young age as a leukocoria. In the past, it was not uncommon that these eyes were removed as a consequence of misdiagnosis of retinoblastoma. This is still an important diagnostic concern.

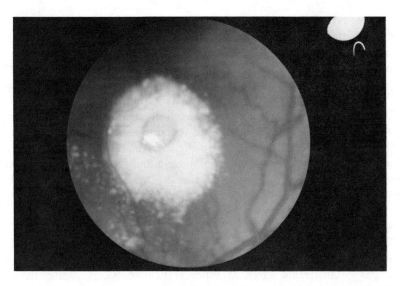

Figure 8.7 This Coat's disease patient exhibits the typical retinal telangiectasia that is sometimes described as a "light bulb" lesion. These telangiectasia tend to leak subretinal exudates, which may becomes so massive that the patient first presents with a leukocoria.

The primary retinal lesion is a telangiectatic retinal vessel or vessels in the periphery that are highly permeable. Vessels may show aneurysms, beading, anomalous A-V (arteriovenous) communications, and loss of the surrounding capillary beds. A "light bulb" lesion may be present. The location of these lesions has some predilection for the superotemporal quadrant of the retina (Egerer et al, 1974). The resulting exudation may be serous, hemorrhagic, or proteinaceous in nature or may be a combination. Typically it turns to a yellowish, subretinal, dense exudate that causes significant visual loss.

Treatment is directed at sealing off the telangiectatic vessels as early as possible with laser photocoagulation and cryotherapy. Retinal detachment is a not infrequent sequela of fulminant disease. Not too surprisingly, eyes with less geographic involvement show the best results of treatment. Early, aggressive treatment can prevent serious visual loss.

Retinal Vascular Disease

Many of the retinal vascular diseases that affect adults may also be found in children although the circumstances may be quite different. For example, hypertensive retinopathy is not an eye disease that most pediatric practitioners would be concerned with. Children and even infants with congenital or acquired severe kidney disease, however, may show the typical retinal signs of hypertension. The same may be true for diabetic retinopathy. Insulin-dependent juvenile onset diabetics may develop severe retinal disease at a young age, occasionally more rapidly than might their adult counterparts. This is due in large part to poor control. There are many female adolescent insulin-dependent diabetics who are out of control for long periods of time and develop severe diabetic retinopathy by the age of 15–20 years. This leads to blindness or severe visual impairment. Retinal vascular occlusive disease can be caused by conditions that affect children as well as adults. Leukemia, Eales' disease, Behcet's disease, lupus erythematosus, sickle-cell disease, liver and kidney diseases, and others may all cause retinal arterial and venous obstruction.

This discussion of retinal vascular disease will concentrate on two of the more important pediatric conditions—sickle-cell anemia and retinopathy of prematurity. The more typical adult types of retinal vascular disease are reviewed in general texts on ocular disease.

Hemoglobinopathies

The hemoglobinopathies comprise a group of inherited abnormalities in the structure of the hemoglobin molecule that lead to various vascular problems both in the eye and systematically. Over 25 different hemoglobin molecules have been described. Hemoglobin A is the normal adult type, and F is the normal fetal type. The ophthalmically important types are hemoglobins S, C, and Thal. The genes for the hemoglobins are autosomal, therefore each individual possesses two of these genes. The abnormal genes are mutations of the normal hemoglobin A gene. These mutations have appeared in several geographic areas and tend to affect individuals in specific ethnic groups. Hemoglobins S and C primarily affect Blacks, while hemoglobin Thal primarily affects people with Mediterranean backgrounds. Because of the heterogeneity of the population in the United States, differentiation based on apparent racial characteristics may prove inaccurate.

The presence of only one of the abnormal hemoglobin genes generally causes a mild form of the disease to occur, a sickle-cell trait. Having two abnormal genes causes a more severe form of disease. It is possible to have a mixed form of disease with one gene of one abnormal type, the other gene of another abnormal type. This heterogeneous form occurs fairly often in the United States, in hemoglobin SC disease. The hemoglobin Thal gene is only rarely seen as a heterozygote with S or C due to its different racial incidence. The incidence of the sickle-cell trait (S or C) is estimated to be at least eight to ten percent of the Black population in the United States, and Thal trait is estimated to be present in less than three to five percent of the Italian and Greek population in the United States. In select populations, however, the incidence may be very high, approaching a majority of the population. It has been hypothesized that sickle-cell disease arose as a protection against malaria and associated parasitic diseases. It is known that individuals with sickle-cell disease are afforded certain advantages in surviving the ravages of malaria in the tropical climates of Africa and Asia where malaria is endemic. Very simple and inexpensive blood tests have been developed to test for the specific type of hemoglobins, allowing for mass screening of populations.

The abnormal biochemical makeup of these hemoglobins leads to a sicklelike shape to the red blood cells. These sickle-shaped cells have difficulty passing through the smaller capillaries, leading to the temporary blockages that result in the clinical manifestations of the various types of sickle-cell diseases. These effects on the red blood cells are worsened when the individual has a decreased oxygenation blood level, for example at high altitudes or even on airplanes that do not maintain an unusually high oxygen level. The major systemic manifestation of sickle-cell disease is a so-called *sickle-cell "crisis"* that occurs when there is a blockage in capillary blood flow through the visceral organs, particularly the spleen, resulting in excruciating pain. Patients with full-blown SS disease typically have repetitive episodes of crises, brought on by various factors that may or may not be controllable. SC disease has less severe systemic problems, and the traits of S or C less still. Thal also tends to cause severe systemic manifestations.

There are a number of specific ocular manifestations that vary with the type of hemoglobin present. The most severe one occurs in CC disease, which is quite rare. Of the more frequently seen types in the United States, SC tends to be the most severe, followed by SThal, SS, and the traits respectively. Ocular disease is rare in the S trait, but mild eye disease has been seen in C and Thal traits. The most common lesions are segmented conjunctival dilatations and tortuosities, which do not of themselves cause problems. These are found in virtually all patients with SS and SC disease. This may be a reasonably simple screening modality in the absence of laboratory analysis of blood, for example in remote areas of Third World countries. Most of the retinal lesions are due to vaso-occlusive processes. These tend to occur most often in the peripheral retinal areas, where the oxygenation of blood in the vessels will be lower than in more central areas.

Several typical retinal lesions are seen in the hemoglobinopathies (Figure 8.8). A salmon patch lesion is seen in about 50 percent of patients with SS or SC disease. This is a disciform hemorrhagic retinal lesion with well-defined borders that first appears as bright red, gradually fades to the salmon color, then turns into either a

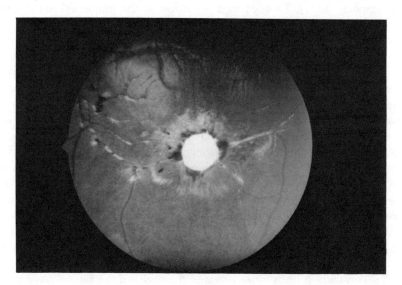

Figure 8.8 An atrophic chorioretinal scar in a patient with sickle-cell SC disease.

whitish atrophic retinal or a shimmering copper-colored area of pigmentation. Occasionally the salmon patches may become very highly pigmented and are called *black sunbursts*. These may be found along with the reddish salmon patches in the posterior pole of the retina. Central retinal artery occlusion may also occur, particularly during a systemic crisis. Occlusion of the perimacular vasculature (Stevens et al, 1974) leading to decreased central vision has been described in about 20 percent of patients. Other variations of nonproliferative retinopathies, including marked tortuosity of the vessels, are also seen.

More serious proliferative retinopathy is found especially with SC disease. A very characteristic retinal lesion is the *sea-fan neovascular tuft* found mostly in SC disease. This neovascular structure is very fragile and can hemorrhage spontaneously, leading to retinal detachment on organization of the bleed. The natural history of patients with sickle-cell disease is for progression of both the nonproliferative and the proliferative retinal lesions (Goldberg, 1971).

Photocoagulation of these sea fans is definitely indicated prior to rupture (Galinos et al, 1975). The nonproliferative lesions are generally left alone. Recently, elucidation of the specific genetic structure of sickle-cell disease has raised the possibility of genetic engineering to counteract the genetic defect. There may be significant change in the natural history of patients with these diseases in the near future.

Retinopathy of Prematurity

Retinopathy of prematurity (ROP)—previously known as *retrolental fibroplasia*—is a retinal vascular disease that is due in most cases to a combination of premature birth, very low birth weight, and the necessity of supplemental oxygenation. The disease was first recognized in the early 1940s (Terry, 1942), and shortly thereafter an association between the use of supplemental oxygenation and ROP was made (Campbell, 1951). This led to a reduction in the frequency and degree of supplemental oxygenation given to neonates that decreased the incidence of ROP but led to increased morbidity and mortality. As the subspecialty of neonatology developed in the 1970s, many infants of low and very low birth weight were kept alive by the emerging technologies, which included greatly increased use and levels of supplemental oxygenation. As a result of these advances, there was a significant increase in the incidence of ROP in these infants. Today there are many more infants with ROP than ever before, and this increase is likely to continue as neonates of lower and lower birth weight are kept alive. In addition, infants born to mothers that are substance abusers (particularly of crack cocaine) during pregnancy have a much greater risk of prematurity. There are recent estimates that up to 40 percent of infants with birth weights of 1 to 1.5 kilograms and up to 80 to 100 percent of neonates weighing under 1 kilogram may develop some degree of ROP. Only a relatively small percentage of these neonates, however, will experience significant visual loss.

The cause of ROP is thought to be due to the effects of high oxygen levels affecting immature retinal vascular tissue. There is an initial vasoconstriction of retinal vessels caused by increased oxygen levels in the blood due to supplemental oxygenation. This constriction leads to occlusion of the vessels if the arterial oxygen levels remain high enough. When a more normal oxygen level returns, there is proliferation of vascular endothelium, leading to neovascularization and the typical clinical appearance of ROP (Patz, 1984). There are also several other theories that have been proposed, but the final mechanism is not as yet certain. Regardless of the cause, there will be more ROP in the future as the tiny premies (premature infants) are kept alive more frequently.

There have been several systems of classifying the appearance and the extent of retinal involvement of patients with ROP. The classification currently used is based on three main parameters: the location, the extent, and the staging of ocular changes brought about by the ROP (Committee for the Classification of ROP, 1984). The location is divided into three circumferential zones with the center being the optic disc. Zone 1 extends just beyond the macula with an equal distance in other directions; zone 2 extends almost up to the ora serrata; and zone 3 is beyond that to the most anterior retina. The extent is based on hours on a clock. The staging is based on the severity of the retinal changes especially at the junction of the temporal avascular retinal zone. Each succeeding stage shows the characteristics of the previous stages in addition to the more severe characteristics of its own. Stage 1 has a flat demarcation line between the vascular and avascular area. Stage 2 has a demarcation line that has mild elevation above the plane of the retina and early neovascular changes posterior to the demarcation line. Stage 3 shows a fibrovascular proliferation posterior to the demarcation line arising into the vitreous. Stage 4 shows partial retinal detachments, and stage 5, total retinal detachments. This system allows for a more exacting classification than did its predecessors.

The classification described above is based on the appearance of the retinal changes that are visible. In actuality, it is often very difficult to perform an adequate examination on a tiny, crying infant. It is always necessary to follow all infants at risk for ROP for six months or more after birth since the retinal changes tend to progress during this time and unapparent retinopathy at an early age may become much more apparent later.

As was already briefly described, there is a junction or demarcation in the temporal retina between the area of vascularized and nonvascularized tissue. This junction tends to advance progressively until the entire retina becomes completely vascularized, which normally occurs in the months after full-term birth. The vascularized retina appears relatively transparent, while the nonvascularized one appears as a translucent or somewhat opaque whitish color. Milder stages of ROP appear as budlike tips to the developing retinal vessels at the demarcation line among a yellowish band of intraretinal tissue. Larger vessels adjacent to the demarcation line may be tortuous at this point. Somewhat more severe ROP shows an elevation of tissue at the demarcation line with neovascularization at this ridge beginning to develop. Fibroplasia and retinal detachments are the most severe manifestations and can lead to the classic appearance of the dragged disc in the temporal direction that is seen in severe cases. In addition to the retinal manifestations of ROP, patients tend to be moderately to severely myopic and have a high incidence of amblyopia, strabismus, cataracts, glaucoma, nystagmus, and corneal problems. ROP is obviously not only a retinal disease but also a more generalized ocular disease.

Several forms of treatment for ROP have been used. The efficacy of Vitamin E has been argued for many years as a means of prophylaxis in neonates at risk for the development of ROP. This is based on the ability of Vitamin E to neutralize oxygen-free radicals that may cause cell damage to the developing retinal vasculature. Premies typically have reduced levels of Vitamin E. Giving supplemental Vitamin E may decrease the level of vascular damage. Several studies have indicated that Vitamin E supplementation significantly reduces the incidence and the degree of damage from ROP (Hittner et al, 1981), but other studies have been less conclusive. In addition, it is known that there is significant risk of toxicity to Vitamin E in premies (Phelps, 1982), including death. This issue is not as yet settled.

Another controversial treatment modality concerns the use of several surgical procedures to treat retinal detachments in the most severe forms of cicatricial ROP. This includes both closed- and open-sky vitrectomies and scleral buckling. Retinal surgeons have advocated these procedures, but the results have been disappointing in patients, with many losing more vision instead of gaining some useful level of acuity as a result. This may be an acceptable treatment in otherwise hopeless patients, however.

A far more promising approach has been the subject of an important multicenter study that was published in 1989 (CRYO-ROP Cooperative Group, 1989). This concerns the use of cryotherapy, which has been shown to decrease the degree of retinal involvement significantly in ROP patients. The study was shown to be so favorable that it was prematurely terminated when it became very evident that it was efficacious. The success was much greater than that anticipated and may herald a new era in the treatment of developing ROP, sparing many infants from serious visual impairment.

NEOPLASTIC EYE DISEASE

Neoplasms of the eye are not common occurrences in the pediatric population with the important exception of retinoblastoma. The prompt diagnosis and treatment of neoplasms are obviously critical to the survival of the patient. Although the treatment of ocular tumors is beyond the scope of optometry, the detection and initial diagnosis is an important responsibility of the pediatric optometrist. Several of the more frequently seen pediatric neoplastic diseases will be discussed in this section. Emphasis will be placed on the diagnostic signs and symptoms and the typical presentations of those disorders. Treatments will only be touched on in the discussion of the specific disease. A number of benign tumors affecting various structures of the eye and adnexa have already been discussed, including orbital and ocular dermoids, capillary hemangiomas, neurofibromas, nevus flammeus, and chalazions.

Retinoblastoma
Heredity and Genetics
Without question, this is the most common and most important pediatric tumor encountered by the optometrist. The incidence of this tumor is estimated at approximately 1 in 15,000 births (Devessa, 1975) in the United States, but there is considerable variability in this incidence in different ethnic populations both inside and

outside the United States. Without treatment, it is invariably fatal. Early detection and treatment before the tumor spreads beyond the eye is associated with a high survival rate (Abramson et al, 1985).

A "two-hit hypothesis" model has been postulated to describe the hereditary basis of retinoblastoma (Knudson et al, 1975). Cases of retinoblastoma arise when two independent mutations occur. When the first mutation occurs in a prezygotic cell, the tendency for the tumor is transmissible, and the second mutation allows the tumor to develop and to then be hereditary. Since there is now present a cell line containing the first mutation, there is a greatly increased likelihood of multiple unilateral or bilateral tumors being caused by multiple second-stage mutations. If the first mutation is postzygotic, the second mutation will not lead to a hereditary tumor, reducing the likelihood of multiple unilateral or bilateral tumors. The hereditary types may have been passed on by a parent or may be a new mutation that will henceforth be transmissible to the patient's offspring. It is currently assumed that the prezygotic retinoblastoma cells in some way either disappear or become inactive after age three or four, explaining why new retinoblastomas rarely develop after this time. There is considerable evidence that the locus of the retinoblastoma gene is on chromosome 13q14. A small number of cases of retinoblastoma appear to be due to deletions of the long arm of chromosome 13 (Sparkes et al, 1979). Recent evidence (Yandell et al, 1989) has even identified the approximate location on the gene responsible for retinoblastoma. This may be very significant in distinguishing hereditary from non-hereditary types of retinoblastoma.

A determination of the hereditary versus nonhereditary nature of retinoblastoma can usually be made based on clinical characteristics and family history. All bilateral cases and all cases having four or more independent tumors in one eye are assumed to be hereditary since the likelihood of multiple unilateral or bilateral tumors in a postzygotic cell line is remote. About 8 to 15 percent of unilateral cases are due to the hereditary form. The hereditary type tends to appear at a younger age (about one year versus two years in nonhereditary tumors according to Knudson and colleagues [1975]). It is important to keep in mind that a second tumor in the other eye may develop at later age, changing the supposition that the tumor was nonhereditary to one hereditary in origin.

An important consideration is the issue of genetic counseling for the family, in particular the likelihood of the parents having another child with retinoblastoma and of that child subsequently having children who have the tumor. If the child has a unilateral tumor without prior family history, there is about a 1 percent chance of another child of those parents having retinoblastoma. This same child with bilateral tumors raises the risk in a sibling to about 8 percent. If there is another sibling with retinoblastoma, then the risk to a third child increases to about 40 percent. A child with a nonhereditary unilateral tumor has about a 10 percent risk of later having a child with retinoblastoma. A child having bilateral tumor has about a 50 percent chance of later having a child with retinoblastoma. There should always be some degree of skepticism about these risk percentages since a particular tumor cannot absolutely be labeled hereditary or non-hereditary in origin at least until chromosome analysis is clinically perfected. It is also important to keep in mind that not all carriers of the retinoblastoma gene manifest the disease (reduced penetrance) and that the form that the disease assumes may vary considerably (variable expressivity).

Presentation

From the optometric point of view, the issue of detection of patients with retinoblastoma is of critical importance. There are a relatively small number of typical presenting signs and symptoms of these patients. A study by Ellsworth (1969) showed that leukocoria was by far the most common (56 percent of the total) presenting sign of retinoblastoma (Figure 8.9), followed by strabismus (20 percent), red, painful eyes with glaucoma (7 percent), and poor vision (5 percent). There were also a number of relatively less common presentations, including orbital cellulitis, pupillary and iris anomalies, and hyphema. A few patients were identified on routine examination.

Although leukocoria is the most common presenting sign of retinoblastoma, it does not always indicate an intraocular tumor. Other diagnoses presenting with leukocoria are persistent hyperplastic primary vitreous, retinopathy of prematurity, cataract, colobomas of the choroid or disc, uveitis, toxocara or other parasitic infections of the eye, congenital retinal folds, Coat's disease, and a host of other rarer conditions. In general, any child presenting with a white pupil, strabismus, or amblyopia must be thoroughly evaluated, including a dilated fundus examination by binocular indirect ophthalmoscopy, for a suspicion of retinoblastoma or other serious eye diseases. Diagnostic imaging should probably also be performed to aid in the diagnosis. The presence of calcifications on CT (computerized tomography) scan is very highly suggestive of retinoblastoma. The optometrist must never assume that any

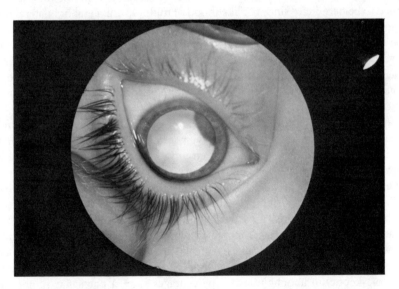

Figure 8.9 This patient has a dense leukocoria resulting from retinoblastoma.

of these signs is due to isolated strabismus or other relatively benign causes. Always assume that there is an ocular disease component to clinical abnormalities until all such diseases have been ruled out.

The tumor may appear as a whitish, almost pearly iridescent mass, either on the surface or adjacent to the retina and extending into the vitreous or as discrete small or large masses in the vitreous itself. The tumors may be necrotic and calcified or may take on a form known as a *rosette*, which is a cluster of tumor cells around a central lumen. The diagnostic criterion that is most predictable concerning patient morbidity and mortality is the extent of tumor growth at the time of diagnosis (Redler & Ellsworth, 1973). Large, multiple tumors are worse than small, singular tumors. The presence of a tumor anterior to the equator carries a less favorable prognosis than does a tumor restricted to the posterior pole. Choroidal involvement is a poorer sign than is the tumor being limited to the retina and vitreous. This choroidal spread makes possible the metastasis through the vasculature to the rest of the body. Spread through the optic nerve is the most common route of all metastases. Spontaneous regression of the tumor has been reported. A small percentage of patients will develop a nonmalignant form of the tumor that has been called a retinoma.

Treatment

The treatment of retinoblastoma has changed greatly in the past decade or so. Formerly most unilateral patients were enucleated, and the poorer eye of bilateral patients was enucleated. Recently there has been an increasing emphasis on treating eyes that are felt to have visual potential with a combination of irradiation, cryotherapy, and chemotherapy. Enucleation is usually restricted to those eyes with massive involvement when there is thought to be little, if any, potential of retaining any useful level of vision. The decision as to the appropriate treatment is based on the size and location of the tumors. Chemotherapy and radiation are given to patients that exhibit spread beyond the eye, but the prognosis remains poor in these patients. It is important to note that the use of radiation may carry significant risk to the patient from the treatment itself. It is now recognized that some patients who survive the treatment of the retinoblastoma will later develop other malignancies, in particular osteogenic sarcoma. It is unclear if this is related to the radiation or if it is another tumor that is related to the underlying genetic disorder that results in the retinoblastoma itself (Abramson et al, 1979). Other types of orbital tumors and cataracts have also been attributed to the use of radiation therapy.

Rhabdomyosarcoma

This is a fairly common tumor of the orbit in children, with an annual incidence in young Caucasian patients of about four cases per million, and it may be slightly more common in Blacks. The average age at onset is 7 to 8 years. Rhabdomyosarcoma is only rarely seen in infants and in patients over the age of 20 years. The primary site of the tumor may be around the eyes or in adjacent areas of the head, especially around the throat. The typical ocular presentation is either a unilateral proptosis, ptosis, or lid mass that progresses rapidly. It may also appear somewhat similar to an orbital or periorbital cellulitis or even to a chalazion or hordeolum. The effect of local trauma around the eye can be confused with the presence of an active tumor, significantly delaying treatment in a patient. Since the hallmark of rhabdomyosarcoma is rapid progression, any lid mass or proptosis that either gets worse or doesn't resolve in the anticipated manner should arouse suspicion. Included in the differential diagnosis are chalazion, hordeola, orbital cellulitis, ocular trauma, dermoids, hemangioma, and neurofibroma. The diagnosis is aided by imaging studies and biopsy. The prognosis is dependent on the size and location of the tumor at the time of diagnosis. The current methods of treatment involve radiation and chemotherapy, especially when the tumor is extensive or has spread. Secondary radiation cataracts often occur.

Gliomas

Gliomas can occur in the eye or in the anterior or posterior visual pathways. There are several different clinical types of gliomas, each with very different prognoses. Histologically gliomas are astrocytic tumors that arise from the optic nerve.

Most gliomas affecting children are considered benign tumors that are fibrous in nature, growing slowly by extension and not by metastasis. They can affect the visual system primarily by extension and compression of adjacent neurological structures. There may be proptosis if the tumor is anterior in location. Reduced visual acuity, optic atrophy, and papilledema are often seen in these patients, depending on the location and size of the tumor (Hoyt & Baghdassarian, 1969). Visual field deficits corresponding to the location of the tumor are present (Glaser et al, 1971), and there may be an afferent pupillary defect. Many of these tumors will stop progressing at some point, making treatment necessary only in those patients that experience progressive vision loss. This variety of optic nerve glioma is associated with neurofibromatosis and may be classified as a hamartoma (Gass, 1965).

The other type of optic nerve glioma is a much more threatening disease that may be rapidly progressive and fatal. These gliomas tend to be located in the posterior chiasm and the hypothalamic or third ventricular area and have been called *posterior gliomas* (Miller et al, 1974) in contrast to the more benign anterior gliomas described by Hoyt and Baghdassarian (1969) and Glaser and associates (1971). These tumors require aggressive treatment. The optometrist may have the opportunity of following patients with the slowly progressive form of anterior optic nerve glioma. Very careful visual field testing is an important component in the long-term follow-up care of these patients.

Leukemia

There have been enormous improvements in the treatment of many types of pediatric leukemias over the past 15 years. Survival rates for the most common type of pediatric leukemia, acute lymphoblastic, have increased from virtually 0 percent to greater than 80 percent and have been rising in recent years (Clavell et al, 1986). Several of the other types of leukemia are still difficult to treat, but in general, wonderful progress has been made in understanding the disease and developing appropriate treatments.

The clinical picture now in children with leukemia is very different from the picture of 15 years ago. Previously these patients would present with massive leukemic infiltrates that were visible in the fundus as whitish exudates, reminiscent of the picture one now sees in Coat's disease. Retinal hemorrhage, leukemic infiltration of the optic nerve, iris and orbit, hyphema, and hypopion were also routinely seen in the eyes of patients with leukemia. Because the central nervous system (CNS) is separated from the rest of the body by the blood/brain barrier, leukemia patients are now occasionally seen with infiltrates in their retinas (because it is a part of the CNS) even when the leukemia is under control elsewhere in their bodies. Most patients today, however, show no ocular evidence of the disease.

Some of the effects of the treatment itself can be seen in many of these patients even years after they are considered to be in remission. The current primary treatment is a combination of chemotherapy and radiation and occasionally bone marrow transplantation. The radiation and chemotherapy may cause posterior subcapsular cataracts in about 50 percent of patients (Hoover et al, 1988b). It is also now recognized that patients who receive radiation may experience reduced tear production as a result of damage to the lacrimal gland and a particular form of punctate keratitis that extends superficially over the entire cornea. These corneal complications may affect the success rate of patients who wear contact lenses, particularly those who become surgically aphakic as a result of secondary cataract formation.

Neuro-ophthalmic Disorders

This is not an exhaustive text on pediatric neuro-optometry. Therefore this section on pediatric neuro-ophthalmic disorders will include only a few of the conditions that are commonly encountered in clinical pediatric optometric practice. Please consult a suitable text for further information on these subjects.

Pediatric neuro-optometry is an exceedingly complex area. The complete diagnosis and treatment of many of these entities may be beyond the scope of office-based optometric practice. The diagnosis of neuro-ophthalmic problems can often be made only tentatively on the apparent clinical signs and symptoms. Diagnostic imaging and complete pediatric neurologic testing is generally required whenever significant disease is present or suspected. Prompt referral to a pediatric ophthalmologist or neurologist at a tertiary care center should be made since these conditions may be life threatening. The pediatric optometrist is an excellent resource for the detection of neurologic disorders that affect the eyes and visual system.

Congenital and Early Acquired Nystagmus

Congenital and early acquired nystagmus has been classified into various categories by different authorities. Some classify nystagmus into *normal* physiologic and *abnormal* pathologic varieties. The normal types include optokinetic, vestibular, and endpoint nystagmus, each of which can be elicited in most normal infants under appropriate testing conditions. The two more commonly used classifications of abnormal or pathological types are based on the suspected etiology (sensory and motor nystagmus) and the appearance (pendular and jerky nystagmus).

Additional classifications depend on motorical characteristics such as the direction of motion, the speed of motion, and the extent of the motion of the eyes, and the specific testing conditions under which the nystagmus is active as opposed to the underlying etiology. There are no universal definitions or standardizations of the various categories of nystagmus, making the appearance of a particular patient's nystagmus difficult to describe to other examiners. Furthermore, the particular etiology of the nystagmus, for example that caused by solely ocular defects as opposed to defects in the brain itself, have significant effect on the appearance and the classification of the nystagmus. Aspects of all of these classification systems will be used in the following discussion of the more clinically important congenital and early acquired types of nystagmus.

Sensory Nystagmus Secondary to Decreased Vision

In general terms, sensory nystagmus is usually thought of as being due to bilaterally reduced central visual acuity that is present at birth or that develops at an early age (Cogan, 1956). This can be due to problems within the eye, along the optic nerve pathways, or in the cortical areas of the brain responsible for the processing of visual information. Clinically, sensory nystagmus is commonly seen in patients with congenital media opacities such as bilateral congenital cataracts and corneal opacities; with geographic retinal problems such as macular colobomas and lesions; with more generalized retinal disorders such as albinism, aniridia, Leber's congenital amaurosis, and achromatopsia; and with optic nerve disorders such as optic nerve hypoplasia (Cogan, 1967).

Sensory nystagmus may be conatal, or it may develop after birth. It may indicate moderately reduced visual acuity or complete blindness. It is usually of a pendular nature, implying equal amplitude and speed from the midpoint of the ocular motion, but it can less commonly be of a jerky character. It is also usually horizontal in orientation even on up and down gaze and only rarely is there a marked vertical or rotatory component. There is a tendency for the amplitude to be larger and coarser when the vision is most severely affected at an early stage, but this does not always hold true. Generally there must be a significant visual acuity deficit before the age of one or two years for the sensory pendular type of nystagmus to develop, but it can develop at a later time under appropriate conditions. The amplitude and speed tend to decrease over time even when the visual acuity does not improve. The nystagmus may decrease significantly, however, if the visual acuity is improved, for example, when bilateral congenital cataracts are successfully treated.

Although sensory pendular nystagmus is seen most frequently under binocular conditions, patients with unilateral disorders may also show the same type of nystagmus under certain conditions. The amplitude of this form of sensory nystagmus is usually smaller than it is in bilateral patients, and there is an increased likelihood of a vertical or rotatory component.

Hereditary Pendular Nystagmus

This is a congenital hereditary nystagmus that occurs in the absence of visible ocular disease or abnormality. The family history is consistent with a dominant or

X-linked hereditary pattern. There is a horizontal pendular nystagmus that is similar in appearance to the typical sensory nystagmus secondary to reduced visual acuity, but no ocular abnormalities appear to be present, and the visual acuity may be essentially normal. There is a tendency for the amplitude of the nystagmus to decrease over time.

Latent Nystagmus

This is a jerky nystagmus commonly found in patients with strabismus and amblyopia, and made more apparent when one eye is occluded (Dell'Osso et al, 1979). Both the fast phase and the greatest amplitude are toward the fixing eye. The nystagmus is often present only when one eye is occluded. When both eyes are open, there is usually no evidence of nystagmus. There is invariably a reduction in measurable visual acuity during occlusion and in the presence of the active latent nystagmus. In order to assess accurately the best potential visual acuity of an eye with latent nystagmus, inserting a moderate strength plus lens or a neutral density lens in front of the fellow eye will usually minimize the latent nystagmus. The nystagmus is generally noted in each occluded eye; the amplitude is often greater, however, in the eye that is more strabismic or amblyopic. This condition may interfere with the treatment of amblyopia by reducing the level of visual acuity beyond that of the amblyopia itself. We have found that occlusion with neutral density filters or occlusive soft contact lenses that are not totally opaque may facilitate the treatment of amblyopia by minimizing the potential for latent nystagmus.

Spasmus Nutans

This is a relatively common form of an early acquired pendular nystagmus that is associated with head nodding and turn or torticollis (Norton & Cogan, 1954). It is not present at birth but develops during the first year of life, often quite suddenly. The child will begin turning or tilting the head, often while nodding the head, and will show a pendular nystagmus simultaneously with the head movements. Parents often assume that this is a type of seizure. The frequency of these episodes varies greatly. The nystagmus tends to be fine in amplitude and rapid in speed. It is often unilateral or asymmetric if it is bilateral. The condition is almost always much reduced in frequency by five years of age. The specific etiology is unknown, but there are apparently no long term sequelae. There have been reports of significant neurologic disease that has occurred coincidentally in patients with spasmus nutans, but these have nothing to do with the condition itself. It is important not to make too hasty a diagnosis of spasmus nutans since more serious neurologic disorders may on occassion mimic the much more benign and isolated spasmus nutans. It is usually worthwhile to have patients undergo a full neurological work-up to rule out this possibility.

Congenital Jerky Nystagmus

This is a jerky type nystagmus with the fast phase toward the position of gaze. There are generally no identifiable ocular abnormalities other than the nystagmus and a secondary form of mild to moderate amblyopia that is due to the nystagmus itself. The nystagmus is present at a very young age, occasionally even at birth, and there is some tendency for the amplitude and speed to decrease over time. Most patients with jerky nystagmus will have a null point, which is a combination of a head and eye position that minimizes the nystagmus and maximizes the visual acuity. This is most often in a position where the better seeing eye is fully adducted and the head is turned in the opposite direction. Patients may assume this head and eye position not during normal activities but rather when maximum visual acuity is required, for example, when looking at a blackboard in school or an eye chart in the doctor's office, the child will assume the compensatory position. Prisms in various combinations are sometimes prescribed to change the apparent null point. Patients that require an extreme null-point position may be aided by a complex muscle operation called a *Kestenbaum procedure*, where the position of both eyes is changed equally to reposition the null point to a more straight-ahead position. Certain patients may also use bilateral convergence to minimize the amplitude of the nystagmus. This may lead to esotropia in a few patients. It is relatively common to see patients with strabismus and amblyopia have both latent nystagmus and a null point for a jerk nystagmus component.

Contact lenses have been used in patients with nystagmus and significant refractive errors to improve visual acuity (Allen & Davies, 1983). The mechanism for this improvement in acuity is uncertain, but it may result from a combination of improved optical correction of the refractive error as the contact lenses move with the eye, reducing optical aberrations and prismatic effects in comparison to spectacles, and from the increased vergence and accommodative effort through the contact lenses. The weight of the lens on the eye may also have a dampening effect on the amplitude of the nystagmus (see Chapter 11).

Table 8.2 Optic disc appearances

Optic nerve pit	*Mini* coloboma; vertically oval; color: gray, yellow, or black; risk of central serous retinal detachment
Optic nerve coloboma	Incomplete closure of fetal fissure; size variable; usually inferonasal
Optic nerve hypoplasia	Maldevelopment of ganglion cells; pigmented double-ring sign; afferent pupillary defect present
Optic atrophy	Degeneration of optic nerve fibers; loss of vascularity; nerve head pale; loss of cupping
Optic neuritis	Inflammation of the optic nerve; visual acuity reduced; may be visible or invisible ophthalmoscopically
Papilledema	Swelling of disc resulting from increased intracranial pressure; margins blurred
Pseudopapilledema	Apparent swelling of disc margins; may be due to glial tissue, refractive error, or drusen
Optic nerve drusen	Hyalin material within the disc causing elevation and indistinct appearance

Neurologic or Pathologic Nystagmus

Jerky or pendular nystagmus may also be caused by a variety of neurological disorders, often affecting the posterior fossa. This may take a great many appearances and can be a diagnostic problem. Since the clinical appearance of neurologic forms of nystagmus may be very similar if not identical to the nonpathologic ocular forms, thorough evaluation by a pediatric ophthalmologist or neurologist should always be considered unless the optometrist is completely certain of its etiology. Even then, referral should be at least considered since the early diagnosis of significant neurologic disease usually improves the prognosis and lessens morbidity and mortality.

Optic Nerve Head Abnormalities

The appearance of the optic nerve head is of great importance in the proper diagnosis of both ocular and systemic disease. The normal appearance of the optic disc is quite variable, and in a typically difficult-to-examine infant or young child, abnormalities may be almost impossible to detect (Table 8.2). The appearance of the optic disc in young infants under six months of age is quite different than it is in adults since it is very pale and without any of the normal pinkish or reddish coloration of the adult disc. Cupping is usually not present. To the inexperienced examiner, all infant discs may look atrophic. This section will describe the appearance of some of the more commonly seen or more clinically important optic nerve head abnormalities and the clinical signs and symptoms of those conditions. Additional ocular and systemic testing may be necessary for a thorough diagnosis of conditions affecting the optic nerve head.

Optic Nerve Coloboma (Figure 8.10)

Like other colobomata of the eye, optic nerve colobomas are the result of incomplete closure of the fetal fissure. The defect may be isolated in the optic nerve

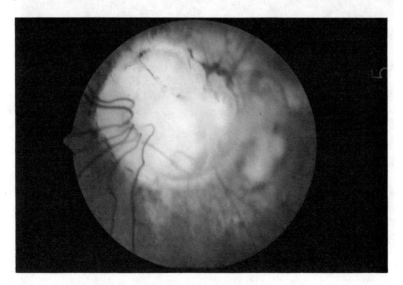

Figure 8.10 Extensive coloboma of the disc with a small area superotemporally spared.

head only, but much more commonly would include colobomata of the adjacent choroid, retina, and sclera. The degree of the defect varies greatly, from relatively minor and occult to extensive in the morning glory syndrome. Likewise, the extent of visual loss varies greatly from mild to complete blindness. Central visual acuity and visual field may be compromised, depending on the location and extent of the coloboma. Although optic nerve colobomas are usually unilateral, they can be bilateral. Rarely there is a family history. Optic nerve colobomas are usually isolated events, not generally associated with other systemic or neurological disorders, but they are seen as part of the CHARGE association and Aicardi's and Wardenburg's syndromes (Pagan, 1981).

Optic Nerve Pits

Optic pits are small, deep holes in the lower temporal quadrant of the optic disc. They are considered by some to be a minimal coloboma of the optic nerve head. There may be deficits of both visual acuity and visual fields depending on the size and location of the pit. An important consequence of optic nerve pits is the association with serous macular detachments during the second and third decades of life. Patients with optic pits located temporally are at increased risk of serous retinal detachments (Brown et al, 1980) (Figure 8.11). There are suggestions that prophylactic laser photocoagulation may be advisable prior to the onset of actual serous detachment.

Optic Nerve Hypoplasia

This condition was formerly thought to be rare, but now is recognized as a major cause of visual loss in infants (Walton & Robb, 1970). It is due to a reduced number

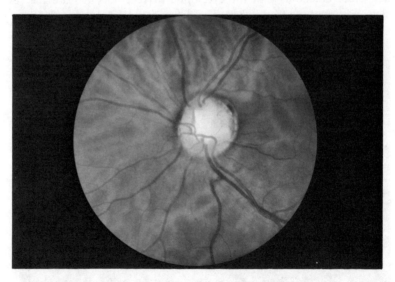

Figure 8.11 Optic pits are often located inferotemporally within the optic disc. Visual-field defects are common, and there is an inceased risk of serous retinal detachments. The depth of the pit is best visualized by a slit lamp exam aided by a Hruby lens.

of retinal ganglion cells and optic nerve fibers. Optic nerve hypoplasia is characterized by a smaller-than-normal optic nerve head that is surrounded by a pigmented ring of sclera that occupies the space between the nerve head and the retina and choroid (Figure 8.12).

The ophthalmoscopic picture is often described as a double-ring sign, with a whitish, atrophic, small disc surrounded by a pigmented ring extending to the edge of normal-looking chorioretinal tissue. Mild cases may be very difficult to diagnose in young children that do not tolerate prolonged examination with the direct ophthalmoscope, which is the preferred method of examination due to the larger image size of the disc in comparison to the binocular indirect ophthalmoscope.

The degree of the optic nerve hypoplasia is variable as is the effect on vision— from minimal visual loss to complete blindness. There is an afferent pupillary defect that matches in degree the relative number of remaining optic nerve fibers. It can be unilateral or bilateral, and it occurs as part of septo-optic dysplasia and a host of other neurological disorders. Other associations have been made with maternal diabetes (Petersen & Walton, 1977) in a partial form of optic nerve hypoplasia, fetal alcohol syndrome, and maternal substance abuse. There is no treatment.

Optic Atrophy

There are many potential causes of optic atrophy in infants and young children. Optic atrophy in young children may be very difficult to visualize during the examination because the appearance of an infant's optic disc normally looks somewhat atrophic and simply getting a good look at the disc may be difficult or impossible in a squirmy child. Optic atrophy in older children usually appears similar to that of

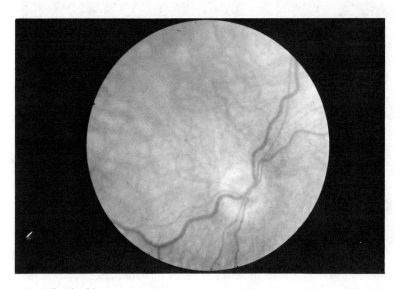

Figure 8.12 The double-ring sign in a patient with optic nerve hypoplasia. The disc itself is small and pale (less than one-half normal size) and is surrounded by a pigmented ring and a whitish area that is scleral in nature. This patient has a hypopigmented fundus as well.

adults, consisting of pallor of the nerve head, a reduction in the capillary content of the disc and adjacent tissue and attenuation of the retinal vasculature, a loss of cupping and a flat appearance to the disc, and glial proliferation that often occurs at a later stage (Figure 8.13). Visual acuity is compromised, nystagmus may be present if the optic atrophy is bilateral (and sometimes even if it is unilateral), and there is an afferent pupillary defect in the affected eye. The ERG is severely reduced in patients with optic atrophy. Since optic atrophy is only a sign of a serious neurological disorder, a complete neurologic evaluation is mandatory in order to assess the child's situation.

Optic Neuritis

Optic neuritis in infants and young children has a similar appearance to that in adults, but its detection and diagnosis is more difficult in the younger patients. The primary signs of optic neuritis are acute visual acuity loss, usually unilateral and painless, and perhaps visual field loss, depending on the cause and location of the optic neuritis (Figure 8.14). If the lesion occurs far enough behind the orbit, there is not likely to be any visible change in appearance of the optic nerve head. If the lesion is more anterior, there may be evidence of disc edema with or without hemorrhages and exudates. Unilateral acute visual acuity loss secondary to optic neuritis in young children is unlikely to be detected early, unless it leads to strabismus or unless there is some other neurological or systemic manifestation that becomes apparent. New methods of testing the visual fields of young children are currently being developed

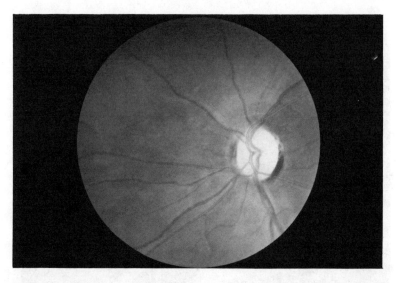

Figure 8.13 The pale appearance of the disc in eyes with optic nerve atrophy is due to a loss of the vasculature, substance, and structure of the optic nerve fibers. Both visual acuity and pupillary function are compromised due to the loss of the nerve fibers.

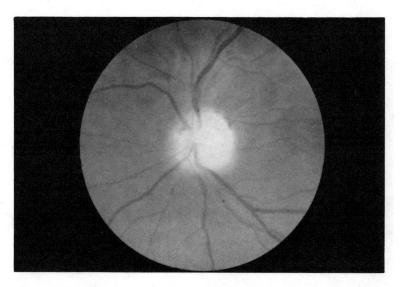

Figure 8.14 The optic nerve head appears white or pale with a loss of visible ophthalmosopic detail. The disc margins may be slightly blurred. Patients will have decreased visual acuity and afferent pupillary defects.

(Mayer et al, 1988) that may in the future aid in the detection of pediatric neuro-ophthalmic disease, but at this time, visual-field testing in young patients is generally not clinically available other than the confrontation fields described in Chapter 4. Therefore, visual-acuity testing will be the primary method of detecting optic neuritis in young children with appropriately suspicious histories. There are a great many potential causes of optic neuritis, but a discussion of the specific etiologies is beyond the scope of this text.

Papilledema and Pseudopapilledema

Papilledema is a swelling of the optic disc that occurs because of an increase in intracranial pressure. There is usually an ophthalmoscopically visible elevation of the optic nerve head with a loss of clarity of the disc margin that is associated with hemorrhages, exudates, and venous congestion adjacent to the disc margin (Figure 8.15). Vision is usually unaffected until later in the course of the disease. This is always an ominous clinical presentation that must precipitate an immediate referral to an appropriate tertiary care setting for complete evaluation by pediatric neurologists. A discussion of the specific causes of papilledema is beyond the scope of this book, but the importance of accurate detection of papilledema is not. Most children presenting with papilledema are already sick. Any ill-appearing or -acting patient that presents to the optometrist's office must have an examination of the optic nerve head to look for the possibility of papilledema.

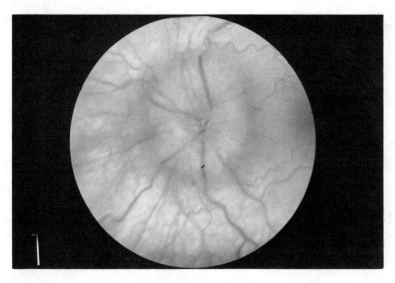

Figure 8.15 This patient has florid papilledema secondary to a posterior fossa tumor. Visual acuity, at least in the early stages before the optic nerve fibers are compromised, is usually relatively unaffected.

Papilledema is a rare condition that many pediatric optometrists will never see in their practice, but the ability to distinguish it from the many causes and appearances of pseudopapilledema is important. Pseudopapilledema is any condition that looks like papilledema but is not. The most common causes of pseudopapilledema are high hyperopia, hyperplastic glial tissue overlying the surface of the disc, and optic nerve drusen. High hyperopia can certainly occur in patients with true papilledema, but its presence should make the optometrist skeptical of its being papilledema. Gliosis often is associated with other, visible anomalies of the hyaloid system such as Bergmeister's papilla. There are, however, no signs of hemorrhage or exudate in the areas adjacent to the disc. Optic nerve drusen are often more difficult to diagnose properly, particularly in young children that will not allow a thorough examination (Figure 8.16). Individual drusen are usually not visible in young children since the hyaloid bodies are buried within the matrix of the nerve head. Their appearance becomes more distinct later (Hoover et al, 1988a). There are a group of patients that show a familial pattern of optic disc drusen, making an exam of all family members very helpful. The degree of disc elevation is variable as is the ophthalmoscopic appearance. An enlarged blind spot on visual field testing is often present. Optic nerve drusen may be a diagnosis of exclusion in certain patients that do not show any evidence of intracranial swelling but that have optic discs that appear somewhat elevated. An exam under anesthesia and complete neurological examination may be required for adequate diagnosis of patients suspected of having disc elevation.

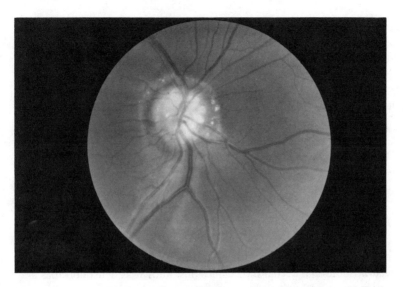

Figure 8.16   The ophthalmoscopic appearance of the disc is usually indistinct in patients with optic nerve drusen, raising suspicion of papilledema. The optic nerve drusen exhibited by this patient are more readily apparent than they are in most patients. Details of this disc are mildly obscurred by the drusen, and there are numerous, quite discrete drusen in the peripapillary area that make this diagnosis straightforward.

Phakomatoses

The phakomatoses (from the Greek word for *birthmark*) are a group of neurological disorders that are related by the presence of *hamartomas*, tumors composed of tissue that is normally present in the involved area but is present to an abnormal degree (Table 8.3). These conditions may be hereditary. Each has important and distinctive effects on the eyes and the visual system as well as more generalized neurological manifestations.

Von Recklinghausen's Disease

Also known as neurofibromatosis, this is a relatively common hereditary disease that has important ocular manifestations. It is dominantly inherited and is reported to have an incidence of about 1 in 3000 births in whites; it is much less common in blacks. There is considerable variation in the phenotypic appearance of the disease in different families. The typical hamartoma is the *neurofibroma*, a proliferation of Schwann cells within nerves, that may greatly affect the function of involved tissue. They can develop in virtually any organ of the body, leading to very variable clinical manifestations.

The cutaneous appearance of at least 6 cafe au lait spots of 15mm diameter are an important criterion in the diagnosis of neurofibromatosis. This is the method by

Table 8.3 The phakomatoses

Tuberous sclerosis Bourneville's disease	Glial hamartomas; "butterfly" facial lesion, shagreen patches, cafe au lait spots; "clumps of tapioca" in retina
Neurofibromatosis Von Recklinghausen's disease	Neurofibromas, cafe au lait spots, plexiform neuromas, lisch nodules; glaucoma; optic nerve glioma
Angiomatosis of the cerebellum and retina Von Hipple-Lindau disease	Hemangioblastomas of cerebellum and retina
Encephalofacial Angiomatosis Sturge-Weber disease	Port wine stains; leptomeningeal angiomas; glaucoma; choroidal hemangioma

which most young patients are identified as having neurofibromatosis by their pediatricians. Additional dermatological lesions, known as neurofibromas and plexiform neuromas, may cause significant disfigurement. Neurofibromas develop within nerve tissue throughout the body, causing disturbance of normal neurologic functioning. There is a wide range of neurological problems that result from the disease, including seizures, mental retardation, and various tumors of the CNS. Of particular ophthalmic importance are gliomas of the optic nerve. There are also a number of skeletal abnormalities, many of which are developmental. Once the diagnosis of neurofibromatosis is made, all patients require periodic neurologic and ophthalmic examination.

There are many ocular manifestations in neurofibromatosis. The sigmoid lid sign is due to a plexiform neuroma of the upper eyelid that produces an s-shaped form of ptosis. Other hamartomas can produce extensive deformation of the face and proptosis. Local involvement of the various nerves, innervating the ocular tissue, may be visible. Of diagnostic importance is the presence of Lisch nodules, which are typically small, discrete, hyperpigmented neurofibromas of the iris stroma although their appearance is variable (Figure 8.17). These tend to develop over time and may not be visible in young children. Optic nerve gliomas will affect the optic disc with manifestations (optic atrophy, optic neuritis, papilledema, visual field defects, visual acuity loss) depending on the site of the tumor. There is also an increased risk of glaucoma from a number of different etiologies. In general, this is a progressive disease. It is not uncommon to follow children with minimal effects from the disease for many years who suddenly develop much more serious neurological and ophthalmic complications. These patients must be followed closely for life.

Encephalofacial Angiomatosis (Sturge-Weber Disease)

The hamartoma in Sturge-Weber disease is a vascular anomaly that can affect the skin, the eyes, and the brain. The classical cutaneous lesion is a nevus flammeus or port wine stain that typically follows the distribution of the trigeminal nerve on only

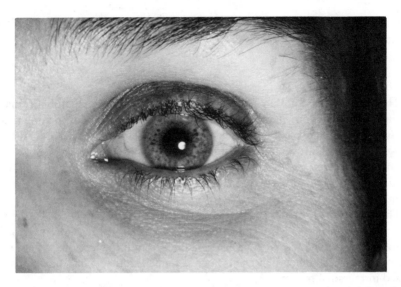

Figure 8.17 Hypo- or hyperpigmented iris nodules that are found in most patients with neurofibromatosis. They do not affect vision but are useful in arriving at the diagnosis of neurofibromatosis.

one side of the face. This is an extensive series of vascular channels that are present at birth and are flat as opposed to the strawberry hemangioma that develops after birth and is quite elevated. The color of the nevus flammeus tends to be a dark reddish-purple and does not darken when crying, unlike strawberry hemangiomas which darken considerably when the patient cries. Many patients with Sturge-Weber disease also have choroidal hemangiomas that may lie under the macula and are difficult if not impossible to see without the aid of the binocular indirect ophthalmoscope (Susac et al, 1974). This choroidal lesion may cause an elevation of the macula above the plane of the retina, leading to an increase in hyperopia. This induced anisometropia can lead to amblyopia if not identified early and treated with appropriate refractive correction.

By far the most important ophthalmic manifestation of Sturge-Weber disease is a particularly difficult-to-treat form of congenital or early onset glaucoma. This always is found in the eye with the nevus flammeus and results from the abnormal vasculature caused by the lesion. It is thought that both the drainage mechanism and the anatomy of the drainage angle itself is disrupted by the vascular lesion (Phelps, 1978). There may also be a increase in the volume of aqueous production. Treatment is usually difficult and ultimately unsuccessful with these eyes eventually going blind.

In addition to the ophthalmic manifestations of Sturge-Weber disease, there are a variety of neurologic problems. One of the hallmarks of the disease are leptomeningeal angiomas, which lead to atrophy, gliosis, and calcification of adjacent cerebral cortex. Seizure disorders, mental retardation, and hemiplegia are among the more common neurological manifestations.

Von Hippel-Lindau Disease

The hamartomas of Von Hippel-Lindau disease are hemangioblastomas of the retina and cerebellum. The hemangioblastomas are tumors comprising masses of thin-walled capillaries and endothelial cells, often associated with dilated larger blood vessels. Von Hippel-Lindau disease may be an AD inherited disorder with mixed penetrance and expressivity and may not become evident until the second or third decade of life. It is very unusual to see significant clinical signs in young children.

The primary neurological manifestation of the disorder are cerebellar hemangioblastomas comprising a large cystic mass with numerous large feeder vessels. The effect of the cyst impinging on adjacent structures within the nervous system is the source of the clinical effects. The neurological signs include ataxia, nystagmus, and increased intracranial pressure.

The retinal hemangioblastomas have variable appearance but usually have a large, dilated vessel passing through the lesion and tend to be reddish in color. They may be unilateral or bilateral and may be multiple. Their size is quite variable. The effect on vision varies as to the size, position, and progression of the lesions. They can lead to retinal hemorrhage and detachment and glaucoma. Current treatment is prophylactic ablation by laser photocoagulation or cryotherapy.

Tuberous Sclerosis

Tuberous sclerosis is also known as Bourneville's disease. It may be inherited in an AD pattern. The hamartoma is called a tuber and is a proliferation of glial tissue. These lesions occur in the cerebrum and the retina along with many other organ systems.

The cutaneous signs of tuberous sclerosis are cafe au lait spots and the adenoma sebaceum, or butterfly rash, of the face. *Shagreen patches*, irregularly pigmented patches that appear on the trunk, face, and extremities, are another characteristic cutaneous sign.

The neurological consequences of tuberous sclerosis are quite severe. The tubers develop in the cerebrum, cerebellum, midbrain, and spine and undergo cystic degeneration and calcification. This leads to a host of neurological signs, including increased intracranial pressure, seizure disorders, mental retardation, and behavioral abnormalities that may present in early childhood and be rapidly progressive.

The hamartomas present within the eye as nodular, cystic masses in the fundus that are described as clumps of tapioca or mulberries, but their appearance is quite variable (Figure 8.18). The ocular lesions are generally of much less importance than are the neurological manifestations, and treatment is usually not necessary. The lesions are, however, of distinct diagnostic importance.

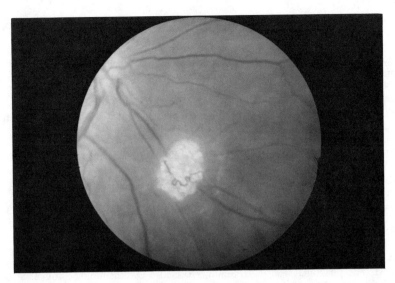

Figure 8.18 The hamartomas of tuberous sclerosis are often described as resembling clumps of tapioca. They appear as whitish, refractile bodies that are usually elevated. The patient has a tortuous vessel traversing the tumor, but others may appear avascular.

REFERENCES

Abramson DH, Ellsworth RM, Grumbach N, et al. Retinoblastoma: Survival, age at detection and comparison 1914–1958, 1958–1983. J Ped Ophthalmol Strab 1985;22:246–250.

Abramson DH, Ronner HJ, Ellsworth RM. Second tumors in nonirradiated bilateral retinoblastoma. Am J Ophthalmol 1979;87:624–627.

Allen ED, Davies PD. Role of contact lenses in the management of congenital nystagmus. Br J Ophthalmol 1983;67:834–836.

Bither PP, Berns LA. Stargardt's disease: A review of the literature. J Am Optom Assoc 1988;59:106–111.

Brown GC, Shields JA, Goldberg RE. Congenital pits of the optic nerve head. II. Clinical studies in humans. Ophthalmology 1980;87:51–65.

Campbell K. Intensive oxygen therapy as a possible cause of retrolental fibroplasia: A clinical approach. Med J Aust 1951;2:48–50.

Clavell LA, Gelber RD, Cohen HJ, et al. Four-agent induction and intensive asparaginase therapy for treatment of childhood acute lymphoblastic leukemia. N Engl J Med 1986;315:657–663.

Cogan DG. Congenital nystagmus. Canad J Ophthalmol 1967;2:4–10.

Cogan DG. Neurology of the Ocular Muscles. Springfield Ill: Charles C Thomas, 1956;189–192.

Committee for the Classification of Retinopathy of Prematurity. An international classification of retinopathy of prematurity. Arch Ophthalmol 1984;102:1130–1134.

Criswick VG, Schepens CL. Familial exudative vitreoretinopathy. Am J Ophthalmol 1969;68:578–594.

CRYO-ROP Cooperative Group. Multicenter trial of cryotherapy for retinopathy of prematurity. Arch Ophthalmol 1989;106:471–479.

Dell'Osso LF, Schmidt D, Daroff RB. Latent, manifest latent, and congenital nystagmus. Arch Ophthalmol 1979;97:1877–1885.

Dennehy PJ, Warman R, Flynn JT, et al. Ocular manifestations in pediatric patients with acquired immunodeficiency syndrome. Arch Ophthalmol 1989;107:978–982.

Desmonts G, Couvreur J. Congenital toxoplasmosis. A prospective study of 378 pregnancies. N Engl J Med 1974;290:1110–1116.

Devessa SS. The incidence of retinoblastoma. Am J Ophthalmol 1975;80:263–265.

Eagle RC, Lucier AC, Bernardino VB, et al. Retinal pigment epithelial abnormalities in fundus flavimaculatus. Ophthalmology 1980;87:1189–1200.

Egerer I, Tasman W, Tomer TL. Coats disease. Ophthalmology 1974;92:109–112.

Ellsworth RM. The practical management of retinoblastoma. Trans Am Ophthalmol Soc 1969;67:463–534.

Foxman SG, Heckenlively JR, Bateman JB, et al. Classification of congenital and early onset retinitis pigmentosa. Arch Ophthalmol 1985;103:1502–1506.

Francois J. Metabolic tapetoretinal degenerations. Survey of Ophthalmol 1982; 26:293–333.

Fulton AB, Craft JL, Howard RO, et al. Human retinal dysplasia. Am J Ophthalmol 1978;85:690–698.

Galinos SO, Asdourian GK, Woolf MB, et al. Choroido-vitreal neovascularization after argon laser photocoagulation. Arch Ophthalmol 1975;93:524–530.

Gass JDM. The phakomatoses. In JL Smith, ed. Neuro-Ophthalmology, vol. 2. St. Louis: Mosby, 1965;223–268.

Glaser JS, Hoyt WF, Corbett J. Visual morbidity with chiasmal glioma. Arch Ophthalmol 1971;85:3–12.

Goldberg MF. Natural history of untreated proliferative sickle retinopathy. Arch Ophthalmol 1971;85:428–437.

Hanshaw JB. Congenital cytomegalovirus infection: A fifteen year perspective. J Infect Dis 1971;123:555–561.

Hittner HM, Godio LB, Rudolph AJ, et al. Retrolental fibroplasia: Efficacy of vitamin E in a double-blind clinical study of preterm infants. N Engl J Med 1981;305:1365–1371.

Hoover DL, Robb RM, Petersen RA. Optic disc drusen in children. J Pediatr Ophthalmol Strab 1988a;25:192–195.

Hoover DL, Smith LEH, Turner SJ, et al. Ophthalmic evaluation of survivors of acute lymphoblastic leukemia. Ophthalmology 1988b;95:151–155.

Hoyt WF, Baghdassarian SA. Optic glioma of childhood. Brit J Ophthalmol 1969;53:793–798.

Karr DJ, Scott WE. Visual acuity results following treatment of persistent hyperplastic primary vitreous. Arch Ophthalmol 1986;104:662–667.

Knudson AG, Hethcote HW, Brown BW. Mutation and childhood cancer: A probabilistic model for the incidence of retinoblastoma. Proc Nat Acad Sci USA 1975;72:5116–5120.

Krill AE. Congenital color vision defects. In Krill AE, ed. Krill's hereditary retinal and choroidal diseases. Hagerstown, Md: Harper & Row, 1977;355–390.

Krill AE, Archer D, Martin D. Sector retinitis pigmentosa. Am J Ophthalmol 1970:69:977–987.

Krill AE, Deutman AF. The various categories of juvenile macular degeneration. Trans Am Ophthalmol Soc 1972;70:220–245.

Lahav M, Albert DM, Wyand S. Clinical and histopathologic classification of retinal dysplasia. Am J Ophthalmol 1973;75:648–667.

Lahav M, Albert DM, Buyukmici, et al. Ocular changes in Laurence Moon Bardet Biedl syndrome: A clinical and histopathologic study of a case. In Landers MB, Wolbarsht ML, Dowling JE, et al., eds. Retinitis Pigmentosa. New York: Plenum, 1976;51–84.

Levin AV, Zeichner S, Duker JS, et al. Cytomegalovirus retinitis in an infant with acquired immunodeficiency syndrome. Pediatrics 1989;84:683–687.

Mayer DL, Fulton AB, Cummings MF. Visual fields of infants assessed with a new perimetric technique. Invest Ophthalmol Vis Sci 1988;29:452–459.

Miller NR, Iliff WJ, Green WR. Evaluation and management of gliomas of the anterior visual pathways. Brain 1974;97:743–754.

Mizuno K, Takei Y, Sears ML, et al. Leber's congenital amaurosis. Am J Ophthalmol 1977;83:32–42.

Nickel B, Hoty CS. Leber's congenital amaurosis: Is mental retardation a frequent associated defect? Arch Ophthalmol 1982;100:1089–1091.

Norton EWD, Cogan DG. Spasmus nutans: A clinical study of twenty cases followed two years or more since onset. Arch Ophthalmol 1954;52:442–446.

O'Connor PS, Tredici: TJ, Ivan DJ, et al. Achromatopsia, clinical diagnosis and treatment. J Clin Neuro-ophthalmol 1982;2:219–226.

Opitz JM. Ocular abnormalities in malformation syndromes. Trans Amer Acad Ophthal Otol 1972;76:1193–1196.

Pagan RA. Ocular coloboma. Survey Ophthalmol 1981;25:223–236.

Pagan RA, Graham JM, Zonana J, et al. Coloboma, congenital heart disease, and choanal atresia with multiple anomalies: CHARGE association. J Pediatr 1981;99:223–229.

Patz A. Current concepts of the effects of oxygen on the developing retina. Curr Eye Res 1984;3:159–163.

Petersen RA, Walton DS. Optic nerve hypoplasia with good visual acuity and visual field defects. Arch Ophthalmol 1977;95:254–258.

Phelps CD. The pathogenesis of glaucoma in Sturge-Weber syndrome. Ophthalmology 1978;85:276–286.

Phelps DL. Vitamin E and retrolental fibroplasia in 1982. Pediatrics 1982;70:420–425.

Pruett RC. The pleomorphism and complications of posterior hyperplastic primary vitreous. Am J Ophthalmol 1975;80:625–629.

Redler LD, and Ellsworth RM. Prognostic importance of choroidal invasion in retinoblastoma. Arch Ophthalmol 1973;90:294–296.

Sparkes RS, Muller H, Klisak I, et al. Retinoblastoma with 13q-chromosomal deletion associated with maternal paracentric inversion of 13q. Science 1979;203:1027–1029.

Stargardt K. Uber familiare, progressive degeneration in der maculagegend des auges. Albrecht von Graefes Arch Klin Exp Ophthalmol 1909;71:534–550.

Stevens TS, Busse B, Lee CB, et al. Sickling hemoglobinopathies: Macular and perimacular vascular abnormalities. Arch Ophthalmol 1974;92:455–463.

Straatsma BR, Heckenlively JR, Foos RY, et al. Myelinated retinal nerve fibers associated with ipsilateral myopia, amblyopia, and strabismus. Am J Ophthalmol 1979;88:506–510.

Susac JO, Smith JL, Scelfo RJ. The "tomato catsup" fundus in Sturge-Weber syndrome. Arch Ophthalmol 1974;92:69–70.

Terry TL. Extreme prematurity and fibroplastic overgrowth or persistent vascular sheath behind each crystalline lens. I. Preliminary report. Am J Ophthalmol 1942; 25:203–205.

Walton DS, Robb RM. Optic nerve hypoplasia. Arch Ophthalmol 1970;84:572–578.

Yandell DW, Campbell TA, Dayton SH, et al. Oncogenic point mutations in the human retinoblastoma gene: Their application to genetic counseling. N Engl J Med 1989;321:1689–1695.

Yanoff M, Rahn EK, Zimmerman LE. Histopathology of juvenile retinoschisis. Arch Ophthalmol 1968;79:49–53.

Yee RD, Herbert PN, Bergsma DR, et al. Atypical retinitis pigmentosa in familial hypobetalipoproteinemia. Am J Ophthalmol 1976;82:64–71.

9

Trauma and Infection

Bruce D. Moore

EXTERNAL EYE DISEASE

The diagnosis and treatment of children with external eye disease is essentially the same as that for adults. Close inspection of the anterior segment, preferably by biomicroscopy, is essential. Cultures and sensitivities by appropriate techniques are important, particularly for the very young patient and for those with severe disease.

The systemic effects on young children of the various antibiotics must always be considered. For example, the use of tetracycline must be avoided because of its adverse effect on dentition and bone structure of young children. Dosage must be determined by the weight of the child. The fragility of the infant's general health should always be kept in mind. A severe eye infection in a baby can have devastating consequences under certain conditions. If systemic problems occur during the treatment of an external eye infection, the child's pediatrician should be notified immediately. An example of this would be a minor eyelid infection that initially appears to be caused by an internal hordeolum, turning out to be a periorbital cellulitis secondary to Haemophilus influenzae with concurrent meningitis.

Internal ocular infections are serious disorders that require intensive medical intervention. They are currently beyond the scope of optometry and are not discussed in this text.

Eyelids

Blepharitis

Chronic blepharitis is a common disorder in children that is often associated with other anterior segment inflammatory processes. Blepharitis is often the result of a combination of bacterial and seborrheic components. One cause may predominate in any one patient, but treatment generally is directed at both simultaneously.

Staphylococcus aureus and staphylococcus epidermis are the most common pathogens associated with blepharitis. Poor hygiene may predispose the patient to chronic staphylococcus blepharitis. Clinical signs of this type of chronic blepharitis

191

include scaling of the eyelids at the base of the lashes, redness of the lid margins, purulent discharge, skin ulceration, and corneal involvement in the form of an inferior punctate keratitis. Additional signs found in long-term chronic cases include madarosis and trichiasis of the lashes, entropion and ectropion of the lids, and a thickening of the lid margins. There is often a concomitant inflammation or infection of the meibomian glands of the upper and lower eyelids.

The most effective treatment is hot compresses applied over the eye with a wash cloth and lid scrubs with baby shampoo to loosen the scales and discharge and physically reduce the population of bacteria along with massage of the eyelids to express any material from inflamed meibomian glands. Topical antibiotic ointments applied several times per day during acute phases may also be considered. Bacitracin and Erythromycin ointments are both effective and rarely cause sensitization. Resorting to antibiotics only in more severe cases is recommended.

The concomitant use of topical steroids is somewhat controversial. Advocates argue that the anti-inflammatory effects of steroids hasten resolution, while critics worry about the adverse effects of the steroids—such as glaucoma, superinfection from resistant organisms, and the potential disaster that may ensue with steroid use on an eye with early herpes keratitis. Steroids should probably be reserved only for those cases where its use is clearly warranted, after less aggressive alternatives have been tried without resolution of the disease, and when good follow-up and careful comanagement with parents is a certainty. Since blepharitis tends to be chronic, treatment is often directed at controlling rather than eliminating the signs and symptoms of the disease.

Blepharitis may also be due to seborrhea of the eyelids alone or to a more generalized condition affecting the face, brow, and scalp. There is often an increase in meibomian secretions with a foamy discharge collecting on the cilia and the lateral canthus. The meibomian glands tend to be full, and an oily discharge is readily expressed with direct pressure on the glands. Cases of pure seborrheic blepharitis will present without any associated keratitis or purulent discharge on the lashes or in the tear film, but there may be a particularly greasy appearance to the lids and lashes. There is usually some bacterial component present in patients with primary seborrheic blepharitis. Acne vulgaris is commonly associated with seborrheic blepharitis in adolescents.

The treatment for seborrheic blepharitis is similar to that for bacterial blepharitis, consisting of hot soaks, strenuous lid scrubs, and massage of the meibomian glands. Topical antibiotics are not required. Steroids may be of some benefit, but care must be exercised in their use. Patients with more generalized seborrheic conditions may need to include systemic tetracyline in the treatment. The use of tetracyline should be limited to adolescents only—definitely not used for infants and toddlers because of the possibility of adverse effects on developing dentition and bone structure. The use in pregnant women should also be avoided because of the possibility of transmission of the drug to the fetus through the placenta. The treatment of blepharitis can turn into a very difficult chronic condition.

It should be noted that patients with Trisomy 21 (Down's syndrome) will often have a chronic form of seborrheic blepharitis that is very resistant to treatment. This may lead to excessive rubbing of the eyes and cause the development of keratoconus in some patients (Pierse & Eustace, 1971). Because of this possibility, it is worthwhile to attempt vigorous treatment of the blepharitis in this group of patients.

There are a number of less common inflammatory conditions of the eyelids that may be seen in children. Patches of impetigo, which is caused by local infection by staphylococcal or streptococcal organisms, may be noted around the eyes. These are usually yellowish in color and vesicular and crusty in appearance. Treatment is with washing, removal of the crusts, and topical antibiotic ointments. Primary herpes simplex blepharitis is usually clinically unapparent, but patients may present with a wet, ulcerative series of vesicles on the eyelids. Antiviral agents may be used to limit the duration of active inflammation. Molluscum contagiosum is a viral infection that presents as a nodular, umbilicated series of small lesions usually at the upper eyelid or brow. They can occasionally precipitate follicular conjunctivitis. Treatment is by incision of the lesions. Acne rosacea is only rarely encountered in the pediatric population.

Hordeolum

These are common, acute infections (often by staphylococcus aureus) of the Meibomian glands or the glands of Zeis and Moll. A hordeolum presents as a local area of redness, pain, and swelling within the eyelid, often at the lid margin. The most effective treatment is simply by hot soaks at least 4 or 5 times per day. Topical antibiotic drops or ointments penetrate the encapsulated lesion poorly, and are of little value, unless there is an associated bacterial blepharoconjunctivititis. A hordeolum typically resolves within about a week, with the lesion spontaneously opening and draining, but occasionally one will form a chalazion if drainage is incomplete. Very rarely, one will progress to a preseptal cellulitis, which requires aggressive medical intervention.

Chalazion

Chalazions are chronic granulomatous inflammations of the meibomian glands and are usually secondary to a hordeolum. They are hard, mobile masses within the tarsus of the lid and are generally not painful. If one is very large, it may press on the globe, temporarily inducing an astigmatic refractive error with the axis perpendicular to the mass. In a young child, this may be amblyogenic if it is present for a long time. Treatment is initially by hot soaks several times per day. If this does not reduce the mass in a reasonable time period, local steroid injection or surgical removal is indicated. Recurrent hordeola and chalazions occur in patients with poor hygiene and chronic seborrheic or infectious blepharitis or meibomianitis. Treatment in these patients must be directed at scrupulous daily lid hygiene.

Parasites

The crab lice (Phthirius pubis) and, less commonly, body and head lice may infect the eyelids and lashes. Sexual activity and poor hygiene may be the direct causes of infestation, but recently large scale infestations have become very common in preschools and elementary schools through casual contact and sharing of articles of clothing by children. Lice cause considerable itching of the lids and less commonly a conjunctivitis secondary to the metabolic waste products of the organism. Treatment is directed at removal of the nits and classically the use of .5 percent eserine ointment to poison the arthropods although virtually any ointment, including bland lubricants and antibiotics, are also effective and have less potential for adverse pharmacologic effects than does eserine. Careful disinfection of contaminated bedding, clothes, and cloth toys with commercially available chemical products is required as well as thorough shampooing with over the counter preparations.

Conjunctivitis

Ophthalmia Neonatorum

Neonatal conjunctivitis and keratoconjunctivitis have been an important ocular problem historically because of infection by Neisseria gonorrhea. Prior to the use of silver nitrate (Crede prophylaxis) about 100 years ago, there was considerable visual morbidity due to corneal infection by Neisseria. With routine use of silver nitrate drops at the time of birth, the incidence of neonatal Neisseria eye infection has been greatly reduced. Today, however, the threat of ophthalmia neonatorum by Neisseria has been partially overshadowed by the greatly increased incidence of neonatal ocular infection caused by Chlamydia.

The incidence of all types of venereal disease in sexually active individuals has recently increased. In spite of routine ocular prophylaxis at the time of birth, there has been an increase in cases of neonatal conjunctivitis due to infection by both Neisseria and Chlamydia. This may be due to improper procedures in the instillation of the medication into the babies' eyes, to premature flushing of the medication from the eye, or to the accidental failure to use the medication at all. In many states, alternatives to the use of silver nitrate, which causes frequent but temporary chemical conjunctivitis of the newborn, include erythromycin and tetracycline ointments (American Academy of Pediatrics, 1980). These ointments have some effectiveness against Chlamydia in the eye but not systemically, and they may have reduced effectiveness against Neisseria. A recent study by Hammerschlag has shown that silver nitrate and both erythromycin and tetracycline ointments are all relatively effective as ocular prophylaxis for Neisseria but are not effective enough ocular prophylaxis for Chlamydia (Hammerschlag et al, 1989). The most effective method of prevention of neonatal Chlamydial conjunctivitis would be universal screening of all women as part of their prenatal care. This is unfortunately not the case at this time in the United States. Ideally all infants born of mothers with either Neisseria or Chlamydial disease should be treated with a full course of systemic antibiotics, but many women with venereal disease go undetected, and the eye infection may not appear in the infant until after discharge from the hospital. Furthermore ocular prophylaxis may have the unintended effect of covering up the ocular clinical signs of Chlamydial infection, allowing the systemic aspects of this disease to progress to a more serious level before systemic treatment is initiated. To summarize, the issue of the best single dose prophylaxis against neonatal eye infection is not as yet completely settled.

All neonatal infections, both ocular and systemic, must be treated as serious medical problems. Preliminary diagnosis can be made on the clinical signs, but cultures and sensitivities should be obtained for confirmation. The clinical signs are not always reliable. It is also possible that the infant may have two or more agents that are responsible for the keratoconjunctivitis. Neonates have an immature immune system and reduced ability to fight off infection. Any infection can rapidly escalate into a life threatening situation. The neonate with an eye infection should be under the care of his pediatrician during all phases of treatment.

Neisseria Gonorrhea

One recent study has shown that in selected populations, up to 10 percent of women are infected with Neisseria (Armstrong et al, 1976) at the time of delivery. Many of these women were asymptomatic and did not receive any pre- or postnatal treatment, and their infants run a high risk of becoming infected during passage through the birth canal. It is clear that the best means of prevention of venereal eye diseases in neonates is by much better prenatal screening and treatment of the mothers (Schachter, 1989).

Neisseria usually causes a bilateral (less commonly a unilateral), hyperacute, purulent infection with lid edema, membrane or pseudomembrane formation, and the possibility of severe keratitis and corneal scarring, leading to visual loss. The infection typically becomes manifest two to four days after birth although onset may be as late as two to three weeks after delivery. In a small percentage of cases, the infection may be much less severe, leading to misdiagnosis, unless culture results are obtained. The infection must be treated very aggressively—usually in an inpatient hospital setting with appropriate systemic and local antibiotics and support therapy. The mother must also be treated, and the appropriate public health authorities must be notified in order to track down the mother's sexual contacts. Neisseria infection is a medical emergency requiring proper medical treatment. Failure to treat may result in severe corneal scarring and decreased vision or even lead to overwhelming systemic infection, leading to increased risk of morbidity and mortality of the infant.

Other Bacterial Conjunctivitis

There are a large number of nongonococcal bacterial organisms that have been isolated from the eyes of newborn infants. Many of these are commensal organisms that do not under normal circumstances cause eye infections. Infants with compromised immune systems (due to various types of congenital immunodeficiencies, medications such as steroids, or HIV infection), however, are at much greater risk of serious sequelae from these usually mild ocular infections. It is also important to note that infants that develop clinical cases of neonatal conjunctivitis may have infection by more than one organism. The use of appropriate antibiotic and supportive therapy must be considered with this in mind. These infections may be picked up during passage through the birth canal or from the hospital environment sometime after birth.

Staphylococcus aureus is a frequent cause of nosocomial infection in newborn nurseries. Although usually fairly mild in severity, compromised infants may have serious complications. Streptococcus pneumoniae and viridans, Escherichia coli, and Haemophilus influenzae may also cause conjunctivitis in newborns (Sandstrom, 1987). Pseudomonas aeruginosa is a rare but serious cause of neonatal conjunctivitis primarily in premature infants. It can lead rapidly to keratitis and a septicemia that may be life threatening. All of these organisms may be associated with a serious generalized systemic infection that requires aggressive medical treatment with appropriate local and systemic antibiotics.

Chlamydia

The leading cause of neonatal conjunctivitis is now considered to be Chlamydia trachomatis. It may be responsible for a third or more of all neonatal conjunctivitis. It is the most common sexually transmitted disease in the United States today (Chlamydia, 1985). Various studies have indicated that up to ½ of infants born to women with cervical Chlamydial infection will become infected during their passage through the birth canal (Hammerschlag et al, 1979).

Chlamydial infection presents as a unilateral or bilateral conjunctivitis of mild to moderate severity and generally less severe than Neisseria infection. There may be lid swelling, redness and chemosis of the bulbar and palpebral conjunctiva, papillary hypertrophy, and mild discharge. Mild corneal pannus and superficial punctate keratitis usually superiorly, along with mild subepithelial infiltrates, may be seen later in the course of the infection.

Even though the initial presentation may be solely ocular, it should definitely be considered a systemic infection and a leading cause of pneumonia, pharyngitis, otitis media, and vaginitis in the infected newborns (Schachter & Grossman, 1981). The infant must be treated with both local and systemic antibiotics (erythromycin is generally used rather than tetracycline because the latter can cause malformations in teeth and bones in infants). The mother and her sexual contacts must also be treated with systemic antibiotics.

Other Causes

Viruses are an infrequent cause of external eye disease in otherwise normal and healthy neonates. Infants, particularly those that are breast fed, obtain a substantial degree of immunity from their mother for the first few months of life. Infants that are immunocompromised are at greatly increased risk of severe, disseminated viral infection. This is totally different than the relatively harmless type of viral conjunctivitis commonly seen in normal children. The same is true for external fungal infections.

Conjunctivitis in Older Children

Bacterial   This conjunctivitis in older children is quite common. There are many organisms that can cause these infections. Most will respond readily to topical antibiotics once the organism has been identified and the appropriate antibiotic agent has been used. Cultures and sensitivities ideally should be obtained in all anterior segment ocular infections prior to the initiation of any treatment, but in practice cultures are gotten only when the infection proves resistant to the initial antibiotic used. Unfortunately by this time, accurate culture results are almost impossible because of the treatment itself.

The use of antibiotic ointments instead of drops is preferable, especially in younger children. It is easier to ascertain that ointment has gotten into the eyes of a struggling child than it is to determine that about drops. Ointments also have a much longer contact time on the eye before being flushed away by the tears, leading to a higher level of drug actually reaching the locus of infection than is possible with drops.

Staphylococcus aureus is the most frequently encountered bacterial cause of conjunctivitis in children. It may present as a mild to moderate acute conjunctivitis with redness, mucopurulent discharge, and crusty lids, especially on awakening. If it is incompletely treated, it may become chronic, causing hordeolum, chalazion, keratitis, and blepharitis. Treatment is with bacitracin, erythromycin, gentamycin, or tobramycin ointments four or five times a day for a week, with a follow-up visit to assess the efficacy of the treatment. Gentamycin is perhaps best not routinely pre-scribed as a first choice antibiotic agent due to its potential toxicity to the corneal epithelium, leading to mild punctate keratitis. Occasionally this may progress to a serious keratitis once the ocular surface is compromised. Since sulfacetamide, even in topical instillation (Genvert et al, 1985), has been linked with Stevens-Johnson disease, some practitioners feel it should not be routinely used to treat mild external eye disease. Chloramphenicol has been implicated as a cause of aplastic anemia in a few individuals, and its use should be restricted to those instances where it is shown by culture and sensitivity to be required. If the conjunctivitis is not completely resolved by the first course of antibiotics, consider switching to another antibiotic since the infectious agent may have developed resistance to that antibiotic. This is a good reason for culturing all bacterial infections before treatment is begun.

Acute hemorrhagic conjunctivitis is caused by Streptococcus pneumoniae and Haemophilus influenza bacteria and several types of adenoviruses. These organisms cause epidemics of hemorrhagic conjunctivitis in preschool and school settings and may be associated with important systemic disease. Although it has been said that Streptococcus pneumoniae is a more common etiology of hemorrhagic conjunctivitis in northern regions of the United States compared to Haemophilus influenza in the south, there is very little conclusive evidence to support this, and either organism can be a causative agent in hemorrhagic conjunctivitis. Haemophilus influenza is a leading cause of periorbital cellulitis and meningitis in young children. A vaccination for Haemophilus influenza is now available and is highly recommended for virtually all young children. Treatment of this infection is by local antibiotics along with systemic antibiotics when it is associated with systemic disease. Hospitalization may be required in the presence of severe systemic disease.

External eye infections may be caused by many other bacteria, particularly in young children or those with chronic, debilitating diseases. Among these organisms are enteric rods such as E. coli, Serratia marscesens, Proteus, Klebsiela, Moraxella, and Pseudomonas. Differentiation of these organisms is generally impossible without accurate cultures since the clinical appearance is often nonspecific. The choice of an antibiotic agent ideally should be based on cultures and sensitivities, but patients may initially be placed on a broad-spectrum antibiotic until the results are obtained.

Recurrent external eye infections in young children should always arouse some suspicion of nasolacrimal duct obstruction. Evaluation for this by the Jones test (instillation of fluorescein onto the surface of the eye and checking for transit through the ducts into the nostril with a cotton-tipped applicator) should be considered. Broad-spectrum antibiotic ointments can be prescribed for acute episodes of conjunctivitis.

Patients with external infectious eye disease that are immunosuppressed, whether from congenital and hereditary causes or acquired due to treatment of underlying disease, must be treated aggressively to guard against superinfection that can have potentially catastrophic results. Included in this category are patients undergoing treatment for various neoplastic diseases (especially following bone marrow transplantation), any of the primary immunodeficiency disorders, and HIV infection.

Viral   In general, viruses are the most common cause of external eye infections in children beyond infancy. Otherwise healthy infants, particularly those that are breast fed, possess a significant immunity passed on from their mother, that provides a considerable level of defense against many of the typical ocular viral diseases. Older children are usually susceptible to frequent viral illnesses of all types once this passive maternally based immunity is lost. Epidemics of various adenoviruses are frequently encountered in schools. Viral conjunctivitis secondary to a systemic viral illness is also common. Less common are primary herpes simplex and molluscum contagiosum infection. Treatment for all viral conjunctivitis except that caused by herpes simplex is palliative in nature. Immunosuppressed patients can develop both external and internal ocular infections from a host of viruses, especially herpes simplex and zoster. Aggressive viral therapy with topical agents such as Viroptic, Vira-A, or Stoxil and systemically with acyclovir is required. Concomitant use of topical and systemic steroids is advocated by some, but not all, authorities.

Sexually Transmitted Diseases   Particularly in older children, the possibility of sexually transmitted diseases such as Chlamydia (Greydanus & McAnarney, 1980), Neisseria, and herpes must always be considered. Eliciting a positive history may be nearly impossible but should be attempted when these diseases are suspected. The presence of a confirmed sexually transmitted eye disease in a younger child should arouse a suspicion of sexual abuse. This must be carefully followed up, and the appropriate social service agency must be contacted. Systemic treatment is essential in all of these diseases. Penicillin is the drug of choice in Neisseria infection. Chlamydia is treated with systemic tetracyline in patients over the age of eight years that are not pregnant, and systemic erythromycin is used in those individuals not able to use tetracyline because of the risk of dental and bone defects in young children from its use.

Allergic   Vernal conjunctivitis is a relatively severe, usually seasonal allergy that primarily affects young males. It is associated with marked itching, burning, and redness of the conjunctiva and a marked papillary response of the upper tarsus and sometimes at the limbus. Initial treatment is with vasoconstrictors and systemic and topical antihistamines, with cromolyn sodium and topical steroids added as needed for more severe cases. The condition usually subsides during late adolescence but may prove almost incapacitating for some patients.

The milder form of atopic conjunctivitis may occur in up to 20 percent of the population. This may be associated with other atopic conditions, including eczema, asthma, and hay fever. Treatment is with topical vasoconstrictors, antihistamines, desensitization, and only rarely with topical steroids. Symptoms are often greater than the clinical appearance of papillae, chemosis, and injection of the conjunctiva would indicate.

Keratitis

Corneal infections may begin as a routine case of conjunctivitis or blepharitis, spreading to the cornea as a result of a compromised corneal epithelium. Prompt treatment of the blepharitis or conjunctivitis may prevent a more serious corneal infection.

The presenting signs of a corneal infection are likely to include discharge, conjunctival injection, tearing, photophobia, and some sort of a behavioral change in the child. There may also be a generalized systemic illness.

Examination of children, particularly of infants and toddlers, will obviously be more difficult than for adults. Adequate slit lamp examination is important, and with persistence is possible on most children, especially if a hand-held portable slit lamp is available. A complete set of cultures is mandatory before any treatment is initiated. If the practitioner is unable to manage this in an office setting, referral to an appropriate source is essential. Serious visual loss may be prevented by prompt diagnosis and treatment.

Bacterial

Staphylococcus aureus is the most common cause of bacterial keratitis. There is often an associated history of blepharitis or conjunctivitis that may have been incompletely treated. Staph keratitis may present in several different ways. Inferior superficial epithelial punctate keratitis is the most common and least severe presentation. Chronic cases may include a marginal corneal ulcer that is mediated by an antigen-antibody type of reaction that is usually sterile—at least initially. These marginal corneal ulcers appear with a so-called *lucid interval*, a clear area of normal corneal tissue between the limbus and the lesion. These lesions can be quite painful, and there may be considerable injection of the adjacent bulbar conjunctiva. A different type of hypersensitivity reaction may cause the formation of a phlyctenule at the limbus. Treatment of these staphylococcus infections is with topical antibiotics and possibly steroids. The most serious form of staphylococcal keratitis is a central corneal ulcer. It is associated with a red painful eye, photophobia, mucopurulent discharge, and sometimes a hypopyon. Aggressive treatment with topical and systemic antibiotics should be started after cultures and scrapings are obtained.

Streptococcus pneumoniae and Haemophilus influenzae both cause hemorrhagic conjunctivitis and less commonly keratitis in children, particularly during the winter months. Pseudomonas aeruginosa keratitis can occur due to the use of contact lenses or contaminated eye drops. Both Neisseria and Pseudomonas can rapidly destroy the cornea, and must be treated very aggressively in an inpatient setting.

Viral

Herpes simplex keratitis is the leading cause of visual-acuity loss due to corneal infection. Many cases of mild herpetic keratitis are made much worse by the inappropriate shotgun use of antibiotic-steroid combinations for red eyes. By the time the child is finally seen by an eye doctor, there is severe dendritic herpes keratitis. Infants have adequate maternal antibody protection for approximately six months after birth. Over the next five years of life, 90 percent of children will develop a systemic or ocular primary herpes infection with only a relatively small percentage going on to develop a secondary ocular infection. Current treatment uses Viroptic and debridement of the ulcer.

Keratitis caused by adenovirus infection is frequently seen in children along with acute follicular conjunctivitis. Systemic involvement commonly includes upper respiratory infection and pharyngitis. Epidemic keratoconjunctivitis causes a punctate keratitis and subepithelial opacities that may linger for months, causing a mild temporarily visual-acuity loss. These lesions may be prolonged by the use of steroids, which should therefore generally be avoided. Varicella keratitis secondary to chickenpox is not uncommon. It may manifest as a mild superficial punctate keratitis, or as limbal vesicles with corneal infiltrates and mild vascularization in adjacent cornea that may progress to a disciform keratitis. Rarely there may be an anterior uveitis. Treatment is generally not required, but topical steroids may be used if symptoms warrant it.

Other Causes of Keratitis

Mycotic infection is occasionally seen in patients that are immunosuppressed. These cases may vary from minor to severe, and some may lead to overwhelming systemic infection and death. The indiscriminant use of topical and systemic steroids may also precipitate mycotic infection of the cornea and conjunctiva. Any infection that proves resistant to standard therapy or is clinically difficult to diagnose should arouse some suspicion of mycotic or amoebic involvement. Acanthamoeba has become a significant concern as a pathogen in patients wearing soft contact lenses, particularly for extended wear, and should be considered in patients presenting with serious keratitis.

TRAUMA
Assessment of the Traumatized Eye

The assessment of a child's traumatized eye is in many ways similar to that of an adult. The major differences concern the obvious difficulty in obtaining information from the patient and the difficulty in examining a child who may be in pain and crying hysterically. A complete evaluation is imperative in order to arrive at the proper diagnosis; an incomplete examination may lead the examiner to a dangerously misleading conclusion. If a thorough assessment is impossible in an office setting, the child must be taken to a hospital emergency room as quickly as possible.

The first step should always be to obtain as thorough a history as possible from the parent or individual that is accompanying the child. If there is any indication of head or systemic injury in addition to the eye trauma, first aid should be applied and the child taken to a hospital for complete neurological and systemic evaluation. Details of the history must be carefully recorded for medicolegal purposes. As always, a good history should lead to an accurate diagnosis, but a history given by the parent or guardian that is not consistent with the physical findings should trigger suspicion of child abuse and that should be investigated appropriately.

An attempt should always be made to assess visual acuity in each eye by an age-appropriate procedure. Infants can be assessed by subjective techniques such as fixation preference and ability to fix and follow or simply by pupillary responses. Objective techniques such as preferential looking, optokinetic nystagmus, and visual evoked potentials may be too time-consuming or impossible on a crying child that is in pain or frightened, but they can be attempted if it is feasible. The child's general mental and physical state should be assessed. A careful evaluation of pupillary responses, eye movements and position, and the integrity of the globe and adnexa and a slit lamp exam of the anterior segment should follow. Do not be quick to dilate the pupils; dilation may hide serious neurologic involvement. Dilation should only be done after it is certain that there are no neurologic complications that must be assessed by a neurologist. A thorough binocular indirect ophthalmoscopy examination should then be performed through the dilated pupil. Intraocular pressure can be obtained by a slit lamp mounted tonometer or a hand-held applanation tonometer. If this proves impossible, a comparison of ocular rigidity by palpation must be done. If it is not possible to examine the child adequately, referral to a hospital and examination under anesthesia should be considered.

Birth Trauma

Estimates of the frequency of ocular injury due to the process of birth range up to 25 percent of all births and up to 50 percent of difficult births (Duke-Elder, 1972). Only a small number of these injuries are apparent; even fewer have any lasting significance; but some may lead to ocular complications and visual loss that may prove difficult to diagnose later.

The most commonly noted ocular sequela of birth is a chemical conjunctivitis that is secondary to the instillation of silver nitrate drops for ocular prophylaxis at birth. The silver nitrate will cause ecchymosis of the eyelids and conjunctivitis, occasionally severe enough to swell the lids shut. This will clear within a few days of birth.

Conjunctival hemorrhages and mild edema and ecchymosis of the eyelids are frequently noted at birth, more often in difficult deliveries, but they are seen even in easy deliveries. Rarely a traumatically induced ptosis of the upper lid may be caused by difficult delivery or by the use of forceps. If the ptosis is severe enough to cause closure of the eyelid, the potential of deprivation amblyopia and induced axial myopia should be considered (Hoyt et al, 1981). Eversion of the lids at birth has been reported. This may resolve spontaneously, or it may require surgical intervention.

Corneal injury from forceps delivery can lead to serious ocular complications. This type of corneal trauma may appear as faint vertical striae or ruptures in Descemet's membrane or as a more generalized denser corneal opacity of large size. This resemblance to congenital glaucoma may complicate the diagnosis. The density of the opacity usually decreases over a period of several weeks, but some degree of scarring and striae usually remain. These opacities can lead to large degrees of corneal astigmatism, myopia, and amblyopia (Angell et al, 1981). Infants with corneal birth trauma must be closely monitored for these refractive problems and should be aggressively treated for amblyopia.

Retinal hemorrhages occur frequently, often even in uncomplicated deliveries. The incidence is lowest in Caesarean sections and greatest in long, traumatic vaginal births. In most cases, they tend to resolve completely within one or two weeks of birth. Rarely a macular hemorrhage in the foveal area may cause amblyopia (Isenberg, 1989). Vitreous hemorrhages have also been reported. The effect of these hemorrhages may mimic that of a congenital cataract if they do not spontaneously resorb soon after birth. Dense vitreous hemorrhages may require early surgical intervention.

Epidemiology of Eye Injuries

Eye injuries are reported about twice as often in boys than they are in girls, probably because of the greater statistical likelihood of boys being involved in sports and in generally rougher play than girls. In a study by Nelson and colleagues (1989), the most frequent cause of eye injury was accidental or intentional trauma by another child, followed by sports-related injuries. Injuries were more frequent during the springtime. Nonperforating anterior globe injuries such as corneal abrasions and foreign bodies and anterior segment contusion injuries were the most common category of injuries, followed by extraocular injuries such as lid lacerations, ecchymosis, and orbital fractures. Perforating injuries to the globe and posterior segment injuries were less frequently noted.

Blow-Out Fracture of the Orbit

Blow-out fractures of the orbit result from serious ocular trauma to the bony areas surrounding the globe. The area most commonly affected is the ethmoidal plate and the area of the infraorbital groove, but any of the surrounding bony structures can be affected as well. Symptoms include pain at the point of injury, pain when the eye is moved, and diplopia and/or blurred vision. Signs include ecchymosis, limitation of eye movements, and ptosis. Nausea and vomiting may occur. It is important to note that there is great variability in the presentation of patients with a blow-out fracture, with some having an essentially occult presentation.

Many patients will experience significant apparent weakness of the inferior rectus muscle due to the mechanical effects of the orbital fractures, including complete incarceration of the muscle. There is often an impairment of elevation and depression of the eye. Strabismus and ptosis may be noted. X-rays are helpful, if not essential, in the diagnosis and treatment of orbital fracture. Surgical intervention is required for many, but not all, patients with blow-out fractures of the orbit. The determination of the appropriate treatment is best left to the surgeon.

Superficial Foreign Bodies

Superficial foreign bodies are among the most common acute pediatric problems that the optometrist will see. The child will present with epiphora, blepharospasm, and crying. Assessment of visual acuity will be greatly aided by the use of an anesthetic eyedrop, but a measurement of visual acuity without an anesthetic should be attempted first for medicolegal reasons. Either slit lamp examination or inspection of the anterior segment with loupes will allow a visualization of the superficial foreign body or a corneal abrasion. Complete eversion of both eyelids is important. Be certain that there is no visible penetration of the globe.

Foreign bodies can be removed by irrigation, cotton swabs, fine gauge needles, or by a spud. Extreme care must be exercised to prevent further ocular trauma to the eye during removal with a sharp instrument. If the child is not controllable, the foreign body removal may need to be performed while the child is under anesthesia, but most children can be steadied by the parents or by ancillary help. A broad-spectrum antibiotic ointment should be applied for prophylaxis against bacterial infection. Pressure patching may reduce the symptoms and increase the rate of epithelialization, but many children object more to the patch than to the eye discomfort. The eye should be rechecked the following day. Scarring is unlikely to occur unless the foreign body penetrates deep into the stroma.

Chemical Burns

Chemical burns are a true ocular emergency requiring immediate first aid in order to minimize the potentially catastrophic results. Regardless of the type of chemical that has gotten onto the eye, the initial treatment is the same, namely copious flushing of the eye with water. Acids tend to precipitate out corneal proteins on contact, which actually limits the amount of damage caused due to both a buffering affect and a physical barrier to further penetration into the corneal tissue.

Alkalies, on the other hand, tend to penetrate very deeply, and can cause necrosis of tissue even days after the initial burn. In general, alkalies cause far more damage to the eye than do acids. The degree of damage is related to the strength of the alkali and the length of time before the alkali is completely neutralized or flushed from the eye. There are four levels of alkali injury to the anterior segment of the eye. Level one shows generalized epithelial involvement and a red eye; level two shows a white eye with blanching of vessels in the conjunctiva. Level three shows a glassy cornea with stromal involvement, and level four a white ground-glass appearance. There is a likelihood of an intraocular pressure rise shortly after the injury. The use of topical steroids is very controversial since they may increase the activity of corneal collagenase, thus increasing the level of corneal damage and also decrease resistance to secondary infection, but steroids do decrease inflammation and corneal pannus. Citrate solution has recently been recommended in the initial stages as a means of increasing collagen development. Extreme care must be taken to avoid secondary infections due to the massively disrupted ocular surface.

Ocular Contusion Injuries

Traumatic Uveitis

Mild ocular contusion can lead to a conjunctival hemorrhage or a traumatic iritis. Both of these tend to resolve spontaneously with little in the way of symptoms and no sequelae. Occasionally the iritis may be more severe with considerable photophobia as a presenting symptom. The pupil may be either miotic or mydriatic and sluggish; cells and flare will be present in varying degrees in the aqueous; and the IOP (intraocular pressure) is usually lower than it is in the nonaffected eye. The examination should include gonioscopy if there is any evidence of an angle recession or if the IOP is increased. The presence of an angle recession raises the prospect of the development of glaucoma at some point in the future. Treatment of uncomplicated traumatic iritis is with a combination of cycloplegic agents and topical steroids with frequent rechecks for hyphema, IOP increases, and secondary infections from corneal abrasions.

Hyphema

More severe contusion to the eye can lead to angle recession and hyphema along with retinal contusion. Hyphema is usually caused by a tear in the iris root or the iris stroma and is often associated with angle recession. The anterior chamber fills with blood, either partially or completely, obscuring the view of the iris (Figure 9.1). In general, the greater the height of blood in the anterior chamber the greater the risk of long-term visual acuity loss. Rebleeding after initial partial or complete resolution of the hyphema also makes the prognosis for full recovery poorer. In the past, children with hyphemas were invariably hospitalized on complete bed rest with both eyes patched, but recently many children are sent home with bed rest alone. These patients must be followed very closely, often daily, until the risk of rebleeding is past (at least one to two weeks). The use of cold compresses in the immediate posttrauma period has been advocated by some, but studies have not confirmed its efficacy.

The use of aspirin has been found to increase the risk of rebleeds greatly, and is no longer used as part of the treatment (Crawford et al, 1975). The use of aminocaproic acid has been advocated by some, but there are significant side effects from the drug, and its routine use in the treatment of hyphema is still uncertain (Kraft et al, 1987). The major complications of hyphema are bloodstaining of the cornea with a reduction in visual acuity and corneal health and sharp rises in intraocular pressure, which can be very difficult to control. This is greatly complicated by the presence of significant degrees of angle recession. The trauma may also be severe enough to cause anterior and posterior synechiae. Less commonly the lens may become subluxated, leading to severe visual acuity loss from optical causes and iris bombe type glaucoma. Cataracts are a fairly frequent sequela of trauma to the eye that may not become

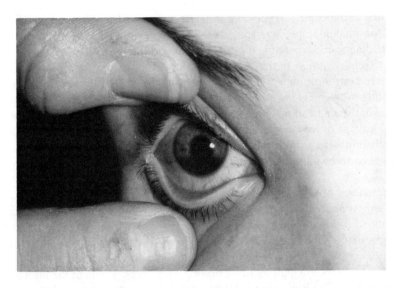

Figure 9.1   Blood in the anterior chamber of this patient is easily visible. Contusion injuries severe enough to cause hyphema place the eye at future risk for angle recession glaucoma. Hyphema may also result in bloodstaining of the cornea, leading to impairment in corneal functioning.

significant until long after the injury. This is perhaps the most common type of acquired cataract in children.

Retinal Trauma

The most frequently seen retinal disorder resulting from ocular contusion injury is Berlin's edema or commotio retinae. This typically appears in the posterior pole region, particularly at the macula, and can result in a significant decrease in visual acuity. The retina in the affected area becomes cloudy with a whitish haze except at the fovea, which usually retains its reddish coloration. This change in fundus appearance is thought to be due to a disruption in the architecture of the outer segments of the photoreceptors and is not due to actual extracellular retinal edema. It is usually easiest to observe the borders of the injury with the surrounding tissue maintaining its normal appearance. Commotio retinae is almost always self-limited with resolution over a period of days or weeks, but there can be retinal pigmentary changes and a loss of vision if the macula is affected. More severe injury to the retina can cause flame-shaped hemorrhage in the nerve fiber layer, rupture of Bruch's membrane leading to large atrophic scars, and rhegmatogenous retinal detachments with its typical sequelae.

Penetrating Ocular Injury

Penetrating injury to the eye is a true ocular emergency. The major risk, in addition to the direct effects of the injury itself, is that of secondary endophthalmitis.

Penetrating intraocular foreign bodies may be seen with a slit lamp or binocular indirect ophthalmoscope, but special imaging techniques may be required for a complete diagnosis. Depending on the material and the location of the foreign body, surgery to remove it may or may not be necessary. Rupture of the globe can be caused by a severe contusion injury. There may be a hyphema in addition to the rupture, significantly worsening the prognosis. Penetration by sharp objects can lead to a variety of injuries, including corneal and scleral lacerations, hyphema, puncture of the lens and leakage of lens material into the aqueous and vitreous, and retinal damage. Endophthalmitis is a serious risk in this situation. First aid can be applied, but these patients need to be admitted to a tertiary care facility for evaluation and treatment.

Prevention of Ocular Injury

The best method of improving the prognosis in all types of ocular trauma is by prevention of the injury itself. Many pediatric eye injuries are easily preventable by the use of adequate eye protection during any activity that puts the eye and the child at risk. For example, in the 1960s, many children in the United States and Canada experienced serious eye injuries while playing ice hockey. Through the efforts of eye doctors such as Dr. Paul Vinger (1981; 1987), protective facemasks were made mandatory for all players, resulting in an enormous decrease in the incidence of eye injuries. Similar results in racquet ball have occurred more recently. There is no excuse for not recommending proper eye protection when it is warranted. It is the responsibility of eye doctors to continue to urge all patients to wear proper protection during both work and play. Excellent fitting protective sport and work eyewear is now readily available in all sizes, and lenses of polycarbonate plastic, a substance extremely resistant to breakage, is in common usage. Patients should be clearly informed of its availability and its importance. Furthermore, any monocular patient should wear such protection at all times. It is important for both legal and ethical reasons that all monocular patients be so informed.

Child Abuse

Any inexplicable or improbable eye injury to a child should lead the optometrist to consider child abuse as a potential cause. The incidence of physical child abuse is now recognized as being much higher than was previously thought. It has been estimated that as many as 40 percent of all children that are physically abused may show ocular signs (Harley, 1980). The specific types of ocular injuries run the gamut from periorbital ecchymosis (black eye), corneal abrasions and lacerations, hyphema and angle recession, and cataracts and dislocated lenses to all sorts of retinal injuries, including total detachments. Suspicion should be aroused when the history does not agree with the physical findings or when the history is inconsistent or illogical. A frequent history of ocular or systemic injuries should also arouse suspicion of abuse. An additional and very important sign of child abuse lies in the child's behavior. As one who comes in contact with large numbers of children, the pediatric optometrist learns through experience when a child's behavior seems questionable. Child abuse may also take the form of sexual and emotional abuse. Unusual behavior patterns are likely to be evident in these children (Smith, 1988). It is very important to pursue suspicions by carefully questioning the child and parent. The optometrist has a legal and a moral responsibility to report those suspicions immediately to the appropriate state or local authorities. Rapid reporting of all suspected child abuse is mandatory, and the reporter is protected by law from any liability in all states.

REFERENCES

American Academy of Pediatrics. Prophylaxis and treatment of neonatal gonococcal infections. *Pediatrics*. 1980;65:1047–1048.

Angell LK, Robb RM, Berson FG. Visual prognosis in patients with ruptures on Descemet's membrane due to forceps injury. Arch Ophthalmol 1981;99:2137–2139.

Armstrong JH, Zacarias F, Rein MF. Ophthalmia neonatorum: A chart review. Pediatrics 1976;57:884–892.

Chlamydia trachomatis infections: Policy guidelines for prevention and control. MMWR 1985;34:Suppl 3S:53S-74S.

Crawford JS, Lewandowski RL, and Chan W. The effect of aspirin on rebleeding in traumatic hyphema. Am J Ophthalmol 1975;80:543–545.

Duke-Elder S. System of ophthalmology, vol 14. St. Louis: Mosby, 1972;9–17.

Genvert GI, Cohen EJ, Donnenfeld ED, et al. Erythema multiforme after the use of topical sulfacetamide. Am J Ophthalmol 1985;99:465–468.

Greydanus DE, McAnarney ER. Chlamydia trachomatis: An important sexually transmitted disease in adolescents and young adults. J Family Practice 1980; 10:611–615.

Hammerschlag MR, Anderka M, Semine DZ, et al. Prospective study of maternal and infantile infection with Chlamydia trachomatis. Pediatrics 1979;64:142–148.

Hammerschlag MR, Cummings C, Roblin PM, et al. Efficacy of neonatal ocular prophylaxis for the prevention of chlamydial and gonococcal conjunctivitis. N Engl J Med 1989;320:769–772.

Harley RD. Ocular manifestations of child abuse. J Ped Ophthalmol Strab 1980;17:5–13.

Hoyt CS, Stone RD, Fromer C, et al. Monocular axial myopia associated with neonatal eyelid closure in human infants. Am J Ophthalmol 1981;91:197–200.

Isenberg SJ. The eye in infancy. Chicago: Year Book Medical Publishers, 1989;381.

Kraft SP, Christianson MD, Crawford JS, et al. Traumatic hyphema in children. Ophthalmol 1987;94:1232–1237.

Nelson LB, Wilson TW, and Jeffers JB. Eye injuries in childhood: Demography, etiology, and prevention. Pediatrics 1989;84:438–441.

Pierse D, Eustace P. Acute keratoconus in mongols. Br J Ophthalmol 1971;55:50–54.

Sandstrom I. Treatment of neonatal conjunctivitis. Arch Ophthalmol 1987;105:925–928.

Schachter J. Editorial: Why we need a program for the control of Chlamydia trachomatis. N Engl J Med 1989;320:802–803.

Schachter J, Grossman M. Chlamydial infections. Ann Rev Med 1981;32:45–61.

Smith SK. Child abuse and neglect: A diagnostic guide for the optometrist. J Am Opt Assoc 1988;59:760–765.

Vinger PF. The eye and sports medicine. In Duane TD, Jaeger EA, eds. Clinical Ophthalmology. Philadelphia: JB Lippincott;1987:1–39.

Vinger PF. Sports injuries, a preventable disease. Ophthalmol. 1981;88:108–113.

10

Ocular Manifestations
of Systemic Disorders

Bruce D. Moore

This section will present brief descriptions of those systemic disorders that have important ocular manifestations. Many of the more commonly seen conditions have already been covered elsewhere in this text. Also included here are a number of conditions that are quite rare and unlikely to be seen in a general practice but are nonetheless important for the clinician to be aware of, and finally, several systemic conditions are included here that are relatively common but have not been discussed elsewhere in the text because they do not easily fall into an anatomic category.

CYSTIC FIBROSIS

This autosomal recessive (AR) hereditary disease is considered to be the most common serious genetically based disorder in white patients. It affects about 1 in 2000 people, and the gene is present in about 5 percent of the white population. It is less common in black and Asian populations.

Many of the organ systems of the body are affected. Pancreatic insufficiency leads to widespread endocrine and exocrine dysfunction, resulting in malabsorption and malnutrition in some individuals. The mucous glands are grossly affected, causing severe and chronic pulmonary problems. The sweat glands are abnormal with hyper-excretion of various minerals. Patients with cystic fibrosis require constant use of antibiotics and respiratory therapy to reduce the greatly increased risk of pneumonia, an important cause of early death in these patients. The life expectancy of cystic fibrosis patients has increased in the past decade through the use of prophylactic measures such as antibiotics, and some patients survive into adulthood and occasionally middle age although earlier death is more common. Recently the specific gene locus has been identified, and there is new hope of treatment with genetic engineering techniques for a definitive cure.

Cystic fibrosis can affect the eyes and visual system in several ways. Malabsorption of vitamin A can lead to xerophthalmia (Poppell & Poirier, 1978) and night blindness (Petersen et al, 1968), which is reversible with vitamin A supplementation. Retinal edema, retinal vascular changes, macular cystic changes, and papilledema have been reported. Because of the abnormal mucous, lipid, and sweat excretions (Sheppard et al, 1989), the constituency of the tear production may be abnormal as well. Cystic fibrosis patients who wear contact lenses tend to have increased levels of deposits on their lenses that appear to be both mucoid and mineral in nature. Vigorous cleaning with an alcohol-based cleaner is helpful in extending the useful life of their lenses.

INFLAMMATORY COLLAGEN AND CONNECTIVE TISSUE DISEASES

By far the most common of these conditions seen in the pediatric population is juvenile rheumatoid arthritis (JRA), which causes a significant percentage of the cases of anterior uveitis in children where a diagnosis can be made. The uveitis is difficult to control and often leads to cataracts and glaucoma. Treatment of this type of uveitis usually is accomplished with topical steroids and cycloplegic agents, but sometimes systemic steroids must be added. Medications are tapered and titrated until the minimal dosage that reduces the cell and flare reaction to an *acceptable* level is maintained. This acceptable level of inflammation is invariably greater than one would really like to see, but a recognition that the medications themselves cause a host of problems and should be minimized to the greatest degree possible must be kept in mind. It is likely that the medications will need to be used over a long period of time, often many years, and that the cumulative effects of long-term steroid use can lead to glaucoma and cataracts in a significant percentage of patients. It is very important that all patients with JRA, particularly the pauciarticular form (affecting 5 or less joints), be followed periodically (at least every four to six months), even in the absence of ocular disease, because of the potential for insidious late onset of eye disease.

Ankylosing spondylitis causes inflammatory disease of the spine, specifically the sacroiliac joints. There may also be a more disseminated arthritis present. Ankylosing spondylitis most commonly affects males in the second decade of life, but the disorder can appear earlier. HLA-B27 antigen is usually present and is very helpful in making the correct diagnosis. The primary ocular involvement is a uveitis. Dry eyes may also be present.

Lupus erythematosus is a necrotic condition affecting various organ systems. There is a very high likelihood of the presence of antinuclear antibodies, indicating that lupus is an autoimmune disease. Females are affected much more frequently than are males. Ocular manifestations include retinal vascular disease and uveitis. Dry eyes may be present.

Reiter's syndrome mostly affects adolescent and young adult males; it is rare in young children and in females. The cause is uncertain, but may be autoimmune. There is thought to be a relationship to prior history of severe diarrhea and venereal diseases, particularly chlamydial and gonococcal diseases. HLA-B27 antigen is often present. The major manifestations of the syndrome include pauciarticular arthritis, urethritis, and conjunctivitis. There may be an associated uveitis and keratitis has also been reported.

Kawasaki Disease

Kawasaki disease is also known as mucocutaneous lymph node syndrome. It was originally described in Japan, where it is diagnosed quite frequently. Recent evidence indicates that it is distributed much more widely around the world but is often misdiagnosed. There may be a greater incidence, however, in orientals than there is in whites or blacks. The condition most commonly affects young children.

It is characterized by a long-lasting high fever, maculopapular truncal rash, *strawberry tongue*, desquamation of the skin at the fingertips, and lymphadenopathy (Rauch, 1989). Perhaps the most serious complication is a form of coronary vasculitis that may lead to death in about 2 percent of patients with the disease. The primary ocular effects are a sometimes severe conjunctival infection without mucopurulent discharge, anterior uveitis, and occasionally a mild vitritis.

The etiology of the disease has remained mysterious. Environmental contaminants have statistically been implicated, particularly a relationship with recently cleaned carpets. Recently, a retrovirus has been tentatively identified as a possible causative agent (Marchette et al, 1987), but there is still much uncertainty about this. A form of toxic shock syndrome has also been theorized as a possible cause. Steroids, gamma globulin, and aspirin are widely used in the treatment of Kawasaki disease. Any young child presenting with fever, rash, reddened tongue, and severe conjunctivitis should be strongly suspected of having Kawasaki disease and should have an immediate work-up for the disease by the pediatrician.

Ehlers-Danlos Syndrome

This is an AR-inherited disorder, the principal features being hyperextensibility of the skin and joints and kyphoscoliosis. There may also be a number of urogenital and vascular abnormalities. The ocular manifestations include epicanthal folds, blue sclera, keratoconus, ectopia lentis, angioid streaks, choroidal hemorrhages, and disciform macular degeneration.

Pseudoxanthoma Elasticum

This AR disease features a yellowish, thickened discoloration of the skin of the neck, orbit, limbs, and abdomen. There may be vascular complications, including telangiectasias, hypertension, and peripheral vascular insufficiency. Typical ocular manifestations include angioid streaks and chorioretinal degenerations.

Marfan's Syndrome

This is an AR-inherited condition that is quite commonly seen in clinical practice and that has significant ocular effects. Patients are generally very tall and thin with frequent and severe kyphoscoliosis and hyperextensibility of the joints. Patients may have aortic aneurysms, which can spontaneously dissect, leading to early sudden death. All patients suspected of having Marfan's syndrome (including any patient with ectopia lentis) should have a cardiologic evaluation for this potential problem. The major ocular manifestations include ectopia lentis, high to extreme myopia, retinal detachments, cataracts, megalocornea, and strabismus.

Weill-Marchesani Syndrome

Ectopia lentis and high myopia are the most common ocular defects in this AR disorder. Patients tend toward short stature in contrast to patients with Marfan's syndrome. There is also a greater likelihood of an anteriorly displaced lens causing pupillary block glaucoma.

ENDOCRINE DISORDERS

There are a number of relatively uncommon disorders of the endocrine system that may have various effects on the eyes and the visual system. Patients with hypopituitarism may present with septo-optic dysplasia, featuring optic nerve hypoplasia. Hyperthyroidism and Graves' disease may occur in teenagers. Hypoparathyroidism can cause bilateral cataracts in young children. Hyperparathyroidism can cause cataracts, and there may be calcific opacities of the cornea and conjunctiva.

Diabetes mellitus is a more common endocrine disorder with potentially serious ocular manifestations in older children. The general clinical manifestations of childhood diabetes are the same as those of adults but are complicated by the increased difficulty of blood sugar control in the adolescent population, mostly due to behavioral considerations. Poor control leads to more rapid onset of cataracts and retinal problems. The management and treatment of adolescent diabetics is quite difficult and is usually best handled by a team emphasizing not only the medical but also the psychosocial problems of adolescents.

SKIN DISORDERS

Ichthyosis

This condition has been classified into several categories based on the hereditary pattern (Katowitz et al, 1974). All of these subtypes present with dry scaly skin. The scaling may be very extensive and appear similar to the scales of fish, giving the condition its name. Ectropion, chronic conjunctivitis, keratinization and papillary hypertrophy of the conjunctiva, corneal stromal opacities, and corneal epithelial opacities have been reported. An extreme form of ichthyosis, found only rarely at the time of birth, has been called the *collodion baby* condition (Orth et al, 1974). There is a parchmentlike membrane that completely covers the neonate at birth, which then desquamates over a period of weeks or months. Visual acuity is usually unaffected in patients with ichthyosis.

Juvenile Xanthogranuloma

Patients with this condition develop yellowish or reddish-brown papules on the skin of the scalp and face during infancy. The ocular manifestations include infiltrates of the uveal tract. This is also a cause of recurrent hyphemas.

Rosacea

Rosacea is a common skin disorder of the skin that primarily affects middle-aged whites. The skin and eyelids present with redness, telangiectasia, papules and pustules, and hyperactive sebaceous glands. There is often blepharitis, meibomitis, and chalazia. The condition may be seen in adolescents and is sometimes confused with the more typical acne vulgaris. The treatment of choice in nonpregnant patients is systemic tetracycline.

Acne Vulgaris

This is the typical form of acne that is so common in adolescents. There are many forms of topical treatments that have been used with varying effectiveness. The use of Retin A (Accutane), a vitamin A analog, has proven very effective for serious cases, but the drug has been shown to be a potent teratogen and must be used very carefully in sexually active female adolescents.

Erythema Multiforme

Erythema multiforme (Stevens-Johnson syndrome) is a disease of uncertain origin that causes a severe, occasionally fatal, inflammatory process primarily affecting the skin and mucous membranes. The condition may be triggered by infection or by the use of drugs and is probably immune-complex mediated. Various sulfa drugs have been specifically implicated, and several cases have been traced to the use of topical sulfacetamide for mild external eye disease (Genvert et al, 1985). The disease may cause severe ocular complications (Arstikaitis, 1973), including ulcerative conjunctival lesions, symblepharon and cicatricial scarring of the conjunctiva, entropion and trichiasis of the lids, and corneal ulceration and opacification. Marked visual loss is not uncommon in severe cases. Treatment is by topical and systemic steroids.

Eczema and Atopic Dermatitis

These important dermatologic conditions have been associated with several types of ocular complications. Among the symptoms of these conditions are itching of the periorbital areas. The itching can lead to vigorous rubbing of the eyes, lids, and periorbita, which can, over a period of time, lead to keratoconus. A particular type of atopic cataract may also occur.

SKELETAL DISORDERS
Craniofacial Abnormalities

This diverse group of craniosynostosis has been discussed in the section on the orbit and whole eye in Chapter 7.

Osteogenesis Imperfecta

This is one of the more common of the fragile bone diseases. These patients experience frequent and sometimes spontaneous fractures of their fragile bones, progressive loss of hearing due to conduction abnormalities, and blue sclera. The blue sclera is due to ectasias of the sclera itself and is not a result of the visible scleral vasculature that is often seen in normal patients. Other ocular manifestations include anterior embryotoxon, cataracts, keratoconus, and megalocornea.

Miscellaneous Skeletal Conditions

The Arnold-Chiari syndrome is a central nervous system (CNS) malformation that often results in hydrocephalus and spina bifida and a *bull-neck* appearance. Down-beat nystagmus and diplopia are among the more common ocular manifestations.

The Klippel-Feil syndrome involves abnormalities of the cervical vertebrae and again a *bull-neck* appearance. Strabismus, nystagmus, and marked disorders of ocular motility are the primary ocular manifestations.

Hallermann-Streiff syndrome results in short stature and marked anomalies of the facies. Bilateral microphthalmus and congenital cataracts are the most severe of the ocular manifestations with nystagmus and strabismus also sometimes present.

METABOLIC DISORDERS

There are a great many uncommon metabolic disorders that may have important ocular manifestations. Some of these disorders have been previously mentioned.

Mucopolysaccharidoses (MPS)

This is a very diverse group of inherited metabolic diseases that all have an abnormal accumulation of mucopolysaccharides, primarily in connective tissue. There is a specific defect in a lysomal enzyme that is responsible for degradation of the particular mucopolysaccharide in each of these disorders. There are currently seven major disorders that have been characterized in the mucopolysaccharidoses (MPS), all of which are AR in their hereditary patterns.

They are classified as:

MPS IH—Hurler's syndrome
MPS IS—Scheie's syndrome
MPS I H/S—Hurler/Scheie compound
MPS II—Hunter's syndrome
MPS III—Sanfilippo's syndrome
MPS IV—Morquio's syndrome; (there currently is no MPS V)
MPS VI—Maroteaux-Lamy syndrome
MPS VII—Sly syndrome

The systemic manifestations of these disorders are very variable but include cardiovascular problems, dwarfism, mental retardation, skeletal abnormalities, and in some cases premature death. The ocular manifestations include progressive corneal clouding, glaucoma, and retinal degenerations in a few of the subtypes.

Mucolipidoses

This is another diverse group of inherited metabolic disorders that affects the storage of both mucopolysaccharides and either sphingolipids or glycolipids. The systemic manifestations include facial and skeletal abnormalities and mental retardation. Ocular manifestations include corneal stromal opacities and a cherry-red spot in the macula.

Fabry's Disease

This condition is due to a storage abnormality of ceramide trihexoside caused by the deficient breakdown enzyme ceramide trihexosidase. It is an X-linked recessive (XR) disease. Female carriers often present only with the ocular characteristics of the disease, but affected males may experience serious or fatal renal and cardiovascular problems. The most apparent ocular abnormality is a striking, whorl-like opacity of the cornea at the level of Bowman's membrane (Sher et al, 1979). There may also be a "propellerlike" lenticular opacity or a spokelike deposit on the posterior lens capsule. Retinal vascular changes in the form of tortuosities and dilatations of the veins and rarely central retinal artery occlusion have also been reported.

Wilson's Disease

This is a hepatolenticular disorder that results in abnormal deposition of copper in the brain, liver, and kidneys and in the cornea and lens of the eye. It is inherited in an AR pattern, with greater expressivity in males than females. It typically presents in the second decade of life, but early signs may appear in childhood.

The characteristic ocular sign of Wilson's disease is a bluish or greenish-brown ring of copper deposits at the limbus, which is called a Kayser-Fleischer ring. It is easily seen in a high percentage of cases on slit lamp examination. A small number of patients may also develop cataracts. Early diagnosis is important as the disease can be effectively treated with a variety of drugs. Any patient that presents with a blue or greenish limbal ring should be referred to a pediatrician for evaluation.

Refsum's Disease

This is a disorder of fatty acid metabolism with an accumulation of phytanic acid in various tissues. The disease manifests several abnormalities, including pigmentary retinopathy, cerebellar ataxia, peripheral polyneuritis, and proteinemia of the cerebrospinal fluid. There may also be dermatologic affects and cardiomyopathy. It is transmitted as an AR pattern.

The ocular signs are important in making the correct diagnosis. The pigmentary retinopathy is initially peripheral with typical bone spicule formation and a salt-and-pepper appearance. The macula may eventually show involvement. Visual fields show peripheral constrictions, and night blindness develops. The clinical appearance in general may be quite similar to classical retinitis pigmentosa (RP). A few patients will develop an atypical retinal appearance also similar to cases of RP. In addition, cataracts, glaucoma, and pupillary anomalies may be found. The electroretinogram (ERG) is usually affected.

The Amino-Acidurias

These include a diverse group of abnormalities of amino-acid metabolism. This is generally due to an aberrant enzyme or pathway. Most are AR with the exception of Lowe's syndrome, which is XR. All have significant ocular manifestations. Only several of the more commonly seen aminoacidurias are discussed here.

Cystinosis

This is an AR inherited disease of amino-acid metabolism that results in deposition of the amino-acid cystine in the tissues of the body. It often leads to early death. There is a characteristic deposition of refractile crystals of cystine in the cornea. Centrally the opacities are located only in the anterior stroma, but peripherally they are fuller in thickness. These opacities are virtually pathognomonic of cystinosis. There is also a peripheral pigmentary retinopathy that gives a salt-and-pepper appearance.

Lowe's Syndrome

Lowe's syndrome is also known as the *oculocerebrorenal syndrome*. Congenital cataracts are almost a universal finding, and many patients have congenital glaucoma. Strabismus, microphakia, nystagmus, miosis, and iris atrophy are also noted. Mental and growth retardation is common as is early death.

Homocystinuria

This is an AR inherited disorder of methionine metabolism caused by a lack of the enzyme responsible for its breakdown and a concomitant increase in the level of homocystine and methionine in the body. Among the important systemic manifestations of homocystinuria are abnormalities of the vascular system and mental retardation. The most important ocular effect is ectopia lentis, often with inferior displacement of the lens. Anterior displacement is more likely in homocystinuria than it is in the other common causes of ectopia lentis. Secondary glaucoma, myopia, cataracts, cystoid retinal degeneration, and optic atrophy may also occur.

Galactosemia

This is a defect in the metabolism of the sugar galactose. It can be caused either by a deficiency in the activity of breakdown enzymes galactose kinase or galactose-1-phosphate uridyl transferase. The latter breakdown enzyme causes a more severe form of the disease. This disorder results in the development of cataracts, hepato-splenomegaly, and mental retardation. Early diagnosis is important because prompt treatment can lead to reversal of the cataract and prevention of further systemic progression. This may be one of the few treatable forms of cataract by other than surgical means.

The Sphingolipidosis

These are a diverse group of disorders of sphingolipid metabolism that leads to premature death. They are sometimes called the amaurotic familial idiocy disorders, indicating the degenerative nature of these disorders. There is a generalized accumulation of lipids within the nerve cells, gradually affecting their functioning. Within the eye, the major defect in Tay-Sachs disease is the appearance of a cherry-red spot at the macula (Figure 10.1). This is caused by a whitening of the retina at the ganglion cell layer with the macula being spared by the anatomical absence of ganglion cells in the area. Optic atrophy eventually develops. Tay-Sachs disease appears first and leads to death by two to four years of age. The disease affects primarily people of Jewish and French-Canadian origin. Bielchowsky-Jansky, Batten-Mayou, Speilmeyer-Vogt, and Kufs disease appear progressively later in life. They do not produce a cherry-red spot as does Tay-Sachs but do cause progressive neurological degeneration. Other causes of cherry-red spots include gangliosidosis, Niemann-Pick disease, Farber's syndrome, and Gaucher's disease.

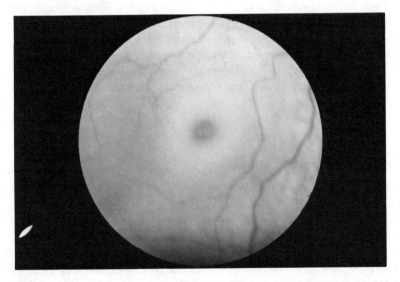

Figure 10.1 The cherry-red spot of the macula is easily differentiated from the rest of the pale fundus that is obscured by abnormal deposition of ganglioside material in the ganglion cell layer of the retina. The normal macular appearance is spared because of the absence of ganglion cells in the macula.

CHROMOSOMAL ABNORMALITIES

This brief discussion concerns the major chromosomal deletions and trisomies that have important ocular affects. A more comprehensive discussion of hereditary factors in pediatric optometry is found in the section on genetic factors in Chapter 2.

Trisomy 13 (Patau Syndrome)

This chromosomal abnormality generally results in the death of the infant in the first few months of life. There are a large number of ocular and systemic anomalies that these infants manifest. Most of these infants have a normal or near normal birth weight but fail to thrive. There are major cardiovascular, urogenital, and neurological abnormalities. The infants are mentally retarded and deaf. The ocular defects include microphthalmus, uveal colobomas, cataracts, retinal dysplasia, intraocular cartilage formation, corneal opacities, and optic nerve hypoplasia. There is an equal incidence in males and females.

Trisomy 18 (Edward's Syndrome)

Most of the infants with Edward's syndrome that survive through birth and delivery are female because most of the males spontaneously abort. Most of these neonates will not survive past the first year of life, are of low birth weight, and exhibit hypertonicity. These infants have a characteristic facial appearance consisting of micrognathia, microstomia, narrow palatal arch, low-set ears, and narrow occiput. The hands and feet are malformed. Severe cardiac and renal defects are present, and they are mentally retarded. The ocular anomalies include epicanthal folds, blepharophimosis, ptosis, hypertelorism, corneal opacities, microphthalmia, glaucoma, and uveal colobomas.

Trisomy 21 (Down Syndrome)

This is considered to be the most common of all of the chromosomal abnormalities. The incidence is estimated to be about 1 in 600 live births (Frynes, 1987), and the incidence increases with increasing maternal age. Patients may have virtually normal lifespans, but premature death is not uncommon. The major systemic abnormalities include mental retardation, characteristic facies, low-set ears, dental hypoplasia, thickened tongue, anomalies of the hands and feet, congenital heart defects, and gastrointestinal anomalies. The ocular defects include epicanthus, Mongolian slant, Brushfield spots (Figure 10.2), strabismus, cataracts, keratoconus, nystagmus, blepharitis, and high refractive errors. All patients with trisomy 21 should have eye examinations at an early age.

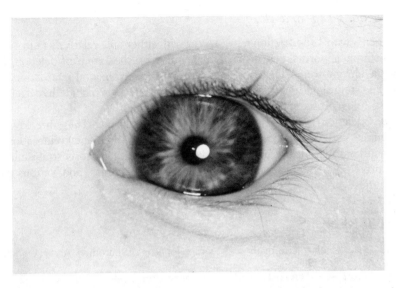

Figure 10.2 Brushfield spots are frequently seen in patients with Trisomy 21 but are also seen occasionally in normal patients. They are areas of normal iris tissue surrounded by hypoplastic iris stroma, and they do not affect vision.

Deletion 5p- (Cri-Du-Chat Syndrome)

This condition is due to a partial deletion of the short arm of chromosome 5. These infants typically are born with low birth weight and are hypotonic. They have a very characteristic cry resembling a cat's cry. Infants are mentally retarded and have characteristic facies and both neurological and cardiovascular abnormalities.

Deletion 11p-

This deletion is strongly associated with aniridia and Wilm's tumor. There is often a series of urogenital abnormalities and mental retardation as well.

Deletion 13q-

These patients manifest characteristic facies, neurological abnormalities, and mental retardation. There is also a strong association with retinoblastoma (Sparkes et al, 1979), and recently there is evidence of the specific location of the *retinoblastoma* gene on chromosome 13 (Yandell et al, 1989). Additional ocular defects include hypertelorism, microphthalmus, epicanthus, ptosis, colobomas, and cataract.

Deletions 18p- and 18q-

Patients with 18p- deletion may present with either only relatively mild or more severe systemic abnormalities, probably depending on the extent of deletion of the arm of the chromosome. This may include microcephaly, mental retardation, short stature, and neurological defects. The ocular manifestations include hypertelorism, epicanthal folds, ptosis, strabismus, and microphthalmia.

18q- deletion is also known as deGrouchy syndrome. These are low birth weight infants with failure to thrive, characteristic facies, and mental retardation. The ocular manifestations include antimongoloid slant, epicanthus, ptosis, strabismus, blue sclera, correctopia, cataracts, color vision defects, colobomas, and various retinal abnormalities.

REFERENCES

Arstikaitis MJ. Ocular aftermath of Stevens-Johnson syndrome. Arch Ophthalmol 1973;90:376–379.

Frynes JP. Chromosomal anomalies and autosomal syndromes. Birth Defects 1987;23:7–32.

Genvert GI, Cohen EJ, Donnenfeld ED, Blecher MH. Erythema multiforme after the use of topical sulfacetamide. Am J Ophthalmol 1985;99:465–468.

Katowitz JA, Yolles EA, Yanoff M. Ichthyosis congenita. Arch Ophthalmol 1974;91:208–210.

Marchette NJ, Ho D, Kihara S, et al. Search for retrovirus etiology of Kawasaki syndrome. Prog Clin Biol Res 1987;250:31–39.

Orth DH, Fretzin DF, Abramson V. Collodion baby with transient bilateral upper lid entropion. Arch Ophthalmol 1974;91:206–207.

Petersen RA, Petersen VS, Robb RM. Vitamin A deficiency with xerophthalmia and night blindness in cystic fibrosis. Am J Dis Child 1968;116:662–665.

Poppell S, Poirier RH. Xerophthalmia in an infant with cystic fibrosis. Metabolic Ophthalmol 1978;2:41–43.

Rauch AM. Kawasaki syndrome: Issues in etiology and treatment. Adv Pediatr Infect Dis 1989;4:163–182.

Sheppard JD, Orenstein DM, Chao CC, et al. Ophthalmol 1989;96:1624–1630.

Sher NA, Letson RD, Desnick RJ. The ocular manifestations in Fabry's disease. Arch Ophthalmol 1979;97:671–676.

Sparkes RS, Muller H, Klisak I, et al. Retinoblastoma with 13q- chromosomal deletion associated with maternal paracentric inversion of 13q. Science 1979;203:1027–1029.

Yandell DW, Campbell TA, Dayton SH, et al. Oncogenic point mutations in the human retinoblastoma gene: Their application to genetic counseling. N Engl J Med 1989;321:1689–1695.

11

Pediatric Contact Lenses

Bruce D. Moore

This chapter is divided into two major sections based on the age of the child. Younger children are defined here as patients under the age of five years. They generally require fitting and management of their contact lenses in a manner quite different than is the procedure with older children. The underlying causes for contact lens wear are often also quite different, most being aphakic and amblyopic. The amblyopia often becomes the major management problem. Sometimes these patients benefit from contact lens treatment of the amblyopia in addition to the underlying etiology.

The older children are more likely to have typical (but high) refractive errors and often can be managed in ways that are not very different from those for adults. Amblyopia may also be an important issue, but it is not usually as dense or as difficult to treat as it is with the younger children. There is obviously a degree of overlap in these two arbitrary age groups, but this dichotomy does have much clinical validity.

YOUNG CHILDREN
Conditions Benefiting from the Use of Contact Lenses

Contact lenses have proven a useful treatment modality for many of the eye problems of young children (Halberg, 1983). High refractive errors and aphakia are the two most obvious pediatric eye conditions benefiting from the use of contact lenses, but patients with amblyopia, cosmetic abnormalities, corneal insult, and photophobia may be helped as well.

Refractive Error
Myopia Young children with high myopia may benefit greatly from the use of contact lenses. It may be difficult for parents to keep a pair of spectacles on their child's face. Peripheral vision is improved through contact lenses, and image size in refractive (as opposed to axial) myopia is more normal with contact lenses than it is with spectacles. These factors may improve the child's visual perceptual and visual motor skills. There is also the issue of improved cosmesis which may be important for some families.

Contact lenses are not used on very young children with only low to moderate degrees of myopia unless there is significant anisometropia and/or amblyopia since their uncorrected visual acuity at the close viewing distances that are of interest to them is generally satisfactory without any correction. Contact lenses may be considered in young children with mild refractive error when spectacle use is difficult due to the child's behavior or to anatomic problems such as a craniofacial anomaly and only when the improved visual acuity is deemed important enough to justify the risk and bother of lens wear.

Hyperopia Patients discovered to have moderate to high degrees of hyperopia require correction at a young age to prevent the possible development of accommodative esotropia or refractive amblyopia. Some children will tolerate correction best with contacts, others with spectacles, and some with a combination of both at different times, but the use of some form of correction is important to reduce this risk of amblyopia and/or strabismus.

Contact lenses may provide additional benefit for young patients with moderate to high degrees of hyperopia and accommodative esotropia by controlling the strabismus more completely than spectacles would (Sampson, 1971). Correction with contact lenses decreases the convergence demand by eliminating the induced base out prismatic effect caused by plus spectacle lenses. Contact lenses also decrease the accommodative demand below that measured through spectacle lenses. This may cause an apparent decrease in the AC/A ratio in contact lens wearers with accommodative esotropia and other milder forms of accommodative and convergence excess, particularly when they have a high AC/A ratio. Bifocal contact lenses should prove even more beneficial in controlling accommodative esotropia in young patients once these lenses are perfected.

Astigmatism Children between about 6 and 24 months of age normally have very variable degrees of both the power and axis of astigmatism (Mohindra et al, 1978; Fulton et al, 1980). This variability in astigmatism usually does not cause any visual problem unless it is associated with high spherical refractive errors and generally need not be corrected unless there is associated strabismus or amblyopia. Since the astigmatism is so variable, the child should be refracted again after several weeks and before prescribing correction whenever it is felt that correction of the refractive error is warranted. It is not unusual to find significant change in the axis or power of the astigmatism after only a few weeks' interval in otherwise normal young patients. Supplying an unnecessary correction may actually cause more harm than good by inducing refractive or anisometropic amblyopia.

When correction by contact lenses is required, custom made gas-permeable or soft-toric lenses can be used. Boston Envision™ aspheric gas-permeable lenses correct considerable degrees of hyperopic astigmatism and can be fit empirically without the benefit of keratometric measurements. Custom-made soft-toric lenses can now be obtained from manufacturers such as CoastVision in virtually any parameter required.

Anisometropia Anisometropia is an important cause of amblyopia in young children. Strabismus may occasionally be the first sign of amblyopia, but often there is no visible deviation. The child may develop a microtropia and amblyopia that will go undiagnosed until full eye examination at a later age, by which time treatment will be more difficult.

When anisometropia is detected early, contact lenses may be useful in correcting the optical portion of the problem. Lenses can be designed to correct any refractive error. The level of compliance with contact lenses may be better in some patients than that level is with spectacles. The optical correction is, however, only the first step in the treatment of anisometropia. Patching to treat the amblyopia is almost always more difficult than maintaining the proper refractive correction. Further discussion of anisometropia and aniseikonia will be found in the section on contact lenses in older children later in this chapter.

Aphakia Cataracts are uncommon in the general population of young children, but they make up a large and important segment of a pediatric contact lens practice. Pediatric cataracts may be unilateral or bilateral and either congenital or acquired. Congenital cataracts until recently were considered very difficult to treat, particularly when they were unilateral (see the section on cataracts in Chapter 7). Cataracts of later onset were thought to be only somewhat more treatable. Problems with surgical techniques, contact lens fitting in young children, and the treatment of amblyopia each played a role in the generally pessimistic outlook in these patients. Techniques to overcome all of these difficulties were developed in the 1980s to the point where they are now considered quite routine (Robb et al, 1987; Mayer et al, 1989).

The prognosis for good vision in young children with cataracts is dependent on a number of factors, including the time of onset, the density of the cataracts, the rapidity of surgery and optical correction after onset, and whether the cataracts are unilateral or bilateral. It is now known that cataract extraction, contact lens correction, and aggressive amblyopia treatment are required before the end of the critical period (thought to be about four to six months of age in human infants) in order to have any reasonable expectation of attaining of good visual acuity in the affected eye (Beller et al, 1981). Cataracts that develop after the critical period do not have as severe an impact on acuity unless they are allowed to remain for too long a period of time.

Bilateral aphakic patients may be fitted with either contact lenses or spectacles. Selected patients may do better with one method of correction than the other, but there are advantages in the use of contact lenses. Contacts cause less magnification than do spectacles (about 20 to 30 percent with spectacles and 8 to 12 percent with contact lenses in a typical pediatric aphakic power), allowing the child to experience a more natural visual perceptual environment. As a result, the child's general development may progress at a more normal level. The normal cosmetic appearance with contacts may enhance the child's social development as compared to the use of thick spectacles. The child may also have difficulty keeping the heavy glasses on the face, particularly in the presence of craniofacial abnormalities. On the other hand, contact lenses may prove difficult for the parent or child to deal with, and the cost of the contacts may be prohibitively greater than that of spectacles, especially in those patients that experience a high rate of lens replacement. Many children with bilateral cataracts do best with both contacts and glasses with the parent and the child deciding on which is best under various conditions over the course of treatment.

For unilateral aphakic patients, contacts are, for the vast majority of patients, a superior form of treatment. Glasses may occasionally work in the small number of patients who are not successful contact lens wearers, but lenses should almost always be tried initially. Intraocular lens implants (IOLs) and surgical procedures such as epikeratophakia should be reserved for those few patients that prove unable to wear contact lenses or spectacles but that tolerate patching for amblyopia when it is required.

Fitting contact lenses to patients with cataracts is an ongoing process. As the eye grows and the prescription changes, lenses must be changed. Constant attention to amblyopia is a major aspect of the treatment. These patients require very intensive levels of care.

Amblyopia (Figure 11.1)

Contact lenses may be used in the treatment of amblyopia in two different ways. High plus lenses can be worn over the normal eye to blur the image quality to a level below that of the amblyopic eye if the degree of amblyopia is not too deep. Surprisingly in many patients treated for early onset cataracts and dense amblyopia, the degree of optical blur achieved with even a +30D contact lens over the normal eye may not be sufficient to induce the child to use the amblyopic eye. High plus lenses may be more useful in patients with milder strabismic or refractive amblyopia.

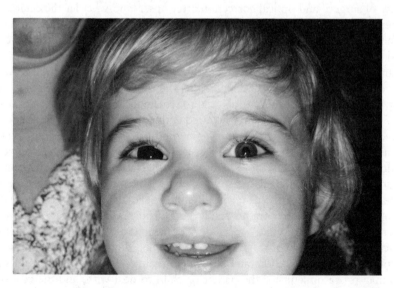

Figure 11.1 This patient with a unilateral congenital cataract is wearing an aphakic soft contact lens on the left eye and an occluder soft contact lens on the right eye in lieu of an eye patch.

Black occluder soft contact lenses have been used on a wide variety of amblyopic patients, including those having congenital and acquired cataracts and strabismic and refractive amblyopia (Moore & Smith, 1984; Moore, 1991). These occluder lenses are most effective in patients already using a contact lens for optical purposes since the patient and the parents do not have to adapt to new techniques of handling or care. Other patients that have had no previous contact lens experience may also do well if the level of parental motivation is high. Evidence is convincing that many young patients object more to the feel of the patch on their face than to the effect of the patch on their vision. Some young patients accept an occluder lens without behavioral problems but object strenuously when a patch is applied over that eye with the occluder lens still in place. The most important negative aspect of use of an occluder contact lens is the risk involved in placing a lens over the normal eye with the possibility, however slight, that a serious problem (such as vision-threatening corneal infection) may develop from the use of the lens. This must be carefully weighed before the use of an occluder contact lens is contemplated. A few children become adept at manipulating the lens off the cornea by hand or by blinking and thus reducing the effectiveness of this modality.

To fit an occluder soft lens, first determine the optimal fit with a clear lens of the same parameters as that of the opaque lens. The lens can then be ordered in opaque form from the supplier (see Appendix B), or ideally opaque lenses may be kept in the practitioner's inventory for immediate fitting and dispensing.

Corneal Masking and Nystagmus

Contact lenses can be used in several ways for the purpose of corneal masking. One use is to cover a disfigured nonseeing eye, for example an eye that has incurred corneal trauma leading to blindness and cosmetic problems for the patient. This is more of an issue with older children because of social pressures related to the appearance of the disfigured eye. These lenses may be obtained from several sources (White Ophthalmic in Calgary, Canada; Narcissus Foundation in California; and Wesley-Jessen in Chicago—see Appendix B) in a variety of colors and patterns. Photos of the normal and damaged eyes may be sent to the manufacturer to aid in the optimal design of the lens. These lenses tend to be quite expensive and may take a considerable period of time to obtain, but the results can be very gratifying for the patient, the family, and the practitioner.

Another use is for patients having severe photophobia. A darkly tinted lens that filters out a significant portion of ambient light may significantly improve vision and comfort. Examples include patients with iris coloboma, aniridia, albinism, or achromatopsia. These lenses particularly benefit patients with achromatopsia.

Patients with marked nystagmus and high refractive error may obtain poor optical correction with spectacles because the visual axis is only intermittently aligned with the optical center of the lens, inducing distortions and prismatic effects. A contact lens will move with the visual axis, reducing these effects. Contact lenses may also reduce the optical blur sufficiently to improve visual acuity and decrease the magnitude of the nystagmus in cases of sensory nystagmus (Allen & Davies, 1983). In addition, there have been anecdotal reports of a dampening effect on the nystagmus by two other mechanisms. One is simply from the weight of the contact lens itself acting as a sort of anchor. The other is caused by the contact lenses dampening nystagmus through a sensory feedback mechanism due to movement of the lens on the eye resulting in increased awareness that the eye is moving. Neither mechanism has been confirmed, however.

Bandage Lens

Bandage lenses of various types may be used on young children for the same reasons as they are used for adults. Corneal healing may be aided with the use of a bandage lens on patients having epithelial abrasions secondary to trauma. Collagen shields are used on adults with a variety of corneal problems, but their efficacy on children has not as yet been reported. There are several rare pediatric dystrophic corneal syndromes that may also be aided by the use of bandage contact lenses.

Mensuration of the Infant Eye

The eyes of a young child are not simply smaller versions of adult eyes. There are distinct differences in the configuration and in the physiology of the ocular surface of the child's eye from that of adults. These differences in configuration should have considerable bearing on the theoretical optimal lens design for children. Unfortunately, however, virtually all of the currently available pediatric contact lenses have been designed for use on adult eyes and are simply scaled up in terms of prescription. This has led to serious problems in the efficacy of contact lenses for younger patients. Many lenses intended for pediatric use simply do not fit the small eyes of infants or are not available in appropriate powers. There are a number of ocular parameters that must be taken into account when designing a lens for a particular category of patient. These parameters are well known and generally accepted for adults and older children but have not been completely determined for younger children although several studies have provided some information (Chase et al, 1984; Enoch, 1972a; Moore, 1987). Lenses for pediatric patients should take these factors into account in order to perform optimally.

Lacrimation

Infant tears have a reduced protein, lipid, mucous, and mineral content and an increased aqueous content in comparison to adults. Infants and young children only rarely have problems with protein, lipid, or mineral deposits on their contact lenses except in the case of silicone elastomer lenses, which can experience severe lipid buildup. The high aqueous content of the tear film of young patients enhances the oxygen supply to the cornea via tear interchange and pumping under the contact lens. This minimizes the risk of eye infections and corneal hypoxia. Lens movement is also enhanced by this relative wetness of the eyes, particularly when the child is awake. Even when the infant is sleeping, the eyes usually appear to be well lubricated, except in the very youngest infants, before normal lacrimation begins at a few weeks of age.

The only clinically important group of young patients with potentially dry eyes are those patients that have received radiation therapy to the head for various types of cancers. The radiation appears to decrease lacrimal gland function and also seems to affect the integrity of the corneal epithelium to resist drying and surface irregularity. Since these patients are at high risk for the development of cataracts, this may lead to decreased success in long-term aphakic contact lens wear. Supplemental ocular lubrication is often necessary in these patients.

Eyelids and Palpebral Aperture

The palpebral aperture of the young child is obviously smaller than is that of adults. This makes insertion and removal of contact lenses more difficult; there is simply less space for an adult hand to work in. Pediatric lenses ideally should be smaller for young children than they are for adults.

The tension of the lids is usually tight when the child is awake but very loose and floppy when the child is sleeping. When the child cries, the lids shut very tightly, possibly preventing insertion or removal of the contact lens. If the parent forcibly tries to open the eyelids of a hysterical child, the lids may evert, and the parent may be forced to wait until the child settles down before reattempting insertion or removal. It may be easier for parents to accomplish insertion or removal when the child is sleeping if the child sleeps deeply enough.

Pupils

The pupillary diameter of a normal, awake infant is quite small, often in the range of two to three millimeters (mm) in diameter. Surgery or trauma to the eye may cause the pupil to become irregular or eccentric. This becomes important when trying to position the optical center of a contact lens over the pupillary aperture. Anatomic abnormalities such as an iris coloboma will also affect the pupil configuration.

Corneal Diameter

The corneal diameter of a normal, full-term infant at birth ranges from 9.25 to 10.50 mm with an average diameter of about 9.8 mm. Premature infants have a smaller corneal diameter. The diameter increases rapidly in the first year of life and then at a slower rate over the next few years until it reaches an adult diameter of around 11.5 to 12 mm by three to four years of age.

Smaller corneal diameters either may indicate a generalized microphthalmia or may be restricted to only the cornea. Most infants with congenital cataracts have smaller corneal diameters than are normal in the affected eye(s). Infants with persistent hyperplastic primary vitreous often have both markedly reduced corneal diameters along with generalized microphthalmia with corneal diameter sometimes as small as six to seven mm. In addition, the rate of growth of these eyes is usually slower than is that of normal eyes. Thus the relative difference in corneal diameters becomes greater as the child ages. This can become a significant cosmetic issue later. It was previously felt that eyes with microcornea or microphthalmia had a very poor visual prognosis, but now it is known that this is not necessarily true for all infants (Karr & Scott, 1986). Small eyes usually require contact lenses that are smaller in diameter than do normal sized eyes.

Larger corneal diameters than normal at birth should immediately arouse a suspicion of congenital glaucoma although there are many less serious causes. Patients with Marfan's syndrome may have megalocorneas up to 14 to 15 mm in diameter along with very high degrees of myopia. These patients may particularly benefit from the use of contact lenses. The large corneal diameter requires very large diameter contact lenses, which may be difficult to obtain.

Corneal Curvature

The central corneal curvature of newborn infants is quite steep. Studies have indicated that it may be as steep as 49.50D in otherwise normal premature infants, 47D in the first one to two months of life in full-term babies, and flattening to normal adult values of 43 to 44D by four years of age. Studies of infant aphakic eyes show similar results (Moore, 1987) with most of the flattening taking place in the first six months of life. This rapid change in corneal curvature during infancy requires appropriate changes in contact lens base curve to maintain proper fit.

Very little is directly known about the configuration of the peripheral cornea in young children. There are indications that it is much flatter than in adults during early infancy but that it begins to steepen somewhat prior to the end of the first year of life. This affects the corneal vault or sagitta to a considerable degree and may be a significant factor in the way contact lenses fit on these young eyes (Enoch, 1979b). A given lens sometimes becomes looser fitting on an infant eye between four to eight months of age, when one would expect the lens to become tighter fitting, due to the rapid flattening of the cornea that occurs by this time (Moore, 1987). The assumption, based on the experience of Enoch, is that the increasing corneal vault (effectively causing the lens to fit in a less stable manner on the eye) becomes a more important factor than is the decrease in central corneal curvature. Optometrists often need to refit a contact lens tighter and steeper in order to counteract this tendency of looser fitting lenses during the second half of the first year of life.

Refractive Error

Refractive error in young children can change quite rapidly. This is particularly true of astigmatism. High hyperopes may appear to have a large increase in refractive error after wearing an optical correction for even a short period of time due to relaxation of accommodation brought about by the correction. Care and repetition are critical to the accurate determination of refractive error in these young patients.

Young children that are aphakic experience dramatic changes in refractive error during the first years of life. Studies have shown the average refractive error at the corneal plane in aphakic infants to decrease from about +31D at one month to +21D at four years (Moore, 1989) (see Figure 11.2), with two-thirds of the change occurring by one and a half years of age. It is essential to monitor these changes in refractive error carefully and make changes in the contact lens, or the patient will potentially be seriously overcorrected.

Lens Materials

Contact lenses are currently made from three basic groups of materials: soft, rigid, and silicone elastomer. There are advantages and disadvantages to each type of material. Characteristics that are unimportant in the adult wearer may be critical for infants and young children and vice versa.

Soft Lenses

Soft lenses currently comprise approximately 80 to 85 percent of the total contact lens market in the United States and are widely used for children. When soft lenses are prescribed for extended wear, the oxygen permeability must be considered carefully. In the strong prescriptions required for many young children, low water content lenses are at best only marginally permeable to oxygen, while the high water content lenses are often too fragile for daily wear. Although high water materials are usually less prone to deposits in children because of their tear composition, giant

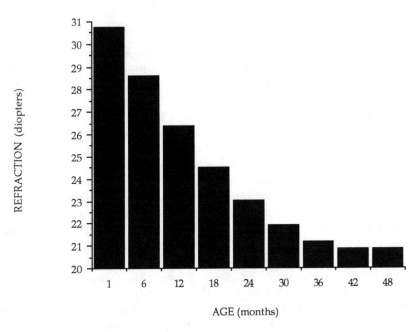

Figure 11.2 Mean spherical equivalent by six-month intervals. Reproduced by permission from Slack Inc. (In Moore BD: Changes in the aphakic refraction of children with unilateral congenital cataracts. J Pediatr Ophthalmol Strab 1989;26:290–295). The mean spherical refractive error obtained longitudinally from a group of 14 infants with unilateral congenital cataracts that were followed from birth to 4 years of age.

papillary conjunctivitis does occur more commonly than with lower water content lenses. The issue of the overall safety of extended-wear soft lenses remains quite controversial.

There are advantages that soft lenses for children offer over other materials. They are generally easy to fit with many experienced practitioners able to fit them in the office setting without special equipment or procedures. The excellent comfort of these lenses makes the adjustment period short. The cost of these lenses varies from about the same as for standard soft lenses to several times that for custom-made products, but it is usually much less than the cost of silicone elastomer lenses. The risk of injury to the infant's eye by improper handling is slight.

The major disadvantage of soft lenses is the difficulty of handling them. This depends greatly on the type of lens, the lens parameters, the abilities of the parent, and cooperation by the child. There are other disadvantages. Soft lenses are more fragile than the other types. The lenses may be rubbed out of the eye fairly easily. Deposits can be a problem for some patients. The risk of infection from poor patient/parent compliance, particularly in extended wear, is greater than it is with the other materials. Availability of soft lenses in pediatric parameters is limited, with some available only on a custom basis, entailing delays in dispensing to the patient. The optics and general quality of these lenses is also sometimes not up to the same level as other materials.

Rigid Gas-Permeable Lenses

Polymethylmethacrylate (PMMA) lenses should not be used on children. Rigid gas-permeable (RGP) lenses have been used with excellent results. In the relatively thick parameters required for aphakic children, they are very durable, but chipping at the edges may occur in some of the highly permeable fluorosilicone acrylate materials. They are easy for parents to handle and care for. Cleaning and disinfection is easier than with soft lenses, and the risk of infection is low. They are the least costly lens material and the most readily available in virtually any design or parameter and from many manufacturers. The lens quality is generally quite good and easy to verify in the office. The oxygen permeability can be excellent in the newer materials, much higher than it is with soft lenses but not as great as is silicone elastomer material. The material is well tolerated by young patients, largely due to their wet eyes.

The major disadvantage of RGP lenses is the difficulty in fitting them to a child's eye. Most practitioners perform the fitting while the patient is under general anesthesia although some practitioners are able to fit the lenses on awake children. These lenses fit in a more individual manner than is the case with other materials, requiring a custom-designed lens for each patient and thereby preventing dispensing at the time of fitting. If the lens that is first ordered does not fit as expected or if a different power is required, additional delays in dispensing will occur. RGP lenses are also more likely to eject or dislodge than are lenses made of other materials, increasing the frequency and expense of replacement. The initial comfort of RGP lenses is poorer than it is for other materials, requiring a longer adaptation period. There is also a greater likelihood of insult to the cornea due to eye rubbing by the child or rough insertion or removal by the parent.

Silicone Elastomer Lenses

There is currently only one silicone elastomer lens available, the B&L Silsoft lens. This lens is made of a silicone rubber material that has a number of properties particularly useful for young aphakic children. It has the best permeability of any contact lens material; studies have shown that the amount of oxygen available to the cornea may actually be greater with the lens on the eye than it is with no lens on at all! In terms of permeability, it is unexcelled as an extended-wear material. They are more durable than are soft lenses and almost as durable as RGP lenses. In addition, these lenses are readily available in a series of stock parameters, making Silsoft fairly easy to fit. Another advantage is that fluorescein can and should be used to help in the fitting and evaluation of the lenses and eye on follow-up visits. The lenses also stay on the young child's eye better than other lenses do.

There are several significant problems with these lenses, however. When it is fit too tightly, one can adhere and become immobile on the eye, leading to serious corneal complications. The material also has an inherent problem with wettability since silicone is a highly hydrophobic material that must have a surface treatment applied in order to be wettable on the eye. If the surface treatment is compromised due to the lens drying out or is cleaned in an inappropriate manner, the surface becomes highly hydrophobic, increasing the likelihood of the lens causing significant corneal problems. The material also has a strong affinity for surface lipid deposits, causing the lens to cloud over and adversely affecting vision, comfort, and corneal health. The use of hand creams and soaps containing lanolin or other greasy ingredients can literally poison the lens surface in this manner. Parental hygiene must be scrupulous. An alcohol-based cleaner such as CibaVision Miraflow must be used to minimize these problems of lipid deposition. (It is worth noting that the FDA [Food and Drug Administration] approved lens care system that B&L recommends in the Silsoft instruction manual is not the best system possible and may cause problems for patients and practitioners. The correct system should be Miraflow cleaner and a rigid lens soaking solution, such as Boston Conditioning Solution for storage of the lens.) The life expectancy of the lens may be very short for certain patients. It is probably the most expensive commercially available lens currently on the market. Silsoft is also an uncomfortable lens due to the edge design and the coating and wetting problems. Children become less tolerant of the lens by the end of the first decade of life, making the lens suitable only for young aphakic children. The lens is currently available only in aphakic parameters. It has been said for the past 15 years that silicone elastomer is the "lens of the future." It still is.

Lens Design in Early Childhood

The following characteristics of the pediatric eye should be addressed in the design of a pediatric contact lens (Enoch, 1979a).

Lens diameter. Since both the corneal diameter and the palpebral aperture of a young child are smaller than those of an adult, the contact lens diameter should also be smaller. Soft lenses should be semi-scleral as they are with adults, but the typical 14 mm diameter is too large. It should usually be about 12.5 to 13 mm in diameter for most infants, smaller for those with microcorneas, a bit larger perhaps for older children. The Allergan Hydron Mini-Lens at 13.0 mm meets this criterion. It has a standard power availability of +20 to −20D, making it suitable for most children other than aphakic infants. Unfortunately the company has curtailed the availability of this design in the higher powers and steeper base curves required for aphakic infants. CoastVision is now producing an excellent design pediatric aphakic soft lens that is readily available. This is undoubtedly the best soft lens currently available for this purpose. RGP aphakic lenses should be a little smaller for children than they are for adults, probably 9.0 to 9.5 mm. Silicone elastomer lenses should be about 11.3 mm, the size presently available, although ideally additional larger and smaller diameters should also be available.

Base curve and sagitta. Base curves for soft and silicone lenses need to be steeper than are those that are currently commercially available. They should be available starting at about 7.0 mm base curve (BC) in both soft and silicone elastomer materials for the steepest eyes with a range up to about 8.1 mm BC. RGP lenses should be fitted a little steeper than the flat K for most patients instead of slightly flatter as is the normal fitting philosophy used on adults. The change in corneal vault or sagitta as the infant gets older should be considered. A range of peripheral curves should be available in order to vary the sagitta of the lens rather than relying on BC exclusively. As was previously mentioned, some infants will develop increased corneal vault over the first year of life, requiring a lens of greater sagitta as they age, which is contrary to what one would expect if the only factor involved in the change in lens fit was the flattening of the cornea.

Lens thickness. Thin lenses are undesirable in young children because of handling and durability problems. Both the center and edge of the lens must be thick enough and in the correct proportion so that insertion is easy and tearing minimal. The only time increased thickness may be undesirable is in extended wear. If there is any doubt about sufficient oxygen permeability for a particular patient with a soft or RGP lens, a silicone elastomer lens should be used.

Optics of the lens. Manufacturers usually keep the size of the optic zone of aphakic and high minus lenses small in order to keep thickness down. Ideally the optic zone should be as large as possible so that vision is relatively unaffected if the lens positions somewhat eccentrically. There is little that the individual practitioner can do to check the quality of the optics before lens insertion. Usually defects become apparent on the eye while performing retinoscopy. The decision to use a single cut or lenticular design is usually left to the laboratory during the manufacture of the lens.

Tint and filtration. It would be useful to have an ultraviolet filter incorporated into every aphakic lens to provide protection for the retina from UV (ultraviolet) light exposure and to reduce the adverse affects of glare.

Currently only a few RGP materials provide UV filtration in aphakic lenses. Visibility tints and neutral density tints are limited or unavailable in the United States in FDA approved soft or silicone materials at this time, but a variety of tints are available internationally. There is no question that these tints (especially UV blockers) would be especially valuable for young aphakic patients.

Handling and comfort. Lens comfort is less important for infants than it is for adults. Infants tolerate lenses that adults will not, for example, the Silsoft lens. When exposed to uncomfortable stimuli, they cry for a short time and then quickly calm down. Children object far more to being held down during insertion or removal of the lens than from the sensation of the lens on the eye. Older children usually tolerate lenses almost as well as do the younger ones.

Young children do require a lens that is more positionally stable than usual. They will rub their eyes frequently for a host of reasons. The lens must maintain its position on the eye, or it will be rubbed off the cornea or out of the eye completely. This requires fitting the lens somewhat tighter than is the case on an adult eye. The lens also needs to be thicker and sturdier to prevent tearing or damage.

The lens must be easy for parents to handle. This is one of the more important requirements of a pediatric lens. If a parent is unable to get the lens onto the child's eye, the treatment will be unsuccessful. Silicone elastomer and RGP lenses have a decided advantage over many of the soft lenses in this respect.

Oxygen permeability. All pediatric lenses should be permeable enough to allow the child to nap safely with them. An insufficiently permeable lens can cause corneal hypoxia, particularly in a closed eye situation. The silicone elastomer lenses excel in their permeability. The newer RGP lenses also provide a sufficient level of oxygen to prevent significant corneal hypoxia. Most soft lenses, even in the higher water contents, provide a marginal level of oxygen to the cornea, especially under closed-eye situations. Extended wear of soft lenses should be pursued only under close supervision and only when other good alternatives do not exist. They are, however, a reasonable choice for use on a daily wear basis. There have not been any significant hypoxic corneal problems with the daily wear of currently available soft lenses, even when they are used routinely through the child's naps.

Contact Lens Fitting Procedures

Fitting under Anesthesia

The preferred method of some pediatric contact lens practitioners for fitting infants and young children is while the child is under general anesthesia. It is the easiest method of obtaining measurements of corneal configuration and refractive power. At that time, a lens may be inserted and its fit evaluated without the child's behavior interfering with the process.

There are, however, several problems with examination under anesthesia. Most important is the finite risk that anesthesia will precipitate a potentially serious medical emergency. The cost of inducing anesthesia is considerable. Another consideration is the probability that the measurements and information obtained under anesthesia are not identical to the conscious state. In the operating room, the child is lying on his back with abnormal lid forces, a virtual absence of lacrimation in a very dry environment, and a completely desensitized cornea.

The intraocular pressure while a patient is under anesthesia may be greatly decreased from normal levels by the effect of the anesthesia drugs themselves, a fact well known to pediatric ophthalmologists who treat congenital glaucoma. This reduction in intraocular pressure may cause the shape of the anterior segment of the eye, including the cornea, to be quite different under anesthesia than it is while the patient is awake. A lens that seems to fit well in the operating room may fit completely differently in the office later the same day. Occurrences of this serve to convince practitioners that the accuracy of lens fitting under anesthesia is questionable at least for some patients. It is best to restrict examination and fitting of contact lenses under anesthesia to instances when anesthesia is indicated for other reasons such as additional ocular or systemic procedures or when an extensive examination is required for a child who would be impossible to examine in the office for medical or behavioral reasons.

When an exam and fitting under anesthesia has been deemed necessary, keratometry, refraction with trial lenses, and measurement by calipers of the corneal diameters should be performed after the induction of the anesthesia (Enoch, 1972b). Then contact lenses of appropriate design and material should be inserted onto the eye. The lens is then evaluated for proper fit by observing the retinoscopic reflex, fluorescein pattern if possible, and the position and movement of the lens, both spontaneously and by actually trying to move the lens through the child's eyelid with a finger. The base curve and diameter should then be modified based on this fit. Once the optimal fit has been achieved, careful refraction should be performed. When high powers are involved, the trial lens should be close to the target spectacle Rx (prescription) to minimize induced error from off-axis retinoscopy or vertex calculations. The eye should then be thoroughly examined with a Koeppe gonioscopy lens and a binocular indirect ophthalmoscope for assessment of ocular health, and the intraocular pressure should be measured. The fit and power of the lens must then be verified on the awake child before dispensing.

Fitting in the Office

It is preferable to fit lenses to young children in an office setting (Moore, 1985); the result will be at least as satisfactory as it is under anesthesia but without the risk. If the initial fit or prescription requires change, it will be detected on subsequent visits, and the lenses can be changed before there is any permanent adverse effect. Measurements of corneal curvature by keratometry are usually not necessary. Retinoscopy with a contact lens on the eye is obtainable if the examiner is patient.

There are six general steps in the office fitting of pediatric contact lenses.

1. A thorough eye exam to make certain that the eye is ready to be fit with a contact lens. This should be performed in conjunction with the infant's surgeon. Most eyes are healed and ready for a lens about one or two weeks after surgery. If the lens is for nonaphakic purposes, a general examination should be performed prior to fitting.

2. Arrive at an initial set of lens parameters for the first trial lens. An estimate of corneal diameter of both eyes should be obtained, and a determination of the initial lens diameter should be made. The initial base curve of a soft or silicone elastomer trial lens should be one step flatter than the steepest lens available in that design. RGP lens base curves can be estimated from keratometry readings or trial lens fitting as is described below.

3. The approximate lens power must now be estimated. Add about two to three diopters more plus power than the mean refractive error for the age of the child as a starting point for the power of the aphakic lens (Moore, 1989) (see Figure 11.2) If the child is nonaphakic, perform retinoscopy with trial lenses, and convert for the vertex distance at the corneal plane for a starting point of the lens power.

4. The fitting characteristics of this first trial lens are then evaluated. Insert a lens of appropriate power and base curve for that design. The position and movement of the lens is then evaluated after the lens has stabilized on the eye. Soft or silicone elastomer lenses should position centrally over the cornea, with slightly less movement than one would prefer for adults. The lens should not decenter more than slightly on the blink or after a finger push on the child's eyelid. If it does, choose a steeper base curve or a different diameter or a lens configuration with a larger corneal vault or sagitta. If there is inadequate movement, choose a flatter base curve or a smaller sagitta. A completely different lens design or material may be necessary if this lens design does not fit properly. RGP lenses should position slightly superiorly, and show an acceptable fluorescein pattern.

5. The final lens power is then determined. After the correct material and base curve have been established, careful retinoscopy should be performed with hand-held lenses over a contact lens as close to the correct power and configuration as possible. In aphakics, the power of the contact lens should be approximately +2.50 to +3.00D greater than the actual refractive error to provide for focusing at the near and intermediate distances that are of prime interest to young children. The power of a nonaphakic lens should be determined in the usual manner.

6. Confirm the correct fit of the lens. The lens should be rechecked several times to be certain that it fits properly and that the power is correct. Changes in lens design or parameter should be made if it is necessary to achieve the ideal fit. The child should be encouraged to rub the eyes to be certain that the lens does not decenter or pop out easily. Pediatric lenses should fit more tightly than they do for adults to minimize the risk of

ejection, but be certain that the parents are able to remove the lens without too much difficulty.

Specific Fitting Characteristics of Each Material
Silicone Elastomer Lens Fitting

Silicone elastomer is the best material for aphakic extended wear and is undoubtedly the most frequently used material for pediatric aphakes. The B&L Silsoft lens is currently the only silicone elastomer lens on the market. The fitting of these lenses is quite straightforward (Cutler et al, 1985). On children less than two years old, simply insert a lens in a high plus power in a 7.7 mm base curve. This lens is only available in the 11.3 mm diameter. Evaluate the centration and movement. The lens should center well and have at least 1.5 mm of movement. If there is less movement, select a flatter base curve; if there is too much movement, select a steeper base curve. It is very important to check the fluorescein pattern. There must be adequate flow of fluorescein under the lens; if there is a sealing off of the fluorescein flow, the lens is too tight. The lens edge is much thinner than the optic zone, and should show several (two to four) *flutes*, small areas of peripheral edge lift, to guarantee tear flow under the lens. If there are no flutes, the lens is too tight and should be flattened. If the flutes are either too large or too numerous, the lens is too flat and should be steepened. Using retinoscopy, adjust the power as required. The Silsoft lens is available in 3 diopter steps between +20 and +32 diopters, and in one diameter, 11.3 mm.

Soft Contact Lens Fitting

The method of fitting soft contact lenses is dependent on the age of the child and the underlying diagnosis (Weissman & Donzis, 1989). Children over four or five years of age are fitted in the same manner as are adults—by refraction, keratometry, and slit lamp evaluation. A lens is then inserted, and after it has settled down, it is evaluated in the usual manner for position, movement, refractive correction, visual acuity, and comfort. Many manufacturers of soft lenses carry a lens series with a base curve that is steep enough, a diameter small enough, and a center thickness thick enough for children age four to five years of age and older who are either hyperopic or myopic. Custom design lenses in spheres and cylinders are available from several sources (see Appendix B). Aphakic lenses in steep enough base curves may be obtained in powers up to +20 D from several manufacturers (Moore, 1990).

Aphakic lenses for younger children can be much more difficult to obtain in the very steep base curves (7.0 to 7.9 mm) and higher plus powers (+20 to +40D) often required. Generally these must be custom ordered, but CoastVision maintains a large inventory in these parameters.

The basic office fitting technique for aphakic children begins with careful trial lens retinoscopy with particular attention to correct vertex distance and on-axis retinoscopy. A trial contact lens is then inserted in a 12.5 to 13 mm diameter and a 7.7 BC (range 7.5 to 7.9 mm BC) in a power as close as possible to that required, taking into account the very significant vertex distance adjustment. After a few minutes, an assessment of the position and movement of the lens is made. The lens should center well and show little lag on movement. It should be fit slightly tighter than is normal. Next retinoscopy should be performed, paying attention not only to the refractive error but also to the quality of the retinoscopic reflex. The appearance of the retinoscopic reflex is the most accurate method of determining the proper fit of the lens. A steeply fitting lens appears as a dark, fluctuating quality central retinoscopic reflex with momentary sharpening of the reflex immediately after the blink. A flat fitting lens appears as a less than sharp retinoscopic reflex, especially toward the periphery, and may look sharpest centrally just before the beginning of the blink. It may be difficult in some children to observe these reflexes as described above because of the child's behavior or the effects of the surgery itself.

The lens is changed until the fit consists of a well-centered lens with a minimal but finite amount of movement and a sharp retinoscopic reflex. The lenticular portion of a well-fitting soft lens may show some mild fluting of the edge of the lens. If this appears excessive, a different base curve or edge design is required to negate the possibility of the lens being kicked by the eyelids and dislodged from the eye. Ideally the power of the lens should be about +2.50 to +3.00 D above neutrality. If the lens fits reasonably well but is of insufficient power, dispense that lens and order the correct power lens. It is better to have a +20D lens on an eye needing a +35D than no lens at all. In addition, the parent and child can begin dealing with the issues of insertion and removal and wear of the lens immediately.

Rigid Gas-Permeable (RGP) Lenses

The technique of fitting gas permeable lenses to children four to five years of age and older is similar to that of adults. Refraction, slit lamp, and keratometry are performed to arrive at a starting point of the rigid lens fitting. Depending on the design and diameter of the lens used, a trial lens can be placed on the eye and evaluated for position, movement, power, and fluorescein pattern. The lens is changed as required, and a final set of lens parameters is determined. The lens is then ordered in the desired material and dispensed after the parents and child are instructed on proper lens care and handling.

In younger and less cooperative patients, keratometry may not be possible to provide a starting point for lens selection (Pratt-Johnson & Tillson, 1985; Saunders & Ellis, 1981). In these patients, simply insert a lens of known configuration, and by assessing position, movement, and fluorescein pattern, a determination is made on the relative fit of the lens. Other lenses can then be inserted that are closer to the desired lens fit. Careful refraction will then determine the final set of lens parameters to be ordered. The Boston Envision design may prove to be an ideal method of rigid lens fitting on young patients. The aspheric back surface design may be easier to fit and more "forgiving" of small irregularities in the geometric relationship to the cornea of young children than are standard designs of rigid lenses. If the child is overly apprehensive of the process of lens fitting or if initial placement of the lens is met with difficulty, a drop of topical anesthetic should be instilled.

Extended Wear or Daily Wear?

Extended wear need only be considered in instances of high refractive error when daily wear of the lens is thought to be too difficult for the parents and the child to manage successfully. There is much controversy over extended-wear contact lenses in all age groups, including infants and young children. Proponents of extended wear contend that it is easier for parents and children to manage than is daily wear and is relatively safe. Opponents argue that its safety is uncertain and it may actually be more difficult to manage over time.

The safety issue cannot be completely answered at this time because of insufficient longitudinal follow-up. The data for adults show that changes do occur in all layers of the cornea in response to extended wear for even short periods of time (Holden et al, 1985). The studies sponsored by the contact lens industry and the Harvard Medical School have clearly shown an increased risk of serious problems with extended wear (Schein et al, 1989; Poggio et al, 1989). This risk may be exacerbated in the thick parameters required for aphakic children in all but the silicone elastomer lenses. In addition, it is not known if constant wear of contact lenses over soft, young corneas may have some lasting effect on the development of the size and shape of the growing eye.

A more important issue to consider is the fact that it is easier to train the parent and condition the child to manage daily insertion and removal of lenses when the child is very young than when the child is older. Even if extended wear works well in the first few years, there is no guarantee that it will still be possible in the future. The child may be unable to continue to wear the original lens design and may require a switch to a lens that cannot be used for extended wear. For example, older children are sometimes unable to continue successful wear of Silsoft lenses that they readily wore when they were younger because of increasing discomfort. Since there are no other good extended-wear options, continued wear of any lens may become difficult or impossible.

It has been said that the major factor in the failure of treatment of aphakic infants is the failure of lens wear. The use of extended-wear lenses is supposed to make the continuation of contact lens wear easier. Experience shows that it is not the problems related to lens wear but rather problems related to patching for amblyopia over the long term that cause much of the failure in the treatment of pediatric cataracts.

If the parent doesn't have the skills to handle the lens easily when the child is older and more difficult to manage, the therapy is more likely to fail. It is preferable to teach parents as soon as possible to handle the lenses, reserving the option of extended wear for those patients with such a small and tight palpebral aperture that daily insertion and removal is simply impossible, or for those patients that fight so vigorously that even the fitter finds it impossible to manage. Even in these situations, extended wear should be considered as only a temporary measure.

Parental Instruction and Follow-Up Care

With regard to young patients, communication with the parents is probably the most critical part of the process of contact lens fitting. The parents must understand fully the goals and objectives of the proposed treatment and the potential benefits and risks of those treatments. The parents need to anticipate the likely day-to-day difficulties, the long duration of care and use of the lenses, and the expenses involved. They must also understand that through their efforts there is the likelihood that their child will be able to see. Their confidence must be enhanced as their expectations are made realistic. They must be taught the skills they will need in order to help in the treatment of their child.

The psychosocial implications of the underlying eye problem their child has must be fully explored. The parents, particularly the mother, may possess hidden guilt feelings about being the cause of their child's eye problem. The mother may believe that some transgression (alcohol, drugs both prescribed and illegal, ultrasound, and so forth) during pregnancy may have precipitated the child's problem. It is best to confront these issues as early as possible during the treatment process to preclude problems later. Warn the parents that by spending so much time and effort with this child, siblings may be affected in various ways. More distant relatives such as grandparents may also play an important role in the treatment and should be considered.

Parents are initially apprehensive about inserting and removing lenses from their child's eyes, but with proper instruction, much encouragement, and lots of patience, most do surprisingly well. Most parents find removal initially easier than insertion. Be certain that the parent is at least reasonably adept at lens removal before sending them home with the lens.

Many children are able to remove, and sometimes also to insert, the lenses themselves by five to six years of age. Encourage children to learn this technique as soon as possible, so that if a lens becomes uncomfortable while they are in school, they can simply remove it without becoming upset or injuring the eye. This allows the child some control over the situation, making parents, children, and schools more comfortable with the treatment.

Lens Care Systems

The basic goal of a lens care system is to keep the lenses clean and disinfected in the simplest and most effective manner possible. Simplicity and safety are key factors for young children. The goal is to minimize the possibility of system failure because the parent may not realize that a mistake or problem has occurred until there is pain, discomfort, or corneal insult to the child. An example might be the improper use of a two-step hydrogen peroxide disinfection system: the lens soaked in hydrogen peroxide and then inserted directly into an infant's eye without first being neutralized, causing corneal irritation. Because of this possibility, The CibaVision Aosept or B&L Renu systems for soft lenses and the Boston Disinfection system for rigid gas permeable lenses are preferred. The AoDisc is changed more frequently than is recommended (every 6 weeks instead of 12 weeks in most patients) to insure its optimal performance. These systems are easy to use, have minimal risk of improper use, and are very effective at cleaning and disinfecting the lenses. Parents are instructed in their proper use and are given simple, clearly written instruction sheets to follow at home. If there are any questions, parents are urged to read the instructions carefully or to telephone the practitioner for further explanation. They are told to use only those solutions they have been given and not to use substitutions unless they consult with the optometrist. There should be very few problems with these strict interpretations of the care systems. In addition, it is advisable to place a duplicate lens care kit with the school nurse in case the lens needs to be removed or cleaned in school.

A modified cleaning and disinfection system for the B&L Silsoft lens should prevent lipid buildup on the lenses. These lenses are particularly sensitive to lipid contamination, which adversely affects the wettability and comfort of the lenses. The parent's hands must be clean and free of any oils (particularly lanolin). Use CibaVision Miraflow cleaner because of the presence of isopropyl alcohol, which effectively cuts through lipid film on the lenses. After thoroughly rinsing the lenses in water or saline, have parents soak them in Boston Conditioning solution overnight to enhance their wettability.

Follow-Up Visits

Frequent follow-up visits are needed to insure that the lenses are performing well and the therapy is proceeding in the desired manner. This frequency is determined by the child's underlying diagnosis, the child's age, the parents' level of competency, how far away the family lives, and the rate of progress of the treatment.

Vision must be measured on each visit. The visual acuity of young children can be measured by visual evoked potentials or by the preferential looking procedure, or at least estimated by other behavioral test. The Teller Acuity Cards are preferred for use on the younger age groups. Older children can be tested by recognition acuity procedures such as Allen Cards, HOTV Cards, Illiterate E Cards, Broken Wheel Cards, or Snellen Letters. An assessment of monocular visual acuity is essential to evaluate the efficacy of amblyopia treatment. The measurement of visual acuity also provides valuable feedback for the parents. They can easily see the improvement in their child's vision from visit to visit when the patching is going well and drop offs in acuity when the patching is lax. The patching for amblyopia is initially with orthoptic eye patches and by occlusive soft contact lenses when patches are not tolerated.

The lens fit must be evaluated on each follow-up visit. Changes in the shape of the eye and the refractive error occur rapidly in infants, affecting the efficacy and fit of the lens. Lenses must be changed as required in order to maintain optimal fit and optical correction. This may need to be done a number of times in the first year. Ocular health must also be assessed on each visit. A hand-held slit lamp or loupes and penlight to inspect the anterior segment are very helpful.

The combination of contact lens wear and amblyopia therapy must be continued until the possibility of regression of acuity is past. This varies in individual patients from ages six to nine years of age. The amount of patching is usually decreased after age five to a level that allows for maintanance of the acuity level. Patching should be increased if acuity drops.

OLDER CHILDREN

In many ways, the fitting and use of contact lenses for older children (roughly defined as children over the age of five or six years) is much the same as it is for adults. These similarities include the types of conditions amenable to treatment, the configuration of the eye, the options in lens materials, and the techniques of fitting and follow-up. There are some important differences, however. The maturity level of the patient, the types of activities under which the lenses will be worn, and the psychological effects of lens wear are all different for children than they are for adults and must be considered carefully during the process of fitting and follow-up.

Mensuration

The human eye reaches adult size for most ocular parameters by three to four years of age. These parameters include corneal diameter, corneal vault, corneal curvature, and palpebral aperture and pupil size. Refractive error, particularly that of myopia, obviously continues to change throughout childhood. There is some tendency for the degree of hyperopia to decrease, except in the patients with accommodative esotropia where the hyperopia usually remains fairly stable. The changes in the magnitude and axis of astigmatism (except in the case of keratoconus) are usually minimal after five or six years of age.

Several other ocular characteristics may undergo change during childhood. The lacrimal apparatus produces more tears in childhood than it does in later life. Naturally occurring dry eye conditions are rare in children unless they are accompanied by ocular or systemic disease such as in Riley-Day syndrome. Dry eyes may be acquired, however, through various types of therapeutic regimens. For example, children that have been treated for neoplastic disease with radiation therapy to the head usually develop dry eyes and a specific form of corneal irritation, and children that are under treatment for allergies with systemic antihistamines also tend to have reduced tear output. Adolescents taking the medication Acutane for the treatment of acne may also have dry eye problems or experience lens intolerance. The composition of the nonaqueous portion of the tear film is different in children than it is in adults with less mucus and lipids in relation to the aqueous portion in children. Clinically, lenses tend to coat with protein and lipids far less frequently with children than with adults unless the patient has ocular or systemic allergies or certain systemic diseases such as cystic fibrosis, which results in abnormally thick lipid and mucous secretion.

Corneal sensitivity may also clinically appear to be reduced in children in comparison to adults, but this is more likely explained in terms of behavior than of physiology. Lid forces tend to be greater in children than they are in adults. This may affect the position and movement of lenses. Pupil size is often greater in children than it is in the elderly, possibly necessitating larger optic zones, especially in rigid lenses.

Conditions Amenable to Treatment
Refractive Error

The most common conditions in older children that will be treated with contact lenses are *normal* refractive errors, in comparison to the younger children who are usually aphakic.

Myopia Without question, the majority of older children interested in contact lenses will be myopic. These young myopic patients will request contacts in lieu of spectacles, but each patient should always have a backup pair of spectacles in a reasonably current prescription for use before and after lens insertion and in case lenses are lost, torn, or can't be worn because of eye infection or general illness. Contact lenses are an excellent mode of correction for myopic youngsters, providing improved physical appearance and flexibility in athletic participation. Recent studies have indicated that RGPs may exert some effect in limiting the rate of progression of myopia. This is discussed more fully in Chapter 17.

Astigmatism Most authorities believe that astigmatism reaches essentially adult levels by about three to four years of age after being very changeable in degree and axis at younger ages. Usually only significant levels of astigmatism (perhaps over 2.5D or so) should be corrected before age three to five years unless they are accompanied by high spherical refractive error, anisometropia, strabismus, or amblyopia that requires optical correction anyway. Contact lenses to correct astigmatism are not ordinarily the first method of correction to consider in early school-aged children but are quite suitable for teenagers because of cosmetic, visual, and social issues.

Mild to moderate degrees of astigmatism, especially when they are associated with spherical refractive error, may be corrected with a variety of readily available soft toric and RGP contact lenses. Moderate to high degrees of with-the-rule astigmatism may best be corrected with the Boston Envision rigid lens design. The specific choice will depend on individual considerations of the patient and the skill and philosophy of the practitioner. Equally good cases can be made for both rigid and soft lenses.

Hyperopia The thick spectacle lenses that are required in patients with significant degrees of hyperopia can be an impediment to their use by many adolescent patients. The nonuse of refractive correction may cause a host of both visual and functional problems for these patients. Contact lenses may be an acceptable alternative to spectacles. In addition to the obvious cosmetic improvement that contact lenses can provide to the hyperopic patient is the additional important advantage gained in young patients with both hyperopia and accommodative esotropia (Sampson, 1971), as previously discussed.

Anisometropia Contact lenses may prove very useful in patients with anisometropia. Unequal refractive error creates retinal images of unequal clarity. This may lead to suppression of the less clear image, the first step in the development of amblyopia. When this unequal refractive error is later optically corrected, aniseikonia, or unequal image size, is created at the retinal plane, further compromising the potential for fusion.

Knapp's Law states that there is no magnification effect in axial ametropes if they are corrected with spectacles and that there is no image size change in refractive ametropes if they are corrected with contact lenses. This has been the theoretical basis of the treatment of aniseikonia for some time. There is evidence, however, that this is not the entire story. Clinically it has been shown that contact lens correction of axial myopia results in both improved visual performance and optical correction than would be expected solely on the basis of Knapp's Law. Romano (1985) has suggested a mechanism for this finding that is based on stretching of the retinal elements in unilateral high myopes, which produces a relative micropsia and increased aniseikonia, and is best compensated for with contact lenses instead of spectacles. Further experimental evidence has been recently reported in birds to confirm Romano's earlier hypothesis. Moreover the reduction in vertical prismatic imbalance with contact lenses may be a greater contribution to fusion than is the theoretical impediment of aniseikoia in axial ametropias. The use of contact lenses in this situation probably has great efficacy for most patients, especially those with unilateral high myopia, and should be the treatment of choice.

Aniseikonic correction, using both contact lenses and spectacles, may prove very beneficial in patients having unilateral aphakia or high myopia, especially in the presence of diplopia caused by the induced aniseikonia. A regular or reverse Galilean telescope can help to equalize the images, sizes and promote fusion. A reverse Galilean telescope uses an overcorrection of a plus power (or less minus power) contact lens and a resultant overcorrection with minus-powered spectacle lenses to reduce the image size. A regular Galilean telescope incorporates the use of less plus or more minus in a contact lens and a resulting increase in plus power (or less minus) in the spectacle lens to give an increase in image size (Enoch, 1976; Enoch & Hamer, 1983).

Aphakia The contact lens treatment of acquired aphakia in older children is usually less difficult than it is in younger children because deprivation amblyopia is not a factor. There is invariably, however, some degree of refractive, anisometropic, or strabismic amblyopia that results from any childhood cataract in comparison to a patient with a typical senile cataract, where amblyopia does not develop.

Cataracts during childhood may be caused by developmental factors, ocular or systemic disease, or trauma. The underlying causes of the cataract must be investigated medically before treatment of the cataract and amblyopia is initiated. The surgical procedures to extract cataracts in older children are more similar to those employed in younger children than they are to those of adults and generally involve aspiration techniques. The period of healing of the surgical wound is very rapid, and fitting a contact lens can be scheduled within a week to a month after surgery. As was discussed in Chapter 7 in the section on cataracts in infants, arguments have been made to correct the aphakia by methods other than contact lenses such as IOLs and epikeratophakia. The reasons for not doing so are explained in the section on cataracts in infants. It is usually easier to fit a contact lens to older patients than it is to do so to infants, so there is little reason to consider other treatment alternatives.

These older aphakic children can best be fitted with daily wear lenses in either soft or RGP materials. The Silsoft silicone elastomer lens is not as good an option in these older children because of its significantly poorer comfort for them. This is due to its poor edge design and the hydrophobic surface characteristics that compromise comfort, especially after it has been worn for a few months, and is due in part to lipid buildup on the surface of the lens. Particularly in the case of corneal trauma resulting in an irregular corneal surface, rigid lenses may result in a better level of visual acuity and may reduce the threat of amblyopia below that for soft lenses.

Amblyopia must always be a prime consideration in any aphakic child, even in those over the age of ten, when many practitioners mistakenly assume that amblyopia cannot develop. Amblyopia can develop at this late age, and it is mandatory to watch closely for it in all young patients regardless of age. The treatment of this amblyopia can be by orthoptic eye patches or by occluder soft lenses, depending on the patient and the circumstances. It is also very important to consider the effects of aniseikonia in monocular aphakic patients as described in the section on anisometropia earlier in this chapter.

Cosmesis The issue of cosmesis is obviously more important in older children than it is in infants. A blind, disfigured eye can become a serious impediment to the normal socialization of the older child and may result in behavioral and psychological problems. Less severely affected eyes may also cause problems for the child. Contact lenses used for the purpose of masking disfigured eyes may have dramatic effects for these patients and should be aggressively considered as a treatment.

Until recently, these lenses have been both very expensive and difficult to obtain in optimal configurations and designs from the few suppliers willing to manufacture them. Wesley-Jessen recently modified their line of Durasoft Colors lenses to make it possible to use them for corneal masking. They are still relatively expensive but are now at least readily available and very reproducible. The normal eye can be fitted with a standard W-J Durasoft Colors lens to provide a near perfect match. It is also possible to take close-up photographs of both of the patient's eyes and send them to the two custom manufacturers (White and Narcissus) for color matching. Trial lenses should first be fitted to the eye to be certain of a stable fit and position. This may be difficult because many of these eyes will be the result of trauma or pythysis, and the fitting relationships seen in most normal patients may be impossible to achieve on these irregularly shaped eyes. Generally these cosmetic lenses should be fit tighter than normal to prevent anomalous position and movement or loss when worn. It is usually necessary to have the appearance or fit of the first lens ordered modified at least once before a satisfactory result is obtained. The patient's expectation of exact matching of appearance between the lens and the normal eye must be tempered somewhat as it is almost impossible to get an exact match. Many patients may be hypercritical of small differences in appearance that the practitioner finds acceptable. There is always a long delay in receiving these lenses after they are ordered. The three main sources of these custom lenses in North America are White Ophthalmic Company in Calgary, Canada; Wesley-Jessen in Chicago; and the Narcissus Foundation in Daly City, California (see Appendix B). There may be additional sources.

Another type of cosmetic lens that may be considered is a neutral density filter lens whose purpose is to block out a significant degree of light in patients with severe photophobia. Patients in this category include those with achromatopsia, albinism, aniridia, pupil abnormalities, and iris colobomas. There can be particular benefit in patients with achromatopsia. These lenses can be obtained in various configurations from White. Many patients with these underlying etiologies will have high refractive errors and nystagmus and may obtain a much improved optical effect from contact lenses as compared to spectacles since the optical center of the contacts remains in much better alignment with the pupillary axis than would be the case with spectacles. There may be substantial improvement in vision both objectively and subjectively with these tinted soft contact lenses.

Bandage Lenses   Various types of bandage lenses may be used on pediatric patients in the same manner as they are used for adults. They are most useful in patients with recurrent corneal erosions and certain rare types of corneal epithelial dystrophies. The lenses may also aid in the healing of the cornea from trauma. Recently collagen shields have been used to aid the healing process in a wide range of corneal problems in adults—with considerable success. There have not been any published reports on their specific use in the pediatric population, but they probably dissolve at a faster rate on the wetter eyes of children, and they may be more easily rubbed out of the eyes of children. This may affect their potential efficacy in children. Disposable extended-wear lenses may also be used as inexpensive bandage lenses.

Conditions under Which Lenses Are Worn

Adults and children do not necessarily use their contact lenses under the same conditions and in the same ways. This is due in small part to differences in ocular physiology and in larger part to differences in general behavior and interests. Lenses that will be used for children must meet the special needs of children.

There are little data concerning the oxygen requirements of the cornea in children, but the much faster rate of general metabolism in children suggests that pediatric corneas need more oxygen than adult corneas. Young children tend to nap. Any contact lens used on a child that naps must be permeable enough to be worn under occasional closed-eye conditions. It is obviously much less likely that this will be an issue for adolescents. However, it makes sense to use lenses that have as high a permeability to oxygen as possible on any child.

Children are usually more physically active than are most adults. They are also sometimes more *unthinking* in their behavior when the lenses are worn. Contact lenses need to be positionally more stable on the eye and less likely to decenter off the cornea or eye when worn by children than when adults wear them. This often requires a tighter fitting lens relationship, something that should be avoided generally in adults because of the possibility of inducing corneal hypoxia or worse. Lenses can be safely fitted in a somewhat tighter manner in children because they invariably have wetter eyes than adults do. This increased aqueous component of the tear film prevents further tightening of the lens, especially if the eyes become drier late in the day or under dry environmental conditions.

Pediatric lenses should be quite durable and easy to handle. Although this is a desirable attribute for any contact lens, adolescents require even sturdier lens than do adults, because of rougher handling and wear. Teens may wear their lenses more often than adults do when they are involved in sports. Larger diameter soft contact lenses may be indicated for these activities such as lenses from CoastVision and the SBH Sport Mate series. The lenses need to stay in place and resist popping out or decentering off the cornea under active conditions, making RGP lenses a less ideal option than soft lenses are for some active patients. Patients that swim a great deal may forget to remove lenses before going in the water. Even though lenses should not be worn under those conditions (especially in fresh water due to the risk of acanthamoeba infection), lenses with better adherence to the eye may be advisable when lenses must be worn in aphakes or high myopes with a preference for soft lenses over rigid lenses.

Extended Wear Versus Daily Wear

Patients and parents may ask about the option of extended-wear lenses. They may assume that they are easier to care for, somehow cause less trouble than daily-wear lenses because of less handling or that they are even safer because of greater oxygen permeability. Practitioners are very aware, however, of the increased risk of extended-wear lenses and generally do not recommend them to most young patients. Extended-wear lenses should be used for young people only under unusual circumstances.

There are a number of reasons for this reluctance to fit extended wear in children. Adolescents are constantly testing the limits of adult authority. The doctor's recommendation to wear extended-wear lenses for a week or less invites the young-ster's attempts to wear it longer than was recommended. Youngsters' negligence in personal hygiene, that is, keeping hands and face clean, increases the risk of infection. There is also an increased legal threat. If a child develops a corneal ulcer resulting in decreased vision as a result of extended wear of contact lenses, the practitioner will find it very difficult to defend against malpractice. Courts are much more likely to find against the doctor than against a child, even when the patient's negligence is a contributing factor.

There is very little good that can be said for the use of extended-wear lenses in young people, except in the possible case of aphakia, but even in this instance, the disadvantages outweigh the advantages. It is best for children to develop the proper habits of caring for their lenses on a daily basis, and assume full responsibility for their lenses. Extended wear allows the child to avoid this responsibility on a routine, daily basis. Therefore it is best to avoid the issue completely and limit the use of extended-wear lenses to unusual cases of aphakia or very high refractive errors. Cosmetic extended wear in children under the age of 10 or 12 years is generally unacceptable.

This having been said, exceptions can be made from time to time. Patients that have proven themselves with daily wear may be able to make a case for extended wear at some point, for example, when they go off to college. They may find that their wearing time may prove excessive with daily-wear lenses when they are studying late into the night and that they prefer at least the option of extended wear. Use disposable lenses in this situation if the lenses fit properly and adequate follow-up can be guaranteed. If standard extended-wear lenses are chosen, frequent replacement should be strongly considered. Patients must continue to prove satisfactory wearing and care habits, or extended wear should be curtailed in the interest of safety.

Psychology of Lens Wear in Adolescents

There are certain psychological benefits to the use of contact lenses over spectacles in adolescents. Even though spectacle use in children is not considered unusual or *nerdy* as it was 20 or 30 years ago and though there are many very fashionable eyeglass frames available, it may still be thought of in negative terms by the child. There may be some degree of social stigma attached to the use of glasses. Children may be subjected to verbal or nonverbal harassment in school that in some cases may reach serious levels, affecting the child's self image and well-being. There are undoubtedly major differences in these perceptions between boys and girls. Some children may simply not wear their glasses when they are around their peers, removing them as soon as they are no longer around their parents, and therefore becoming visually compromised. Switching to contact lenses may have surprisingly great effect on their self-image and behavior.

Contact lenses may be a necessity for individuals involved in sports or the performing arts. Spectacles may be inappropriate in a child who is acting, dancing, or wearing a football or hockey helmet. The alternative for some of these patients is simply to not wear their spectacles. This may make it difficult or impossible to perform as required.

Fitting Technique

The technique of fitting contact lenses to children older than 5 or 6 years of age need be little different than that used with adults. Some authorities do feel, however, that special attention and procedures ought to be applied to these young contact lens wearers (Ryan, 1990). These practitioners prefer to familiarize the child to the exam room and exam procedures in a separate appointment before the actual fitting of the lenses. This may cause more anxiety for the patient than simply proceeding with the fitting on the first visit without giving the child time to fret over thoughts of pain and discomfort. All procedures should be thoroughly explained to the patient as the fitting progresses, but this is not really different than it should be with any other patient.

Prior to the actual fitting of the contact lenses, each patient should have a thorough examination, including history, ocular motility and binocularity, external and internal ocular health evaluation, refraction, and a careful case analysis. Once it has been determined that contact lenses may be a suitable treatment modality, the parents and the child should decide along with the practitioner to proceed with the fitting. This may be performed on the same day as the initial examination, or it may be deferred to a later time. Additional tests beyond the standard examination should include keratometry and evaluation of the tear film and blink pattern.

The child's level of maturity and responsibility must be carefully evaluated. This is probably the single most important part of the prefitting assessment. Parents will often ask how old a child must be before contact lenses should be prescribed. This is actually a moot point. Of much greater importance is the child's ability to take full responsibility for every aspect of lens wear and the motivation for lens wear. This may be somewhat difficult to assess on only a single visit, but any suggestion that the child is not yet ready to assume the appropriate level of responsibility should preclude fitting at this time. It is far better to err on the side of caution than to fit a child before that child is mature enough. The parents and the child must also understand that any evidence of lack of responsibility at any time during or after the fitting is grounds for immediate discontinuation of lens wear. This should not merely be an idle threat. In fact, it should probably be the case for patients of any age, including adults.

Once the evaluation is complete, a suitable lens should be inserted onto the child's eye. It may prove useful to instill a drop of topical ophthalmic anesthetic onto the eye prior to actual lens insertion in order to make the very first experience at lens wear a comfortable one. Some patients may be so nervous at the thought of a lens on the eye that even minimal lens sensation on insertion may color their perception of wear and make adaptation much more difficult. The anesthetic will allow the first experience to be comfortable, and the gradual normalization of lens sensation will make the patient more adaptable to wearing contacts. The anesthetic is especially useful when RGP lenses are to be used. The idea of using an anesthetic may be unacceptable to many practitioners, and its use is certainly optional. Speed in lens insertion is important. It is best to not give the child the chance to procrastinate before the actual insertion of the lens.

Once the lens has settled down on the child's eyes, the position, movement, and fit of the lens should be evaluated much as it is with older patients. The lens design should be changed if the fit does not appear optimal, but as has been explained, the fit can be a little tighter (especially with soft lenses) than would be customary for adults. The final step in the fitting process is to determine the proper refractive correction.

The patient must then be fully trained in insertion and removal and lens care. Some older children, who have narrow palpebral apertures and squeeze their lids apprehensively, may do well with a smaller diameter lens such as the Allergan Hydron Mini-Lens. The practitioner must be certain that the patient is capable of handling and caring for the lenses. Any suggestion that the child is not ready to have the lenses dispensed at this time should necessitate another visit with further instruction before dispensing. Having the parent present during the initial instruction on handling the lenses may make some children apprehensive. It may be advisable to bring the parent in for a demonstration of the proper procedures only after the child has mastered the techniques. Our guidelines for selecting lens disinfection systems are the same as those applied to younger children. It is highly recommended that the patient be given clear written instructions on insertion and removal of the lenses and on the lens care system. The patient should have an appointment scheduled for follow-up visits, and finally the patient should have a telephone number to call if problems of any type occur or if the patient is unclear about any instructions.

Follow-Up Care

The follow-up care of children wearing contact lenses is, like the process of lens fitting, quite similar to that of adults. A follow-up appointment should be made for the patient one or two weeks after the lenses are dispensed. The patient should then be closely questioned about the handling and care being given to the lenses, and any questions or problems that have arisen should be resolved. It is probably a good idea to corroborate the child's responses with the parents' perceptions and observations. If there are discrepancies, further investigation should follow, and the patient must be made to understand what is expected.

The follow-up examination should include an assessment of visual acuity, corneal health, refraction, binocularity, and lens fit. Evaluation of the movement, the position, the appearance, and the cleanliness of the lenses is essential. Fluorescein staining, particularly in the case of RGP lenses, is advised.

If the prescription or the fit of the lens needs modification, the lenses should be changed at this time. Patients having handling problems with thin, floppy soft lenses may require a switch to a thicker soft lens with better handling characteristics or even to a rigid lens if further instruction does not alleviate the handling problems. Patients experiencing repeated lens ejection may benefit by a tighter (steeper) lens of the same type or by a different design completely. Patients with hyperopia and accommodative esotropia may require a stronger prescription than was initially thought. This is especially true if there is residual esotropia at near or if the hyperopic correction causes a further relaxing of the level of accommodation and additional residual hyperopia is present. Patients with moderate to high degrees of myopia who initially may have complained of asthenopia at near should by now have adapted to their new accommodative and convergence demands, but if they are still having complaints, the prescription may need modification. At least one or two additional follow-up exams should be scheduled over the next month or two to confirm the success of lens wear and patient compliance, and procedures or the fit should be modified as required.

Problems

Although most young patients that are fitted with contact lenses will have a very good experience with them, there will invariably be problems. These problems will range from the trivial to the serious, potentially even resulting in loss of vision. The best way to avoid problems is to educate patients and to provide comprehensive follow-up care. Even in the best of circumstances, however, unintended sequelae are to be expected and should be prepared for in advance. During the process of fitting the contact lenses to the child, the optometrist must be certain to warn patients and parents of the potential for lens-related problems. This is important for professional, ethical, and legal reasons. Failure to give these warnings adequately may constitute malpractice.

Many of the problems that will be faced during follow-up examinations are related to a lack of understanding of the correct procedures on the part of the patient and parents. Included in this category are problems related to handling and proper care of the lenses. This is undoubtedly the largest group of problems that will be faced. Usually clear explanations to the patient, along with written instructions and possibly audiovisual aids, will minimize the potential for these problems. Sometimes the problem is related to lenses that are either not performing as anticipated or are simply fitting badly. A change in lens design will usually solve this sort of problem.

Of greater concern are lenses that have produced a physiologic or pathologic response on the eyes that requires treatment and may result in permanent sequelae. This may range from corneal hypoxia to severe ocular inflammation or infection. The first step in remediation is correct diagnosis of the underlying problem, which may not be easy. If the problem is severe enough and the diagnosis is unclear, the patient should be referred to a corneal specialist. In any event, lens wear should not be attempted again until the problem is completely resolved. These patients must then be followed even closer than is usual, until it is certain that the lenses and the eye are performing correctly.

Corneal ulceration is the most severe form of contact lens-related problem. Any treatment must be preceded by complete culturing of the cornea, including aerobic and anaerobic culture media and gram staining. Initial treatment should be appropriate to the clinical appearance and should be modified when culture and gram stain reports are available or if the initial treatment appears ineffective. Usually the first choice antibiotics are gentamycin or tobramycin drops at least every other hour and ointments instilled frequently overnight. A highly effective gram positive agent such as bacitracin ointment should be included if it is indicated by the results of lab tests or if clinically it appears that staph or strep is a likely cause. Steroids should not be used initially, particularly if there is any possibility of herpes simplex keratitis infection. Patients must be seen again the following day, or under certain circumstances, the patients may even require hospitalization to make certain that the medications are used correctly and the infection is resolving. It may make more sense to refer these patients immediately either to a corneal specialist or a pediatric ophthalmologist.

Various other problems may also be encountered on follow-up. Sensitivities to various components of the cleaning and disinfecting systems seem to occur less frequently now than was the case in the past, but may occasionally still be seen. Patients will report conjunctival injection, a foreign body sensation, and an increasing level of contact lens intolerance. Treatment consists of discontinuing lens wear until the inflammation has abated and switching to a different set of solutions. A new pair of lenses may also be helpful. Giant papillary conjunctivitis (GPC) can occur even in young contact lens wearers. GPC should be treated initially with discontinuation of lens wear and the use of cromolyn sodium eyedrops until the papillae reduce in size and the eye becomes quiescent. Lens wear can then be attempted with new lenses. A switch to either RGP lenses or disposable daily-wear lenses may prove very helpful although these patients will always have a predilection for recurrence of the GPC.

There are also lens-induced problems that may occur. Patients may either develop an abrasion from rough handling or wear or a recurrent corneal erosion that more likely is caused by a non-contact lens-related cause that is misdiagnosed as lens-related. The most common problem of all will be repeated lens loss or tearing. Parents will complain loudest over this problem. A change to a different lens design may alleviate the problem, and patients should be reinstructed on the proper techniques of lens handling. Lenses may also develop deposits that affect vision or comfort. Again, a change in lens design or solutions, along with a review of procedures, may solve this problem. Rigid lenses may be the best solution of all, however. The patient's behavior may be the cause of any of these lens-related problems. It is possible that the patient is simply not taking adequate responsibility for the lenses, resulting in many of the problems that have just been discussed. The optometrist should make every attempt to determine if this might be the ultimate cause of the patient's problems.

REFERENCES

Allen ED, Davies PD. Role of contact lenses in the management of congenital nystagmus. Br J Ophthalmol 1983;67:834–836.

Beller R, Hoyt CS, Marg E, et al. Good visual function after neonatal surgery for congenital monocular cataracts. Am J Ophthalmol 1981;91:559–565.

Chase WW, Fronk SJ, Micheals BA. A theoretical infant schematic eye. Paper presented at annual meeting of American Academy of Optometry, St Louis, 1984.

Cutler SI, Nelson LB, Calhoun JH. Extended wear contact lenses in pediatric aphakia. J Pediatr Ophthalmol Strab 1985;22:86–91.

Enoch JM. Fitting parameters which need to be considered when designing soft contact lenses for the neonate. Contact Intraocul Lens Med J 1979a;5:31–37.

Enoch JM. Techniques for evaluating scleral curvature and corneal vault. Contact Lens J 1979b;8:19–31.

Enoch JM. Use of inverted telescopic corrections incorporating soft contact lens in the (partial) correction of aniseikonia in cases of unilateral aphakia. Advanc Ophthal 1976;32:54–66.

Enoch JM. The fitting of hydrophilic (soft) contact lenses to infants and young children. I. Mensuration data on aphakic eyes of children born with congenital cataracts. Contact Lens Med Bull 1972a;5:36–40.

Enoch JM. The fitting of hydrophilic (soft) contact lenses to infants and young children. II. Fitting techniques and initial results on aphakic children. Contact Lens Med Bull 1972b;5:41–47.

Enoch JM, Hamer RD. Image size correction of the unilateral aphakic infant. Ophthalmic Ped Genetics 1983;2:153–165.

Fulton AB, Dobson V, Salem D, et al. Cycloplegic refractions in infants and young children. Am J Ophthalmol 1980;90:239–47.

Halberg GP. Contact lenses for infants and children. In Harley RD, ed. Pediatric ophthalmology. Philadelphia: Saunders, 1983;1280–1288.

Holden BA, Sweeney DF, Vannas A, et al. Effects of long-term extended contact lens wear on the human cornea. Invest Ophthalmol Vis Sci 1985;26:1489–1501.

Karr DJ, Scott WE. Visual acuity results following treatment of persistent hyperplastic primary vitreous. Arch Ophthalmol 1986;104:662–667.

Mayer DL, Moore BD, Robb RM. Assessment of vision and amblyopia by preferential looking tests after early surgery for unilateral congenital cataracts. J Pediatr Ophthalmol Strab 1989;26:61–68.

Mohindra I, Held R, Gwiazda J, et al. Astigmatism in infants. Science 1978;202:329–331.

Moore BD. Contact lens therapy for amblyopia. In Rutstein R, ed. Problems in optometry; amblyopia, vol 3. Philadelphia: Lippincott, 1991;355–368.

Moore BD. Contact lens problems and management in infants, toddlers, and preschool children. In Scheiman M, ed. Problems in optometry; pediatric optometry, vol 2. Philadelphia: Lippincott 1990;365–393.

Moore BD. Changes in aphakic refraction of children with unilateral congenital cataracts. J Pediatr Ophthalmol Strab 1989;26:290–295.

Moore BD. Mensuration data in infant eyes with unilateral congenital cataracts. Am J Optom & Physiol Optics 1987;64:204–210.

Moore BD. The fitting of contact lenses in aphakic infants. J Am Optom Assoc 1985;56:180–183.

Moore BD, Smith L. Occluder soft contact lenses in the treatment of amblyopia in young children. Paper presented at the annual meeting of the American Academy of Optometry, St. Louis, 1984.

Poggio EC, Glynn RJ, Schein OD, et al. The incidence of ulcerative keratitis among users of daily-wear and extended-wear soft contact lenses. N Engl J Med 1989;321:779–783.

Pratt-Johnson JA, Tillson G. Hard contact lenses in the management of congenital cataracts. J Pediatr Ophthalmol Strab 1985;22:94–96.

Robb RM, Mayer DL, Moore BD. Results of early treatment of unilateral congenital cataracts. J Pediatr Ophthalmol Strab 1987;24:178–181.

Romano PE. An exception to Knapp's Law: Unilateral axial high myopia. 1985;1:166–170.

Ryan JB. Fitting younger patients. Contact Lens Forum, August 1990; pp 19–21.

Sampson WG. Correction of refractive errors: effect on accommodation and convergence. Trans Am Acad Ophth and Otol 1971;75:124–132.

Saunders RA, Ellis FD. Empirical fitting of hard contact lenses in infants and young children. Ophthalmology 1981;88:127–130.

Schein OD, Glynn RJ, Poggio EC, et al. The relative risk of ulcerative keratitis among users of daily-wear and extended-wear soft contact lenses. N Engl J Med 1989;321:773–778.

Weissman BA, Donzis PB. Contact lens application after infantile cataract surgery. In Isenberg SJ, ed. The eye in infancy. Chicago: Year Book Medical Publishers, 1989;320–326.

12

Prescribing and Fitting of Children's Eyewear

Leonard J. Press

There are numerous factors to consider in prescribing eyewear for children. Among these are the power and form of lens prescribed, the type of frame selected, and the monitoring of their proper usage. These factors vary considerably dependent on the age, individual needs, maturity, and personality of the child as well as on the disposition and prior experiences of the parent.

INDICATIONS FOR PRESCRIBING EYEWEAR

Many parents question the need for a child's first prescriptive lenses. When optometrists first present the case summary, the response is often: "Do you really think it's necessary?" Parents have four major expressed or unspoken concerns:

1. They believe that wearing glasses will accelerate a deterioration in the child's vision.
2. They are not confident that the child will accept wearing glasses.
3. They dislike the idea of hiding their child's beautiful eyes behind a pair of glasses.
4. They have financial constraints.

The balance of this section will address conditions for which the optometrist should prescribe aggressively and circumstances in which prescribing should be tempered.

Refractive Amblyopia

The most important element in treating refractive amblyopia, particularly in young children, is to prescribe the full prescription (Rx). This should be done expeditiously, and the prescription should be worn as much as possible. In bilateral refractive amblyopia secondary to high isometropic refractive error, spectacles are optically adequate. If there is anisometropia in excess of three diopters, contact lenses should be encouraged irrespective of the axial or refractive nature of the ametropia. From a clinical standpoint, the induced prismatic imbalance from spectacle lenses is a greater impediment to binocularity than are theoretical considerations of aniseiko-nia. If contact lenses are not feasible or cannot be tolerated, spectacle correction is prescribed in the interim. With aggressive use of the prescription at a young age, maximum acuity can be obtained in the amblyopic eye; the less the glasses are worn, the less likely that maximum acuity will be obtained. The child can be told: "The more you wear your glasses now, the less you'll need to wear them when you are older." This is true because, once a child has passed age nine and has attained maximum acuity in the amblyopic eye, there is little concern that acuity will drop in the amblyopic eye if the Rx is not worn consistently.

There are different amblyogenic parameters in hyperopic, myopic, and astig-matic anisometropia that need to be considered when tempering the prescription. These factors are discussed in the respective sections on hyperopia, myopia, and astigmatism.

Accommodative Esotropia

With young children, the same concern exists for full-time use of the prescrip-tion as in refractive amblyopia. In this instance, prescribing eyewear is imperative to maximize use of the two eyes together at a time when the development of this capability is at a sensitive stage. There are two primary manifestations of accommo-dative esotropia. In cases of high bilateral isometropic hyperopia, the deviation is usually not present unless the eyewear is removed. Parents should be reassured that this is normal. The greater the AC/A ratio, the more this discrepancy will be apparent. When the ametropia is high, the demand on accommodative convergence is less with contact lenses as was discussed in Chapter 11.

The other manifestation of accommodative esotropia occurs when there is low ametropia but a noticeably greater deviation at near than at distance. In this instance, a bifocal is imperative. The power of the bifocal add can be arbitrarily selected at +2.50. The effect of the add in reducing the near angle should be documented for future comparison. Even if the add does not initially reduce the near angle, it should be given on a trial basis. Since children have a short Harmon distance, one need not be concerned about overplussing the add. The examiner should be careful to differentiate accommodative esotropia from V pattern esotropia. I have seen numerous cases where the patient was diagnosed as accommodative esotropia when there was no accommodative component. Rather the child exhibited more esotropia at near because the distance cover test was performed in primary gaze and the near cover test was performed in a more downward position with the child pumped up in the chair. The near angle should therefore be assessed in primary gaze as well as in downgaze.

Parents must be educated as to the difference between wearing lenses for clear vision and wearing lenses to minimize the eye turn. Parents should be encouraged, if they know that wearing glasses, particularly bifocals, is not necessarily a lifelong endeavor for the child. The same strategy for aggressive wearing of the glasses can be applied as was stated for refractive amblyopia.

Hyperopia

We know from refractive trends that hyperopia is normal and even desirable in early childhood. There seems little justification for prescribing lenses under + 2.00 for isometropic infants or preschoolers with normal binocular function (Ciner, 1990). For the school-aged child, particularly when there is esophoric shift, accommodative hysteresis, or complaint of asthenopia, compensation of low-grade hyperopia is indicated. Some children experience initial discomfort with moderate plus lens prescriptions but adapt within several days. One way of gaining more immediate acceptance is by instilling one percent cyclopentolate when dispensing of the eyewear (Silbert & Alexander, 1987). When binocularity is normal and the child is asymptomatic, there is little virtue in pushing the full Rx. General guidelines for plus lens correction in latent hyperopia are given in Table 5.1.

In instances of anisometropic hyperopia, prescribing is directed toward minimizing refractive amblyopia rather than "pushing the plus" on both eyes. Refractive amblyopia is likely to ensue when the anisometropia is greater than one diopter. If the child has been previously uncorrected, the probability is that the child will not tolerate a good portion of the full correction. Consider the following example:

Retinoscopy:	OD: + 2.00 (20/50)	OS: + 3.25 (20/60)
Subjective:	OD: Plano (20/20)	OS: + 1.50 (20/30)
Initial Rx:	OD: + 0.50	OS: + 1.75

Certain performance measures can be used to temper the prescription such as its effect on stereopsis and the lag of accommodation. Do not prescribe a bifocal in the initial Rx, as the carrier Rx itself requires an adaptation. Independent of all clinical wisdom, convention, and findings, there is no substitute for placing the lenses in a trial frame and asking the patient how things look and feel, especially if the child is sufficiently cognitive and sensitive.

Myopia

Conventional wisdom suggests that children with progressive myopia should be undercompensated by 0.50 to 0.75D (Grosvenor, 1991) although this is not universally accepted (Carter, 1967). When the case history reveals that the child is presenting due to failure of a school vision screening, it is usually impractical to underprescribe to the extent that the child would still fail the screening if immediately retested. We therefore adhere to the conventional wisdom and underprescribe only to the extent that the child can at least read the 20/40 Snellen line at distance. Some parents, themselves myopic, wonder whether prescribing the glasses will make the child's vision deteriorate more rapidly. Considerations in myopic progression are discussed in Chapter 17. In considering the final power of the prescription, the practitioner must take into account the child's previous Rx and age, the ability to manage undercorrection through preferential seating in the classroom, and the potential for myopia containment therapy.

As contrasted with hyperopic anisometropia, myopic anisometropia is usually not amblyogenic until it exceeds four diopters. This is because the natural monovision process insures that the child will have had adequate stimulation of the more myopic eye. Indeed, the more myopic eye is the preferred eye at short viewing distances. For this reason one should be conservative with the initial Rx and underprescribe for the more myopic eye. Keeping the myopic anisometropia to a minimum will also aid fusion. If refractive amblyopia is already exhibited, the Rx for the amblyopic eye should be full power with aggressive therapy as will be discussed in Chapter 16.

Astigmatism

Refractive trends in children under the age of three years show that astigmatism is labile (Atkinson et al 1980). Astigmatic refraction less than two diopters, therefore, need not be compensated. Indeed, unnecessary or premature prescribing of lenses may interfere with the emmetropization process. Higher powers should be prescribed to the extent that leaving a blurred image might be amblyogenic. As suggested by Ciner (1990), oblique cylinder greater than 1.25D persisting beyond age two should be prescribed and closely monitored. Children have more plasticity and do not generally experience the spatial distortion or asthenopia common to adults who are prescribed higher cylindrical powers.

Isometropic and lesser amounts of cylinder usually warrant straightforward prescribing when they are accompanied by visual complaints. There is a school of thought in behavioral optometry to underprescribe for low or moderate amounts of against-the-rule cylinder with school-aged children because it is likely to be stress-induced (Birnbaum, 1978). A general guide is the extent that the cylinder in the subjective matches with Javal's rule. If keratometry shows spherical Ks, -0.50 against-the-rule cylinder is expected, and it should be prescribed accordingly. If K readings are with-the-rule, withhold the against-the-rule cylinder.

Plus Lenses for Nearpoint

The optimal plus lens for nearpoint is determined by the clinical profile of plus lens acceptance. This includes a higher NRA (negative relative accommodation) than PRA (positive relative accommodation), a high lag of accommodation, improved performance measures, a maintained Harmon distance (distance from first mid-knuckle to elbow) through the tentative add, and subjective acceptance of the trial-framed lenses. OEP (Optometric Extension Program) analysis includes formulations for determining when to prescribe or cut plus lens additions at near (Apell & Streff, 1962). When they are indiscriminately applied, nearpoint adds can do more harm than good (Press, 1985). When applied judiciously, they exert effects far beyond their magnifying and AC/A properties (Press, 1991).

The use of added convex power at nearpoint has widespread application for children. Such prescriptions can be classified as: developmental, preventive, training, remedial, and compensatory (Apell & Streff, 1961). Applications of bifocals to myopia, latent hyperopia, and esodeviations are discussed in their respective sections earlier in this chapter. Bifocals for children who do not as yet have acuity or binocular problems are best termed *learning lenses* (Apell, 1976).

Prismatic Lenses

Base-in or base-out prism for compensating nonstrabismic binocular anomalies in children can be applied sparingly with the proper differential diagnosis. This includes the use of prism adaptation testing and consideration of the prospects for successful vision therapy. If prism is prescribed as an alternative to vision therapy because of time or financial constraints, it is important to project the anticipated course of progression. A child with convergence insufficiency who is given base-in prism may have increasing symptoms of diplopia or loss of place with need for progressive increases in prism power. There have been cases where patients were caught up in this spiral during their teenage years, ultimately arriving at the need for occlusion to maintain single vision.

Yoked prism can be used for active or passive vision therapy (Press, 1989). Small amounts of prism, typically under five prism diopters yoked bases up or down, have been used prescriptively to influence refractive status. Introverted children can be observed to look up and outward based on prescriptive amounts of yoked bases down prism. Larger amounts of prism, typically greater than ten prism diopters yoked bases up, down, left, or right, have been used disruptively to reorient visual-spatial judgement.

Placebo Lenses

There is as much a place for placebo lenses in optometry as there is for placebo medication in medicine (Skjerdal, 1987). It is the optical analog of artificial tears for phantom eye irritation. In the case of a child, the placebo may be as much for the parent as for the patient. As was discussed in Chapter 10, low-power plus lenses can be used for juvenile hysterical amblyopia.

When Not to Prescribe

There are instances when it is not advisable to prescribe lenses, even if they are ostensibly indicated. High on this list is the child who is resistant to wearing glasses. Excuse the parent from the examination room and ask the child: "Just between you and me, if I give you glasses that would make it easier for you to see, would you like that?" If the answer is an emphatic no, this is a time to be holistic. The negative psychological impact of glasses on a child can outweigh the salient visual benefits. Particularly with myopia, the child can be accommodated by preferential seating in the classroom. As was mentioned earlier, however, be more aggressive in bribing the child to wear the Rx in cases of refractive amblyopia and accommodative esotropia.

OPHTHALMIC LENS OPTIONS
Crown Glass Lenses

Lenses made of crown glass have no place in children's eyewear. At one time such lenses were prescribed with the thought that children scratch CR-39 (plastic) lenses so readily as to make them impractical. Current thought is that it is too dangerous to prescribe glass because of the possibility that the lenses can shatter.

CR-39 (Plastic) Lenses

CR-39 is the material most often prescribed for children. It is unlikely to shatter or splinter on impact. It is lightweight, which helps keep the lenses from sliding downward on small and active children. Its drawback is its propensity toward scratching, particularly through the carelessness with which most children handle their eyewear. For this reason, scratch-resistant coatings are imperative (Dowaliby & Dowaliby, 1981).

Although children scratch their lenses readily, the need for replacement is usually more the parent's concern about appearance than actual disturbance of the optical quality. The exception to this is the dense scratches that occur in the center of the lenses when children have repeatedly placed their eyewear on a table surface with the front surface downward.

Scratch-Resistant Coating

High quality, multilayer coating should be standard on all children's lenses. The explanation to parents is: "We're prescribing plastic lenses for Adam because they won't shatter like glass. Of course, they'll have a scratch-resistant coating applied. This doesn't mean they can't scratch, but if we didn't have it applied, it would wind up looking like you cleaned them with steel wool."

Coatings supplied by the manufacturer in the lens blank are more effective than are those applied locally. One example is Silor's Super Shield, which has an effective patient education pamphlet. In addition, parents are assuaged by products that have "The Good Housekeeping Seal of Approval" and replacement guarantees.

Polycarbonate Lenses

Polycarbonate or similar high index material offers maximum resistance to breakage. It is considerably more expensive and scratches more readily than does plastic. Traditionally these lenses have been reserved for situations in which eye protection is of particular concern such as in contact sports or when vision is poor in one eye (Dowaliby, 1988b). We appear now to be moving in the direction of recommending polycarbonate lenses for all children. Should this be adopted as the standard in the field, documenting the recommendation of polycarbonate lenses to the parent will have medicolegal implications.

Multifocal Lenses

When children under the age of 12 are prescribed lenses, a Kryptok is a suitable choice. Most frames with eye sizes under 50 will afford adequate seg height for a Kryptok and provide the child with a "near invisible" bifocal. Seamless or blended bifocals can be used with older children. Progressive lenses have been used successfully with children, who adapt more readily to peripheral distortion than adults do (Cho & Wild, 1990). In view of the cost differential, I would have difficulty encouraging the child of needy parents to obtain a progressive if a Kryptok can suffice. Conversely if the child needs to use a computer for extended periods of time, a progressive would be the lens of choice to allow incremental plus lens application for all distances.

The practice of prescribing executive bifocals with the seg height splitting the pupil is overkill in most instances, based more on theoretical considerations than on practical experience. When a Kryptok is inadequate or a progressive is prohibitive, use a flat-top 35 over an executive because of its lighter weight and improved appearance. The functional reading area is more than adequate.

Ultraviolet (UV) Protection

There has been a concerted effort in the ophthalmic industry to educate the public about the potential hazards of UV radiation. Paradoxically, parents have traditionally discouraged children from wearing sunlenses or tints because of a concern that they would become dependent on them. From evidence to date (Tucker et al, 1985), it would appear that optometrists should counsel the parents about the potential benefits of UV protective lenses for their children to at least the same extent that they would do so for the parents. There is currently a company that produces sunwear exclusively for infants and young children (see Appendix A).

Tinted Lenses

If a child is enthusiastic about a tint for cosmetic purposes or is light sensitive, select a light gradient tint. This can reduce overhead glare yet provide comfortable amounts of light for near work. As photochromic lenses become more widely available in CR-39, they will be a popular option for children.

Antireflective Coating

There is little justification for antireflective coating because children smudge them so readily, even with the newer hydrophobic coatings. There have been instances where parents were concerned about the cosmesis of higher powered lenses and agreed to accept the positive attributes of the antireflective coating along with its drawbacks. In special instances such as modeling, the child can have a pair of antireflective coated lenses for photographic purposes.

OPHTHALMIC FRAME OPTIONS

Parents and children rarely share the same opinion about frames. To illustrate this point, consider the mother who became entrepreneurial with the process of frames. After having visited her local optician to select eyewear for her two daughters, she decided that frames were not designed with children's tastes in mind. She held a contest at a local school to have children design their own eyewear. After compiling their drawings, she collaborated with a manufacturer to develop her own line of eyewear. The eyewear was cute with wild colors and interesting shapes. The children who came into our optical area were attracted to them. There was only one problem: the parent would say, "I'll be darned if I'm going to let her walk around in those."

There are frames available that strike a compromise between the novel features that appeal to children and the subtlety desired by parents. As examples, Marcolin model 7019 has a small butterfly with a diamond on the top of the eyewire, and Lux de Paris Tann's model 808 has small novelty eyes that wiggle in the upper corners.

Some infants and preschoolers will not tolerate anything on their faces, and balk at the process of frame selection. This becomes a time of reason and compromise. Parents should be reminded that it is the child who must wear the glasses. For children who are mature enough to have strong self-images, decisions such as color should be made with their input (Dowaliby, 1988).

Metal Frames

Metal frames are attractive choices for young children because they provide flexibility in adjustment at the bridge of the nose. In addition, they are thinner and less conspicuous than most zyl frames. They are contraindicated for contact sports since they bend easily. A new titanium alloy used by Marchon in its Autoflex and Accuflex frames is a welcome addition because they provide ultimate flexibility in material.

Nonmetal Frames

Zyl or carbon frames are preferred by most parents because they perceive them to be sturdier and safer than metal frames. Some zyl frames are available with adjustable nosepads, making them a good compromise choice. One example is the Starwalker (Martin-Copeland) available in eye sizes from 40 through 49.

Spring Hinges

Spring hinges are strongly recommended for all children's frames. They not only offer greater resistance to breakage, but they also provide a margin of flexibility for growth.

Design Features for Infants and Preschoolers

Infants and preschoolers have flat bridges. To minimize slippage, infants require frames with a low bridge and riding bow comfort cables (Drew, 1989). Frames meeting these two criteria are listed in Table 12.1. Straps that secure the frame behind the head are helpful in keeping frames with skull temples in place (Figure 12.1).

Product Identification

Children and their parents have a more positive image of eyewear when they are associated with a popular commodity. Young children relate to toys or cartoon characters. Adolescents identify with clothing names. In either event, parents want to be reassured about safety and durability. There are many current examples of eyewear lines that have capitalized on this concept. Disney characters have timeless and universal appeal and are prominently displayed on Marchon frames. The Fisher-Price line by Clear Vision appeals to parents because of the association with durable

Table 12.1 Frames under 40 eye size with low bridge

Manufacturer	Model	Spring Hinge	Riding Bow Cable
A&A Optical	Curly	x	x
Avante Garde	Tots 2	—	x
Berdel	Youth 206	x	x
Classic Optical	Star	—	x
Denver International	Ann/Andy 5	x	—
Fashion Optical	Jenny/Ricky	—	x
Fisher-Price	Little One	x	x
Fisher-Price	Primary	x	x
L'Amy	Noel	—	x
Marine	Tweety	x	x
Nordic International	Bamby Cable	—	x
Optical Import	Riri	—	x
Pathway	Toddle Goggle	—	x
Poriss	Cupcake/Tiger	—	x
Preview	Baby	—	—
Pumuckl	Special Baby 01*	—	Headband strap
Society Optiks	M348	—	x
Windsor	Talpy	—	x

*Very small eye size.

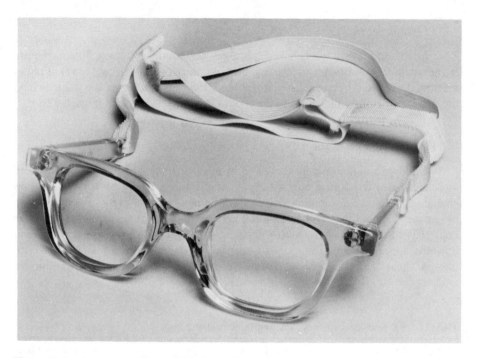

Figure 12.1 A commercially available frame (New Luv by Renaissance) comes with a harness strap to secure the eyewear on the infant's head.

children's products. Older children find it offensive to wear frames with a logo of a cartoon character or an association with children's toys. They lean toward clothing lines such as Bennetton.

Several companies have created independent ophthalmic product identification. Clear Vision has attractive frame display boards and contests "Just For Kids." Several of the companies have story books that accompany their eyewear to reinforce the positive aspects of wearing glasses. The Tann's line of Lux de Paris has beautiful strap cases and calculators as accessories to complement their eyewear. In addition, they have distinctive color combinations for their metal frames.

Eyewear Warranty

Children frequently damage their eyewear. It is a nuisance for the parent and inefficient for the staff to service the eyewear repeatedly. A well-made frame that will retain its adjustment and resist breakage is worth the investment. The practitioner should warranty the eyewear for a one year period.

DISPENSING OF EYEWEAR

On dispensing, temples should be securely adjusted and support on the bridge distributed well. If the child is hyperactive and a comfort cable is unavailable, a long skull temple can be wrapped into a riding bow form around the ear (Weber, 1985). The child should be allowed to select an attractive case for the eyewear. Parents tend to prefer hard cases to minimize scratches and loosening of the lens. Do not forget to shower the child with compliments.

REFERENCES

Apell RJ. The role of lenses in development of visual perceptual skills. In Greenstein TN, ed. Vision and learning disability. St. Louis: American Optometric Association, 1976:223–239.

Apell RJ, Streff JW. Four reasons for using lenses. Child Vision Care 1961;34(2):5–8.

Apell RJ, Streff JW. Lens prescribing: Considerations, evaluations, and predictive values. Child Vision Care 1962;35(1):1–4.

Atkinson J, Braddick O, French J. Infant astigmatism: Its disappearance with age. Vision Res 1980;20:891–893.

Birnbaum MH: Functional relationship between myopia, accommodative stress and against-the-rule astigmatism: A hypothesis. J Am Optom Assoc 1978;49:911–4.

Carter DB, ed. Special Report. Symposium on conventional wisdom in optometry. Am J Optom & Arch Am Acad Optom 1967;44:731–745.

Cho MH, Wild BW. Spectacles for children. In Rosenbloom AA, Morgan MW, eds. Principles and practice of pediatric optometry. Philadelphia: Lippincott, 1990;192–206.

Ciner EB. Management of refractive error in infants, toddlers, and preschool children. In Scheiman MM, ed. Problems in optometry: Pediatric optometry 1990;2:394–419.

Dowaliby M. Eye fashions for kids. Optom Management 1988a;Jan:79–82.

Dowaliby M. Practical aspects of ophthalmic optics. 3d ed. New York: The Professional Press, 1988b;151.

Dowaliby M, Dowaliby P. Healthy eyes for your child. Chicago: The Professional Press, 1981;26.

Drew R. Young people and eyewear. Optom Management 1989;Aug:107–109.

Grosvenor T. Management of myopia: Functional methods. In Grosvenor T, Flom MC, eds. Refractive anomalies: Research and clinical applications. Boston: Butterworth-Heinemann, 1991.

Press LJ. Do plus lenses work? Ped Optom Vis Ther 1991;1(1):4–7.

Press LJ. Lenses and behavior. J Optom Vis Devel 1989;20:5–18.

Press LJ. Physiological effects of plus lens application. Am J Optom Physiol Opt 1985;62(6):392–397.

Silbert JA, Alexander A. Cyclotherapy in the treatment of symptomatic latent hyperopia. J Am Optom Assoc 1987;58:40–46.

Skjerdal AM. Organic vs. psychogenic factors in visual dysfunction. J Am Optom Assoc 1987;58:108–111.

Tucker MA, Shields JA, Hartge P, et al. Sunlight exposure as a risk factor for intraocular malignant melanoma. New England J Med 1985;313:789–792.

Weber J. Dispensing glasses to children. Op-Topics 1985;1:4.

13

Amblyopia and Strabismus

Leonard J. Press

The two visual anomalies that draw universal attention in infancy and childhood are amblyopia and strabismus. The plasticity of the visual system in the early years is a dual-edged sword, rendering the child vulnerable to the effects of visual deprivation yet malleable to therapeutic intervention. Amblyopia and strabismus can be conceptualized as two interrelated anomalies in a continuum of neurodevelopmental abnormality and are clinically intertwined in childhood (Press, 1988; Flynn, 1991). This chapter addresses the differential diagnosis and prognosis for amblyopia and strabismus. The treatment of these two conditions is elaborated in Chapters 14, 15 and 16.

Classification

The clinician must be vigilant to the probability that strabismus and amblyopia coexist. Flynn and Cassady (1978) reported that amblyopia was associated with strabismus in 80 percent of their clinical cases; the remaining 20 percent were anisometropic. This is a higher proportion of strabismic amblyopes than is usually reported because they carefully differentiated microtropia, a condition frequently undetected as a strabismic entity (Ciuffreda et al, 1991). It is therefore a better indication of the extent to which strabismus and amblyopia coexist. Because of the comingling of these two conditions, one can consider the overall prevalence rate of strabismus and amblyopia to be 3 percent. Amblyopia is usually classified according to its etiologies as listed in Table 13.1. Strabismus is usually classified according to its characteristics as listed in Table 13.2.

DIAGNOSIS

The diagnosis of strabismus and amblyopia was discussed in Chapters 3, 4, and 5. Its significance warrants independent discussion and amplification.

Case History

As was discussed in Chapter 1, the parent is asked: Has the child had any previous visual care? The child with refractive amblyopia will rarely exhibit symptoms and is usually not detected unless a screening or examination has been performed.

Table 13.1 Classification of amblyopia

Strabismic	Organic
Refractive	Optic nerve hypoplasia/degeneration
Spherical anisometropia	Retinal hypoplasia/degeneration
Meridional amblyopia	Delayed myelinization
High bilateral uncompensated error	Cortical damage
Deprivation	Nonmalingering (bilateral)
Ptosis/hemangioma	Psychogenic (hysterical)
Corneal opacity	Stress-induced (Streff syndrome)
Cataract	
Obstructed media	
Nystagmus	
Occlusion induced	

Other questions to the parent are: If there has been prior treatment through glasses, patching, medication, or vision therapy, at what age was this conducted and for what length of time? Most importantly, was the child compliant with the treatment program? Parents or children may confide that they had been given glasses or patches but rarely used them as prescribed. In this instance, verbal reporting is more insightful than a review of previous clinical records.

The history related to strabismus is usually more definitive as compared with the history of amblyopia. With an angle of reasonable magnitude, the concern of the parents in detecting the eye turn often precedes the clinical diagnosis of the condition. It is relatively rare that we examine a child with an eye turn greater than 15 prism diopters and surprise the parents with news that there is a strabismus. Conversely there are false alarms that occur in cases of epicanthus as was discussed in Chapter 3. It is sometimes even difficult for nonophthalmic practitioners to differentiate true, small-angle esotropia from epicanthus.

In view of the physical signs by which parents can gauge its presence, the onset and course of strabismus can be more readily reviewed than the results of prior treatment of amblyopia. In addition, there are specific clinical signs that serve as strong

Table 13.2 Classification of strabismus

Age of onset	Magnitude
Congenital	Microtropia
Infantile	Small angle
Early onset	Moderate angle
Constancy	Large angle
Intermittent	Refractive influence
Constant	Accommodative component
Laterality	Comitancy
Unilateral	Correspondence
Alternating	Organicity (association with disease)

clues that the strabismus is early onset or long-standing. This information is useful in differential diagnosis and prognosis.

Clinical Diagnosis: Amblyopia
Visual Acuity

The principal clinical finding that serves as the barometer for amblyopia is the extent of acuity difference between the two eyes (Duke-Elder & Wybar, 1973). Children have trouble attending to an acuity chart selectively, so it is common practice for the clinician to present isolated pictures or alphanumerics to maximize attention. This tends to mask interocular differences in acuity (Rodier et al, 1985). There are several approaches to minimizing this problem:

1. Have an entire chart of symbols exposed, but have an assistant direct the child's attention with a pointer to specific rows or symbols.
2. Use a Good-lite box (see Appendix A) with a sliding aperture that permits exposure of isolated lines or letters.
3. Use acuity cards that have some degree of contour interaction such as the Broken Wheel Acuity Test (Richman et al, 1984).
4. Use the Flom Psychometric Acuity Chart (Flom et al, 1963) which controls for contour interaction in conjunction with a demonstrator Landolt "C." Children can use the "C" in the same manner as they use a tumbling "E."
5. Use the LH Visual Acuity Test System (Figure 13.1). This test, developed by Hyvarinen and colleagues (1980) for use with preschoolers, has numerous features including the log MAR acuity chart format of the Bailey-Lovie design.
6. As was discussed in Chapter 4, the B-VAT system (Mentor, Inc., Appendix A) electronically presents a variety of optotypes and configurations including contour interaction bars around isolated letters.

Nonacuity Factors

Additional clinical findings used in the diagnosis of amblyopia are listed in Table 13.3. Performance should be recorded for the amblyopic eye for comparison with the nonamblyopic eye. The more abnormalities that are noted in the amblyopic eye as compared with the fellow eye *and* the greater the extent of abnormality, the more difficult it will be to gain improvement through therapy. The reader is referred to the recent text on amblyopia by Ciuffreda and associates (1991) for a detailed discussion on testing of contrast sensitivity, accommodative, and ocular motor functions in amblyopia.

London and Silver (1991) presented a concise overview of pathologic causes of amblyopia in children. As they noted, functional amblyopia can be superimposed on pathological amblyopia. Once the practitioner ascertains that any pathologic element of the case has been identified or monitored, treatment can be instituted for the functional component. Issues and techniques in amblyopia therapy will be discussed in Chapter 13.

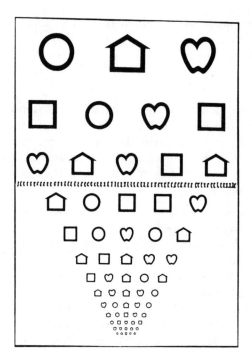

Figure 13.1 A preschool acuity chart with logMAR scale designed by Hyvarinen (see LVI, Appendix A).

Random dot stereopsis tests have been promulgated as fail-safe methods for amblyopia or strabismus detection with young children (Reinecke & Simons, 1974). Recent reports signal caution in overreliance on these procedures. Peli (1983) reported on a patient with 20/200 anisometropic amblyopia who attained 20 seconds of arc stereoacuity on the Randot Test. Garzia and Richman (1985) reported obtaining stereopsis on the Random Dot "E" with a small-angle esotropic amblyope.

Streff Syndrome

One entity infrequently cited in ophthalmic literature is juvenile bilateral amblyopia (Streff nonmalingering syndrome). This is paradoxical, as it is a well-known clinical entity among behavioral optometrists (Bosse, 1990). The syndrome consists of bilaterally, symmetrically reduced acuity in the range of 20/30 to 20/100 in the

Table 13.3 Diagnostic testing of amblyopia

Visual acuity	Fixation status
Recognition symbols (picture cards or objects)	Objective: visuoscopy
Resolution charts (psychometric charts)	Subjective: M.I.T./Haidinger Brush
Contrast sensitivity	Spatial localization (stick in straw)
Accommodative amplitude	Eye movement accuracy (saccadic
Accommodative facility	fixator)
	Binocular status (strabismus elevation)

absence of appreciable refractive error. Increased lag of accommodation and reduced stereopsis has been reported (Maino, 1987). It is usually encountered in children around the age of puberty who are susceptible to stress-induced disorders. This syndrome is easily differentiated from bilateral refractive amblyopia as there is no manifest refractive component. It is probably a less extreme form of hysterical amblyopia, which has a tubular visual field. The condition tends to be self-limiting though its resolution may be accelerated through the application of plus lens addition at nearpoint, accommodative-convergence flexibility training, and stress-reduction techniques.

Clinical Diagnosis: Strabismus

Clinical findings of significance in strabismus are principally those related to the items in Table 13.2. Strabismic amblyopia occurs when one eye is constantly deviated and results in a typically more profound acuity loss than is the case with refractive amblyopia. When the strabismus is alternating without fixation preference, amblyopia is rare.

Sensory Phenomena

Anomalous correspondence (ARC), a condition in which the foveal projection of one eye does not correspond to the foveal projection of the fellow eye, is a purposeful, time-related sensorial adaptation to shield the child from diplopia. The child with early onset strabismus usually develops ARC and is unaware of diplopia in contrast with the adolescent or teen who acquires strabismus and is likely to report diplopia. ARC is a sign that the strabismus is long-standing and has implications in therapy that will be discussed in Chapter 16.

Motor Phenomena

In addition to sensory phenomena that are time-related, there are also several motor signs that are time-related. These are associated with infantile esotropia, which occurs at a prevalence rate of 75 percent among cases of infantile strabismus (von Noorden, 1990). The hallmark features of infantile esotropia are bilateral overacting inferior obliques (OAIO), double dissociated hyperdeviation (DVD), and latent nystagmus. The mechanisms for DVD and latent nystagmus are poorly understood although they share the common property of being manifest only when one eye is covered. The most interesting aspect of these signs is their time of onset. DVD and latent nystagmus do not make their initial appearance until approximately 19–24 months of age. Furthermore, they do not seem related to the degree of eye turn nor are they influenced by strabismus surgery or vision therapy. Whereas they do not interfere with visual function when both eyes are open, they signal important clues that the child has infantile strabismus. This is particularly relevant when the child is older or adopted, and there is vague clinical history about the time of onset of the condition.

When not associated with other ocular disease, noncomitant strabismus is usually congenital. A head tilt or turn is a sign that the noncomitancy is long-standing.

The tilt is usually in the direction that will allow the child to fuse more easily. Occasionally one will see a child whose compensatory head posture is in the direction that maximizes suppression of the strabismic eye. If the child fuses habitually, such as in Duane's or Brown's syndromes, the prognosis for improved binocular function through vision therapy is good. If the child has paretic strabismus in which fusion cannot be obtained other than in a limited position of gaze, a surgical consult should be sought as early as possible.

Nystagmus blockage syndrome is another specific, adaptive ocular-motor abnormality (Dell'Osso et al, 1983). This is esotropia that results from purposeful and persistent overconvergence to dampen nystagmus. Any intervention to lessen the esotropia must take the nystagmus into account. For this reason, surgical intervention is the treatment of choice (Shuckett et al, 1981).

PROGNOSIS

The prognosis for the remediation of any clinical condition is related to the criteria established for its cure. There are, to date, no universally accepted criteria for cure of amblyopia or strabismus. Useful clinical guidelines have been suggested, and although they are present independently, they are interrelated.

Amblyopia

There are two extreme positions that have been espoused in the treatment of amblyopia, neither of which is clinically justifiable. One view holds that amblyopia cannot be successfully treated after age seven or eight; the other professes that it is never too late to treat amblyopia. The former view is held principally by ophthalmologists who adhere to the laboratory model of critical periods of visual development during conditions of extreme deprivation.

The error in this dogmatic approach is twofold. First, it is relatively rare to encounter conditions of extreme deprivation clinically. This is seen only in congenital conditions of obstruction such as cataract or in image degradation such as high uncompensated unilateral myopia. It is more likely that one encounters a more subtle form of amblyopia secondary to strabismus or moderate ametropia. These conditions are certainly responsive to amblyopia therapy beyond the critical period.

The second fallacy in this approach is the value judgement that it is not worth undertaking amblyopia therapy unless acuity can be normalized. We know that visual acuity is very labile in the child from birth until 4 years of age. For example, at 3 years of age, as brief a period as three weeks of constant direct occlusion can bring a strabismic amblyope from 20/1000 to 20/20. If occlusion is abruptly terminated without binocular integration, however, the acuity will revert to 20/1000. It is therefore justifiable to state that more can be accomplished in a shorter time frame when occlusion is implemented prior to age 7 or 8. Indeed an age will be reached at which the child can no longer attain near 20/20 visual acuity in the amblyopic eye despite any and all means of intervention. This does not mean, however, that it is not worthwhile at age 14 to take a child from 20/400 to 20/70.

Conversely the evidence that success in amblyopia therapy can be attained at older ages (Birnbaum et al, 1977) stems from clinical experience in vision therapy. This is bolstered by controlled studies in older amblyopes (Ciuffreda, 1986) as well as case reports of spontaneous recovery of the functionally amblyopic eye when the contralateral eye experiences a precipitous loss in acuity secondary to acquired ocular disease (Hamed et al, 1991). Moreover laboratory evidence exists that the visual cortex is still modifiable long after the critical period through noradrenergic stimulation of the locus coeruleus (Kasamatsu et al, 1983). This bolsters the clinical impression that the cooperation of the child with therapy is almost as important a factor as the age of the child. This should not be construed as a license for overzealous treatment, however, when the prognosis for improvement is dismal.

One is therefore led to the conclusion that the cost-benefit ratio of instituting amblyopia therapy should be considered carefully with the older child on an individual basis. A 12-year-old asymptomatic, unmotivated child with dense amblyopia secondary to previously uncorrected high unilateral myopia may be better left alone than subjected to a protracted period of vision therapy. The positive prognostic factors for amblyopia are summarized in Table 13.4.

Strabismus

As with amblyopia, the prognosis for successful outcome of intervention in strabismus is related to the criteria established for the cure. Two widely recognized criteria for the cure of strabismus are those expounded by Flom (1963) and von Noorden (1988). Von Noorden considered his results in the context of postsurgical results with young children who had infantile esotropia (Table 13.5). He concluded that, although the data show that surgery prior to age two yields superior results, a functionally useful form of binocular vision can ensue when surgical treatment is concluded after the age of four years.

Flom (1990) recently reviewed his criteria for cure of strabismus. As von Noorden, he implies acceptance of treatment outcome with less than ideal results (Table 13.6) Indeed his terminology has appropriately changed from functional *cure* to functional *correction*. His primary differentiation of the functional correction of strabismus lies in the maintenance of bifoveal fixation in everyday situations of life, even though a "reasonable amount" of prismatic correction in spectacle form may be required to accomplish this. The probability of functional correction of the various types of strabismus from most favorable to least favorable is given in Table 13.7.

Table 13.4 Positive prognostic factors in amblyopia

Central fixation
Refractive amblyopia
Good acuity on laser interferometry
Normal VEP waveform
Improvement in acuity through telescope greater than predicted by the magnification factor
Cooperative patient under the age of 10

Table 13.5 Von Noorden's classification of postsurgical results

	Class 1: Subnormal	Class 2: Microtropia
Phoria	Asymptomatic phoria	Inconspicuous or no shift on cover test
Acuity	Normal in both eyes	Mild amblyopia
Fusion Ranges	Present	Present
Correspondence	NRC	ARC
Suppression	Foveal when binocular	Relative to ARC
Alignment	Stable	Usually stablea

von Noorden GK. A reassessment of infantile esotropia. Am J Ophthalmol 1988;105:1–10.

Table 13.6 Flom's criteria for cure of strabismus

	Functional Cure	Almost Cured
Bifoveal fixation	99% of the time	Less than 99% of the time
Alignment	May require approximately 5 prism diopters to attain fusion	May require larger amounts of prism to attain fusion
Stereopsis	May be lacking	May be lacking

MC Flom. Issues in the clinical management of binocular anomalies. In Rosenbloom AA, Morgan MW, eds. Principles and practice of pediatric optometry. Philadelphia: Lippincott, 1990; 219.

Table 13.7 Rank-ordered probability of functional cure in strabismus

Motor Status	Sensory Status	Probability Factor for Cure
Intermittent exotropia	NRC	0.8
Intermittent exotropia	ARC	0.7
Intermittent esotropia	NRC	0.6
Intermittent esotropia	ARC	0.5
Constant exotropia	NRC	0.5
Constant exotropia	ARC	0.4
Constant esotropia	NRC	0.3
Constant esotropia	ARC	0.1

Adapted from MC Flom. Issues in the clinical management of binocular anomalies. Rosenbloom AA, Morgan MW, eds. Principles and practice of pediatric optometry. Philadelphia: Lippincott, 1990; 219.

As with amblyopia therapy, the cognitive abilities and level of compliance of the child with the therapy program influence the outcome of intervention to at least as great an extent as do positive or negative clinical findings.

REFERENCES

Birnbaum MH, Koslowe K, Sanet R. Success in amblyopia therapy as a function of age: A literature survey. Am J Optom Physiol Opt 1977;54:267–275.

Bosse J. Streff non-malingering syndrome. J Optom Vis Devel 1990; 21(4):1–2.

Ciuffreda KJ. Visual system plasticity in human amblyopia. In Hiller SR, Sheffield JB, eds. Development of order in the visual system. New York: Springer-Verlag, 1986;211–244.

Ciuffreda KJ, Levi DM, Selenow A. Amblyopia: Basic and clinical aspects. Boston: Butterworth–Heinemann, 1991.

Dell'Osso LF, Ellenberger C, Abel LA, et al. The nystagmus blockage syndrome: Congenital nystagmus, manifest latent nystagmus, or both? Invest Ophthalmol Vis Sci 1983;24:1580–1587.

Duke-Elder S, Wybar K. System of ophthalmology. Vol. 6: Ocular motility and strabismus. St. Louis: Mosby, 1973.

Flom MC. Issues in the clinical management of binocular anomalies. In Rosenbloom AA, Morgan MW, eds. Principles and practice of pediatric optometry. Philadelphia: Lippincott, 1990;219.

Flom MC. Treatment of binocular anomalies of vision. In Hirsch MJ, Wick RE, eds. Vision of children. Philadelphia: Chilton, 1963;210–212.

Flom MC, Weymouth FW, Kahnemann D. Visual resolution and contour interaction. J Opt Soc Am 1963;53:1026–1032.

Flynn JT. Strabismus: A neurodevelopmental approach: Nature's experiment. New York: Springer-Verlag, 1991.

Flynn JT, Cassady JC. Current trends in amblyopia therapy. Ophthalmology 1978;85:428–450.

Garzia RP, Richman JE. Stereopsis in an amblyopic small angle esotrope. J Am Optom Assoc 1985;56:400–404.

Hamed LM, Glaser JS, Schatz NJ. Improvement of vision in the amblyopic eye following visual loss in the contralateral normal eye: A report of 3 cases. Binoc Vis Quarterly 1991;6:97–100.

Hyvarinen L, Nasanen R, Laurinen P. New visual acuity test for pre-school children. Acta Ophthalmol (Copenh) 1980;58:507–511.

Kasamatsu T, Watabe K, Scholler E, et al. Restoration of neuronal plasticity in cat visual cortex by electrical stimulation of the locus coeruleus. Neuroscience Abstracts 1983;9:911.

London R, Silver JL. Diagnosis of amblyopia: Emphasis on nonacuity factors. Problems in Optometry 1991;3:258–275.

Maino JH. Ocular hysteria and malingering. In Amos JF, ed. Diagnosis and management in vision care. Boston: Butterworth–Heinemann;1987:419.

von Noorden GK. Binocular vision and ocular motility: Theory and management of strabismus. 4th ed. St. Louis: Mosby, 1990.

von Noorden GK. A reassessment of infantile esotropia. Am J Ophthalmol 1988;105:1–10.

Peli E. Normal stereo acuity despite anisometropic amblyopia. J Am Optom Assoc 1983;54:919–921.

Press LJ. Amblyopia. J Optom Vis Devel 1988;19(1):2–15.

Reinecke RD, Simons K. A new stereoscopic test for amblyopia screening. Am J Ophthalmol 1974;78:714.

Richman JE, Petito GT, Cron MT. Broken wheel acuity test: A new and valid test for preschool and exceptional children. J Am Optom Assoc 1984;55:561–565.

Rodier DW, Mayer DL, Fulton AB. Assessment of young amblyopes: Array vs. single picture acuities. Ophthalmology (Rochester) 1985;92:1197–1202.

Shuckett EP, Hiles DA, Biglan AW, et al. Posterior fixation suture operation (fadenoperation). Ophthalmic Surg 1981;12:578–585.

14

Comanagement of the Strabismic Child

Leonard J. Press
Brian Altman

OPTOMETRIC CONSIDERATIONS IN SURGICAL REFERRAL

The traditional optometric approach to strabismus surgery is either protagonist or antagonist. A middle ground, comanaging patients with a pediatric ophthalmologist when surgery is in the patient's best interest is preferrable. Consideration of surgery to reduce the magnitude of deviation is part of a continuum in the sequential management of strabismic patients (Figures 14.1 and 14.2). Comanagement of the strabismic child should parallel the optometric-ophthalmologic symbiosis that has proven successful with the adult cataract patient.

This section reflects the position of the optometrist as case manager. This appears less attainable in institutional settings or when the optometrist is not a partner in the practice, in which case the optometrist may not have full control over the timing of surgical intervention. Although the skill of the surgeon with whom the optometrist will deal is the key element in immediate mechanical success, knowledge of general outcomes of strabismus surgery, as was discussed in Chapter 13, is helpful in guiding the patient. Three recent broad literature reviews have been conducted (Table 14.1), which quantify the results of surgery for various types of strabismus. A useful, overall clinical guide remains the observation by Scobee (1951) that some form of fusion is attainable in approximately 50 percent of patients who are treated with a combination of lens and/or prismatic compensation, medication, or surgery when postsurgical alignment is good. The addition of formal orthoptics to the therapeutic regimen improves the success rate to 80 percent.

Although the reader may be aware of optometric support for a conservative approach to strabismus surgery when the capacity for fusion can be demonstrated (Scheiman & Ciner, 1987), the American Academy of Ophthalmology (1987) supports a conservative approach as evidenced by:

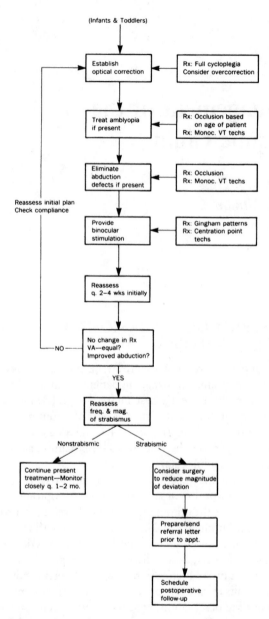

Figure 14.1 Flow diagrams for sequential management of infants and toddlers with strabismus. Flowchart emphasizing sequential management principles for infantile esotropes 24 months of age or less (Rx = prescription/prescribe, VT = vision therapy, q = each/every, VA = visual acuity, Freq = frequency, Mag = magnitude, post-op = after surgery). (Reprinted with permission of the publisher from GN Christensen et al. Management of infantile-onset estropia. J Am Opt Assoc 1990;61:559–572.)

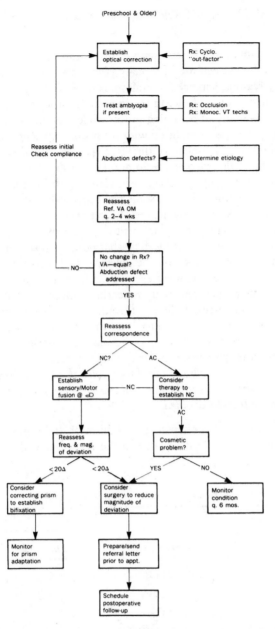

Figure 14.2 Flow diagram for sequential management of preschool and school children with strabismus. Flowchart emphasizing sequential management principles for patients greater than 24 months of age with suspected early onset esotropia (Rx = prescription/prescribe, VT = vision therapy, Ref = refraction, VA = visual acuity, OM = ocular motility, q = each/every, NC = normal correspondence, AC = anomalous correspondence, H = objective angle of strabismus, Freq = frequency, Mag = magnitude, Post-op = after surgery). (Reprinted with permission of the publisher from GN Christenson et al. Management of infantile-onset esotropia. J Am Opt Assoc 1990;61:559–572.)

The prism adaptation test represents a formalization of a simple clinical practice which has been used for many years, especially in Europe. There, for a variety of reasons, surgery for strabismus is often delayed until the second half of the first decade of life. In the interim, in order to provide the child with some possibility of obtaining fusion while awaiting surgical alignment of his eye, the patient is often fitted with prisms of sufficient magnitude to permit orthotropic alignment of the visual axes on the object of regard. In many cases this will provoke a restoration of sensory binocular cooperation in a form of fusion and even stereopsis. Carrying this out is actually then a clinical trial of orthotropia with some predictive value of whether or not, when the patient is surgically aligned, fusion may be restored. In addition, some patients respond to the placement of prisms by increasing their deviation. In such cases it may well be that peripheral fusion and anomalous retinal correspondence based on the objective angle drive the eyes to maintain this adaptive alignment even in the face of prismatic correction. One will see the patient return after wearing such prisms with a greater angle of deviation corresponding to the addition of the prisms. In the vernacular such patients are said to "eat" their prisms. Casual observations have suggested that patients who do this may require significantly more surgery than other patients in order to obtain correction of their deviation. *In some cases, patients who obtain fusion with this prism therapy may simply be weaned off the prisms if the angle of their deviation is not too large and surgery may be thereby avoided.*

When the optometrist is discussing the option of strabismus surgery, the goals of the parents must be clearly delineated in the record, and the objectives of the

Table 14.1 Literature review of surgical success rates in strabismus

Type of Strabismus	Number of Cases	Percentage	
		Functional	Cosmetic
Infantile Esotropia	2113		63
	1286[a]	22[a]	
Acquired Esotropia	1473		43
	1170[b]	15[b]	
Intermittent Exotropia	919		57
	571[c]	34[c]	

[a]M Scheiman, E Ciner, M Gallaway. Surgical success rates in infantile esotropia. J Am Optom Assoc 1989;60:22–30.
[b]M Scheiman, E Ciner. Surgical success rates in acquired, comitant, partially accommodative and nonaccommodative estropia. J Am Optom Assoc 1987;58:556–561.
[c]N Flax, A Selenow. Results of surgical treatment of intermittent divergent strabismus. Am J Optom Physiol Opt 1985;62:100–104.

optometrist must address these goals. If the parents are looking for cosmetic improvement and the optometrist measures progress in other terms, the parents will be dissatisfied. Conversely if the parents are looking primarily for performance changes in school but the optometrist addresses success only in terms of the magnitude of deviation and the level of fusion, another gap in communication will ensue.

In summary, the optometrist should address the option of strabismus surgery when a treatment plan is presented for three basic reasons.

1. Parents are usually aware that the child has strabismus prior to the examination and have been exposed to the possibility of surgery through friends, relatives, or other professionals.
2. Parents will guide the optometrist about their feelings toward surgery. Some will want to know why surgery as the initial approach is not recommended. Others have already made the decision to pursue a nonsurgical approach and are seeking reinforcement.
3. Vision therapy should be positioned as a treatment of first choice with surgery a fallback position. Even for those parents who seek only a cosmetic cure, therapy can be complementary to surgery in paving a stronger foundation and stabilizing the postsurgical results.

Presenting the Role of the Surgeon

When the decision has been made to suggest that the parents consult with a surgeon, the role of the surgeon should be clearly defined. Few have placed the role of surgery into better perspective than Duke-Elder and Wybar (1973):

> The aim of surgery in general is to place the eyes in a position as nearly as possible approaching normal so that the normal binocular reflexes may develop either as the result of the constant impact of natural stimuli or those of specifically applied orthoptic treatment. Insofar as the cure of squint is measured in terms of the restoration of binocular vision, operation cannot by itself effect a cure; it is merely a mechanical expedient to orientate the eyes by placing them in a position approximating orthotropia from which an adequate range of fusional movements is possible so that the neuro-muscular mechanism subserving binocular vision can become effective.

Explain to the parents that in this regard the surgeon is a skilled technician who will put their child's eyes in a position that will make it easier for them to begin to work together. The surgeon will not be the one who determines the need for eyeglasses. Nor will the surgeon be the one who will determine the need for vision therapy or the duration of that therapy. In other words, the optometrist should not plan or administer the surgical procedure, and the surgeon should not manage the optical or visual components. Explain further to the parents that much as you can give them a feel for what is involved in surgery on muscles of the eye and what to expect, surgeons may comment on their impressions of the need for optical or visual treatment before or after surgery. However, the surgeons are the experts in deciding on what needs to be done in surgery, and the optometrists should abide by their judgement. Similarly the optometrist should consider the surgeon's input on the need for lenses, prisms, or vision therapy but should exercise independent skilled judgment in these matters.

Timing of the Surgical Referral

The decision to refer a child for strabismus surgery hinges in part on the age of onset as well as the magnitude of the problem. If it is established that the strabismus was constant prior to 6 months of age and the child is less than age 3, vision therapy and lenses for a trial period of 3 months are recommended (see Chapter 16). If results show significant reduction in the angle or desired performance changes, surgery should be deferred, and therapy should be continued. If there is little or no movement, a surgical consult should be arranged. If the child is 3 to 6 years of age, project a trial period of 6 months. If the child is above age 6, project a period of 12 months. The older the child and the longer the duration of the strabismus, the longer is the expected time frame for altering sensory-motor status. Particularly for older children in whom ARC (anomalous correspondence) is probably manifest when the strabismus is long-standing, establishing NRC (normal correspondence) prior to surgery is a distinct advantage.

When the onset of strabismus is documented to have been after one year of age, particularly when there is a strong accommodative component, parents should be counseled that there is no rush to do surgery. The shorter the duration of the strabismus, the better the prognosis that binocular vision can be restored without the need for surgical intervention.

The Comanagement Concept

The best model for comanagement of the strabismic child comes from the current concept of comanagement of the cataract patient. A symbiotic relationship has evolved where the optometrist is the gatekeeper who decides when decrement in visual function warrants surgical intervention and who retains management responsibilities in postoperative care. This cooperative relationship breeds mutual respect and serves the optimal needs in patient care and the delivery of services. If the optometrist learns that the surgeon has stepped into the nonsurgical domain of patient care, the optometrist will probably seek a new surgeon who better understands the division of labor.

In this regard the optometrist should become acquainted with the philosophy and reputation of the surgeon to whom the majority of the optometrist's patients will be directed. It is appropriate to give the parents a choice of surgeons but to indicate which one you would select were it your child going to surgery. It is not uncommon that parents will seek more than one opinion when they are considering surgery for their child.

It is preferable when one can find a surgeon with a conservative approach toward strabismus surgery so that parents do not feel pressured into action. Prepare parents for the possibility that the surgeon may suggest deferring surgery until after medication has been tried or when there are contra-indications as will be reviewed later in this chapter.

Optometric Postsurgical Follow-Up

The ophthalmologist sees the child for immediate postoperative care. The child's eyes are engorged and chemotic after surgery, which precludes immediate vision therapy. As will be explained in this chapter, each surgeon has a timetable for postsurgical checkups.

The optometrist should reevaluate the child within one week after surgery. If extensive vision therapy had been done prior to surgery, specifically if a centration range had been established in esotropia or a compensated exotropic angle had been sensorially massaged through lenses, prism, or instrumentation, a good postsurgical result is anticipated. When presurgical sensory fusion is weak or nonexistent, the optometrist should insist on seeing the patient before readaptation ensues. The optometrist should be conversant with the surgeon's approach for particular procedures. For example, if the child is left with an intentional overcorrection under 10 prism diopters following bilateral recession for divergence excess, the optometrist should know that it is desirable to see the child with this deviation because it will tend to orthotropize in time. Conversely a residual postsurgical amblyopia puts the presurgical esotropic patient at high risk for developing consecutive exotropia (Folk et al, 1983). The onset of the postsurgical exotropia may take years to develop, underscoring the importance of continual care.

The remaining sections in this chapter present an overview of surgical treatment of the strabismic child to acquaint the optometrist with ophthalmologic thought processes in extraocular muscle surgery. Insight into the actual procedures aids the role of the optometrist in prereferral counseling of the family and facilitates the comanagement concept.

SURGICAL TREATMENT OF STRABISMUS

In the hands of an experienced strabismologist, eye muscle surgery is the quickest, most reliable way to improve ocular alignment. Benefits include improved appearance and function and hopefully binocularity. Issues related to postsurgical sensory motor results are discussed in detail in Chapter 10. The purpose of this section is to give the optometrist an "over-the-shoulder" view of strabismus surgery.

Preoperative Planning

The patient is given a full external and internal eye examination including, but not limited to, distance and near visual acuity, visual fields when possible, tests of binocularity and color vision, refraction slit lamp, and fundus examination. Ocular alignment is measured in distance, in near viewing positions, and in the nine cardinal positions of gaze. Often full cycloplegic correction is employed to measure alignment of esotropes and full myopic correction in exotropes. Amblyopia should be treated as much as possible before surgery, so the patient has the best chance to maintain binocularity postsurgically.

Infants and retarded patients present special challenges. Often estimations of the strabismus angle have to be made as was discussed in Chapter 3. Strabismus surgeons have used approximate tables of millimeters of muscle recession or resection to correspond to degrees or diopters of misalignment (Table 14.2), but each person has a group of "fudge factors" to slightly alter the measurements. Pediatric ophthalmologists are constantly trying to improve surgical results and determine new contributing factors. Not everyone agrees on what procedure is best in a given case. Often a surgeon's personal experience guides his judgement and selection. For instance, for many years Dr. Arthur Jampolsky and the "Western school" have advocated unilateral recess-resect procedures as the procedure of first choice for an infantile esotrope whereas Dr. Marshall Parks and the "Eastern school" have been in favor of an initial bilateral medial rectus recession. There is not necessarily a "right" answer, but each surgeon has a first choice for a number of reasons. We feel that the recession procedure is better because a recession is more predictable and the child maintains the full muscle present should subsequent procedures be required. Once a muscle is shortened, it is difficult to subsequently lengthen it.

It is advantageous to have NRC (normal correspondence) when eye muscle surgery is being done, but the lack of this sensory status is not a contraindication to surgery. As was discussed in Chapter 13, it does appear to lessen the probability for a full functional cure.

Informed Consent

When deciding on strabismus surgery, the surgeon certainly wants to improve the patient's ocular status with the minimum possible risk. A discussion with the patient and family includes an explanation of the procedure, its purpose, and alternative methods of treatment or nontreatment. Possible risks, such as anesthesia

Table 14.2 Estimate of the amount of muscle alteration to achieve alignment in esotropia

Prism Diopters	Recess MR OU (mm)	Resect LR OU (mm)
15	3	5
20	3.5	6
25	4	7
30	4.5	8
35	5	—
50	6	—

Source: JH Calhoun, LB Nelson, D Harley. Atlas of pediatric ophthalmic surgery. Philadelphia: Saunders, 1987.

problems, possible infection, new ocular alignment positions, and associated diplopia are reviewed. For many years, eye muscle procedures have been performed mostly at hospital short procedure units or at surgicenters, where experienced, competent anesthesia and nursing staff are available. The possibility of a second surgical procedure should be mentioned, since the surgeon cannot guarantee the stability of postoperative alignment.

Which Muscles Need Surgery?

Often the answer to this question is obvious. In an infant with esotropia, it is usual to recess the medial recti. Suppose, though, that there is a sixth nerve or lateral rectus palsy present. In this case, a medial rectus recession alone would not be likely to result in improved ocular alignment and motility. The weak lateral muscle would have to be strengthened with a resection or even a muscle transposition procedure to improve the eye's abducting ability. In these situations especially, there is no uniform "correct" procedure, and the surgeon strives for the most optimal results with his operation of choice.

If patients have superior oblique palsy, they may be helped by superior oblique tucks or similar shortening procedures. If they have developed compensatory inferior oblique overaction, inferior oblique recessions may be done. Sometimes the vertical recti may need corrective surgery too, and combined procedures may help.

For patients with unilateral poor vision, try to operate unilaterally if possible even if a resection is used. Although a young infant's eye is smaller than an adult's, the amount of muscle movement for a given amount of strabismus correction appears to be the same.

Contraindications to Surgery

For any surgical procedure and patient, there are absolute and relative contraindications and precautions. A person with poor general medical status may be subjected to undue risk if strabismus surgery is performed. If the cardiovascular or respiratory system would be jeopardized, surgery should be deferred. In the past, anesthesiologists were uncomfortable about very young infants being given anesthesia. Now, however, it is routine to operate on strabismus patients who are only a few months of age.

There is controversy today about the laboratory data necessary for patients undergoing surgery. The surgeon arrives at a compromise position between tests that are desirable and tests that are essential for preoperative evaluation of patients.

The child's physician should clear the child medically with a general history and examination, elicit any personal or family history of medication and anesthesia allergies, and obtain a complete blood count and urinalysis. If there is a history of unusual or prolonged bleeding, prothrombin time, partial thromboplastin time, and bleeding time are requested. Patients on medication are often permitted at least a portion of their morning dose before surgery.

Preoperative Procedures

It is safest to keep the patient's stomach empty of food for several hours prior to surgery. Early morning surgery is best. Some surgeons prefer certain preoperative medications for pain, sedation, and induction of drowsiness, but this is entirely up to the ophthalmologist and the anesthesia staff. Avoid presurgical narcotics because they predispose the child to recurrent bouts of postsurgical vomiting. A family who can calmly prepare a child for surgery and an understanding staff can often do as much as or more than all types of preoperative drugs, especially if the medications are given by injection.

Have the child anesthetized by mask; then an IV (intravenous injection) is begun once he is asleep. Older children and adults are sometimes given medications by IV to induce their anesthesia. It helps to speak soothingly to virtually all patients of any age as they are put to sleep.

Surgical Procedures

Over the past centuries, many surgical techniques have evolved for the realignment of extraocular muscles. The following is an overview of some of these procedures.

Incisions

The six extraocular muscles all attach to the glove several millimeters behind the limbus. They can be approached in various ways. A limbal incision is easy to initiate, and approach to the muscle is often well visualized. Usually 60 to 120 degrees of conjunctiva is dissected free from the corneal limbus while the assistant aids in muscle exposure and homeostasis. The main disadvantage is postoperative discomfort and visualization of the incisional scars by the patient and his family. A direct approach over the muscle was popularized by Kenneth Swan, but a great deal of scarring, including the muscle, made this method lose favor.

Frank Costenbader and Marshall Parks developed the *cul-de-sac* approach (Figure 14.3), which initially is more difficult to perform and assist but which has the advantage of being behind the lids so the patient is very comfortable without postoperative patches or bandages. Scarring is kept away from the muscles. This is the preferred method whenever possible. Spatula needles are used to lessen the risk of perforation for these procedures. Topical and/or local anesthetics have been used for strabismus surgery, particularly in surgery on adults.

Rectus Muscle Recession (Weakening)

This is the most common procedure done. After a lid speculum is inserted that holds the lids apart, a cul-de-sac incision is made for the lateral muscle. The inferior rectus may be operated from the same incisions if necessary. The incisions may be made superiorly for simultaneous superior rectus access. A small, then medium, then self-retaining, muscle hook is placed beneath the muscle just posterior to its insertion and the muscle is freed from its soft tissue attachments. A double-arm 6-0 vicryl suture

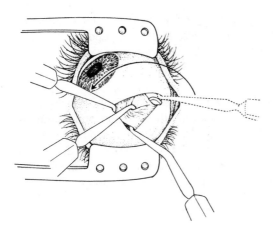

Figure 14.3 The cul-de-sac approach used for incision during extraocular muscle surgery. (Reproduced with permission from Calhoun JH, Nelson LB, Harley D. Atlas of pediatric ophthalmic surgery. Philadelphia: Saunders, 1987.)

is imbricated through the insertion of the muscle and locked at the poles. The muscle is transected from the globe, and bleeders are cauterized. Castroviejo calipers are used to measure back the specified number of millimeters from the original insertion. Needles are placed one-half depth in the sclera in a crossed-swords fashion, and the sutures are tied and cut (Figure 14.4). A variation with loose sutures is called the *hang-back technique*. The conjunctiva is closed with 8-0 collagen sutures that dissolve rapidly within the next few days. A few drops of balanced salt solution are applied to the eye during the procedure. Surgery then proceeds to the other eye if that is necessary. Sulfa-steroid ointment is applied. Two single-armed 5-0 chromic sutures can be placed alternatively around the upper and lower (or medial and lateral) one-third to one-quarter of the muscle at its insertion. The muscle is transected from the globe and resewn a specified distance posterior to the original insertion. They can

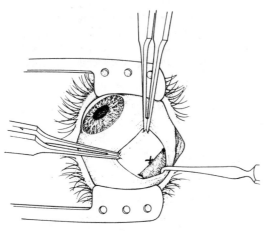

Figure 14.4 Rectus muscle recession with one double-armed suture tied in a crossed-sword fashion. (Reproduced with permission from Calhoun JH, Nelson LB, Harley D. Atlas of pediatric ophthalmic surgery. Philadelphia: Saunders, 1987.)

be resutured to the sclera with short horizontal, vertical, or oblique bites and sewn each to itself. Interrupted plain, chromic, or other sutures are used to close the conjunctiva. Parks does not close with sutures in his recession procedures.

Rectus Muscle Resection

A similar incision is made, and the muscle is isolated on three successive hooks. A measured amount of muscle is determined back from the insertion, and a suture is imbricated half-depth through one-half of the muscle, then locked at the poles. Some surgeons use one suture for the entire muscle; some use two. A muscle resection clamp is placed anterior to the sutures, and the muscle is cut anterior to the clamp (Figure 14.5). The shortened muscle is resewn to the original muscle insertion point on the eye, using varying techniques.

Inferior Oblique Recession

Through the inferolateral cul-de-sac incision a 4-0 black silk suture is passed beneath the elevated lateral rectus near its insertion and used to elevate the eye in adduction. Two small hooks are used to isolate the inferior oblique at its insertion (Figure 14.6). The muscle can be imbricated with a 6-0 vicryl locked at the medial and lateral poles prior to or after the muscle is transected from the globe. The sutures are then placed one-half depth in the sclera at the desired position near the inferior rectus muscle insertion. There are several other inferior oblique weakening procedures, including ablation of its nerve, excision, and extirpation.

Superior Oblique Procedures

The superior oblique can be approached through a superolateral or superomedial incision. The superior rectus has to be identified and protected. The tendon may be partially transposed (Harada-Ito procedure), lengthened, resected, tucked, or transected (tenotomy). A portion may be removed (tenectomy). There are various

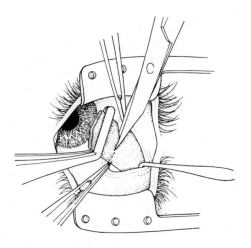

Figure 14.5 Rectus muscle resection with double-armed suture. (Reproduced with permission from Calhoun JH, Nelson LB, Harley D. Atlas of pediatric ophthalmic surgery. Philadelphia: Saunders, 1987.)

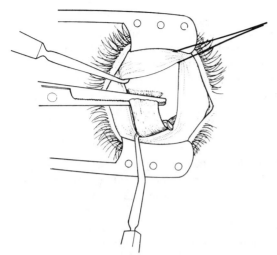

Figure 14.6 A black silk suture passing beneath the elevated lateral rectus muscle allows isolation of the inferior oblique at its insertion. (Reproduced with permission from Calhoun JH, Nelson LB, Harley D. Atlas of pediatric ophthalmic surgery. Philadelphia: Saunders, 1987.)

sutures used for some of these operations, and the incision may or may not be closed with sutures afterwards.

Adjustable Suture Technique

In patients of sufficient age and intellect to participate in this procedure, the muscles may be recessed and tied with a loop or slip knot. Later in the day on which the procedure is performed, the patient may be asked to view a target and the slip knot untied under topical anesthesia. The position of the muscle can be advanced or further recessed according to the patient's verbal report of fusion and/or the surgeon's observation of eye position. A simple screening can be done to see if the child is a suitable candidate for this procedure. A child who is intolerant or fearful of a Q-tip pressing on the bulbar conjunctiva will be a poor candidate (Wright, 1991).

Posterior Fixation (Faden) Sutures

This technique is used when there is a variable amount of strabismus deviation and can be helpful on the medial rectus for a variable amount of accommodative esotropia or on the superior rectus for a variable dissociated hypertropia. Various conjunctival incisions can be used, and the procedure may or may not be done before or after a simultaneous muscle recession. Traction is applied on the muscle insertion so the muscle is exposed 14 to 16 mm posterior to its insertion. This is difficult, and many retractors may be needed. A 5-0 dacron suture on a half-circle spatula needle is optimal. The needle is placed half depth in the sclera and through about one-quarter to one-third of the muscle approximately 14 mm posterior to its insertion. The suture is tied and clamped while another needle and suture are placed through sclera and the other side of the muscle at a similar distance posterior to its insertion. This is tied, and both sutures are cut. The conjunctiva is then closed.

Transposition Procedures

Occasionally a muscle is very weak, and the eye cannot move in its primary field of action. Neighboring muscles or portions of them can be transposed adjacent to the weak muscle, or a nonabsorbable suture can be used to attach the neighboring muscles loosely to the weak muscle. These procedures will not work if there is any mechanical restriction preventing the eye's movement.

Postoperative Procedures

After patients emerge from anesthesia and the vital signs stabilize, they are transported to the recovery room. They receive intravenous fluids and any necessary drugs through an IV until they awaken and are stable. After the vital signs normalize, they are transported to their families where they remain together for awhile in a less intensely monitored area, and subsequently they are allowed to go home.

It is not necessary to patch children after strabismus surgery. There is some ocular seeping for several hours after surgery, and the lids may become matted. Gentle warm soaks can loosen this. A combination sulfa-steroid ointment (Cetapred, Vasocidin, or Blephamide) is recommended as a postoperative medication. If there is a history of sulfa sensitivity, erythromycin or Polysporin ointment with a steroid ointment are used t.i.d. (*ter in di'e*) for 3–5 days, starting the evening after surgery. There is usually not much pain after these procedures, but acetaminophen may be used for the first couple of days. Occasionally vomiting may recur and require medication. When this occurs, sips of clear liquids with a slow progression toward a normal diet often ease this discomfort.

Postsurgical Follow-Up Care

When a family is reliable, the postoperative visits may be timed loosely; otherwise, the patient must be seen on the day following surgery. Look for signs of systemic inflammation and/or infection such as pneumonia or orbital, lid, and extraocular reaction as well as signs of endophthalmitis, hyphema, uveitis, or retinal problems. After a few weeks if the ocular alignment and motility are not satisfactory, the possibility of future surgery should be discussed. A second opinion should always be offered for surgery.

Surgery should be seen as a portion of the ongoing management of the strabismic patient. The child with unilateral strabismus must be corrected for best visual acuity and monitored for amblyopia on an ongoing basis. The parent must be discouraged from the false sense of security of cosmetic alignment with regard to the recurrence or depth of amblyopia. Alternative procedures such as chemodenervation of extraocular muscles merit consideration. Their rightful place in the total approach is evolving as will be reviewed in Chapter 15.

REFERENCES

American Academy of Ophthalmology. Basic science and clinical course, section 6, pediatric ophthalmology and strabismus, 1987–1988. San Francisco: American Academy of Ophthalmology, 1987;224–225.

Calhoun JH, Nelson LB, Harley D. Atlas of pediatric ophthalmic surgery. Philadelphia: Saunders, 1987.

Christensen GN et al. Management of infantile-onset estropia. J Am Opt Assoc 1990;61:559–572.

Duke-Elder SS, Wybar K. Ocular motility and strabismus. In Duke-Elder SS, ed. System of ophthalmology. St. Louis: Mosby, 1973;489.

Flax N, Selenow A. Results of surgical treatment of intermittent divergent strabismus. Am J Optom Physiol Opt 1985;62:100–104.

Folk ER, Miller MY, Chapman L. Consecutive exotropia following surgery. Br J Ophthalmol 1983;67:546–548.

Scheiman M, Ciner E. Surgical success rates in acquired, comitant, partially accommodative and nonaccommodative esotropia. J Am Optom Assoc 1987;58:556–561.

Scheiman M, Ciner E, Gallaway M. Surgical success rates in infantile esotropia. J Am Optom Assoc 1989;60:22–30.

Scobee RG. Disturbances of ocular motility. Rochester: American Acadamy of Ophthalmology and Otolaryngology, 1951;60.

Wright KW. Color atlas of ophthalmic surgery: strabismus. Philadelphia: J.B. Lippincott, 1991;88.

15

Pharmacologic Treatment of Strabismus

Rudolph S. Wagner
Bruce D. Moore

ANTICHOLINERGICS OR CHOLINERGIC ANTAGONISTS
Mechanisms

The mode of action of cholinergic antagonist agents is to block the neurotransmitter acetylcholine at receptor sites of the ciliary body and iris. Ocular anticholinergic agents are used primarily for the diagnostic purposes of cycloplegic refraction and pupillary dilation. They are also often used in conjunction with adrenergic agonists such as phenylephrine hydrochloride. In addition, they are occasionally used for therapeutic purposes in the treatment of strabismus and amblyopia.

The five ophthalmic anticholinergic drugs that are used clinically are atropine, scopolamine, homatropine, cyclopentalate, and tropicamide. Atropine is the only one that is really useful in the treatment of strabismus or amblyopia. Tropicamide has variable and relatively ineffective cycloplegic activity. Homatropine has greater mydriatic than cycloplegic effect. The duration of cyclopentalate is too short. Scopolamine is somewhat less effective and shorter acting than atropine, possessing no attributes that are superior to that of atropine. Atropine, on the other hand, is effective for up to about one week after multiple instillation and provides highly effective and predictable cycloplegia. Thus atropine is the agent of choice in the pharmacologic treatment of amblyopia and strabismus.

Indications

Anticholinergic agents are potentially useful in the treatment of accommodative esotropia by nature of their cycloplegic effects. Their actions mimic the use of maximum plus power spectacle lenses by paralyzing accommodation and convergence. Theoretically atropine could be used by itself without refractive correction to

291

reduce or eliminate accommodative esotropia in affected patients, but because of the significant optical blur caused by the cycloplegia, atropine is almost always used in conjunction with refractive correction. This indication for the use of atropine, however, is only rarely considered today (Rethy, 1971).

A much more common usage of atropine in the treatment of strabismus or amblyopia is to "encourage" the hyperopic child to accept the wearing of high plus power spectacle lenses. This was also discussed in Chapter 6 as cyclotherapies for low and moderate degrees of hyperopia. When high plus spectacles are first dispensed, the child initially may have difficulty in relaxing the level of habitual accommodation and will be quite optically blurred. The child will then reject the use of the correction. In order to facilitate acceptance of the spectacles, atropine may be used for a period of several weeks in both eyes to provide cycloplegia. The only way to obtain clear vision under cycloplegia in the moderate to high hyperope will be through the use of spectacles. This technique can prove very effective in getting the child to accept the spectacles. After acceptance has been gained, the atropine is discontinued. The child will usually continue to wear the spectacles even after the effects of the atropine have completely worn off.

It is important to keep in mind that in patients with significant degrees of hyperopia found under cycloplegia, considerably more hyperopia may be encountered weeks or months later—after the child adapts to the spectacle correction and is re-refracted under cycloplegia. The refractive prescription may then need to be increased, especially if there is still some residual accommodative esotropia.

Another potential use of cycloplegic agents in the treatment of amblyopia is in the technique of penalization (Rutstein, 1991). Atropine (or a shorter acting agent such as cyclopentalate) is instilled in the nonamblyopic eye to blur the acuity of that eye to a level below that of the amblyopic eye. Since the cycloplegia will prevent any accommodation, the eye will be blurred at one or more distances depending on the underlying refractive error. If the patient is hyperopic in the nonamblyopic eye, the drug will blur near vision more than it will far vision, and no correction may be required in the nonamblyopic eye. If the eye is myopic, there will be little, if any, effect beyond that present without the drug. Atropine penalization is useful only when the level of amblyopia is relatively mild. If the amblyopia is severe there is usually little, if any, benefit since the degree of blur brought about by the drug is invariably less than that present in the amblyopic eye. Spectacles are usually used in conjunction with the cycloplegic agent.

CHOLINERGIC AGONISTS OR ANTICHOLINESTERASE AGENTS
Mechanism

There are two long-acting anticholinergic agents that are used in the treatment of accommodative esotropia, diisopropylfluorophosphate (DFP) and echothiophate iodide (phospholine iodide or PI). Their pharmacologic action increases the effectiveness of acetylcholine by inactivation of acetylcholinesterase, thereby stimulating accommodation and miosis as well as increasing aqueous output.

The important effect of this class of drugs on patients with accommodative esotropia is to reduce the AC/A ratio. The reduction in accommodative effort results in a decrease in accommodative convergence, thereby reducing the esotropic deviation at near. There may also be a slight further effect caused by induced miosis increasing the depth of focus of the eye, thereby reducing the stimulus to accommodation, but this has not been confirmed (Ripps et al, 1962).

Indications

Clinically, miotic agents may convert an accommodative esotropia into a phoria, allowing for restoration of binocularity. Most authorities stipulate that miotics should not be continued in the absence of some degree of binocularity. Miotics may be indicated in patients who will not tolerate wearing bifocal spectacles. Some authorities believe that miotics are preferable to spectacles because the patients may become overly reliant on the glasses. This argument seems to ignore the possibility of adverse side effects from the drug itself, especially when it is used over a long period of time.

Patients that potentially may benefit from the use of miotics generally have high AC/A ratios and are usually hyperopes. Such patients should be placed on a trial of the medication for about two weeks. If there is a significant decrease in the angle of deviation at near or especially if there is a restoration of binocularity, a continuation of the medical treatment is warranted if there are no adverse effects from the drug itself. If there is not a significant reduction in the angle of deviation, it is likely that the underlying cause of the esotropia is not accommodative, and miotics are contraindicated.

Because more severe miosis occurs with DFP, PI is usually the drug of choice. The starting dosage is generally 1 drop of .125 percent or .06 percent solution each evening before bedtime. If there is a good response to this dosage, the concentration and the frequency of use can be decreased to the lowest dosage that maintains adequate effect.

Miotics may cause the development of iris cysts. Phenylephrine hydrochloride drops are often used concurrently with the miotic as a method of preventing formation of these cysts. The usual dosage is 1 or 2 drops of 2.5 percent phenylephrine hydrocloride per day although some authorities recommend that the pharmacist formulate a single solution combining both the PI and phenylephrine hydrochloride. Any patient that is on miotic therapy must be monitored frequently for the development of these iris cysts or other adverse side effects as well as for the state of the strabismus and visual acuity.

Side Effects

Anticholinergic agents are potent drugs with a host of potential side effects. As was mentioned above, the formation of iris cysts has been associated with the prolonged use of both drugs but perhaps somewhat more readily with use of DFP. These epithelial cysts are located at the inner margin of the pupil and can extend into the pupillary aperture, occasionally progressing to the point of occluding the pupil if miotic therapy is inadvertently continued over the long term. Phenylephrine hydrochloride has been found to prevent, or at least to minimize, this hypertrophy of the iris.

More worrisome is the effect that anticholinesterase drugs have on cholinesterase levels in red blood cells and in plasma. These agents decrease the rate of hydrolysis of succinylcholine, a drug used to facilitate general anesthesia. If a child who is on miotic therapy undergoes emergency surgery and the use of succinylcholine in the anesthesia, respiratory paralysis may ensue. Parents must be clearly made aware of this potential risk.

Systemic side effects in the form of excessive salivation, lacrimation, urination, defecation or diarrhea, and sweating (SLUDS) may be encountered, but usually are not clinically significant in the absence of overdosage. Ocular effects include iris cysts and the theoretical possibility of retinal detachment and cataracts, which have not been reported in children. Photophobia, headache, and browache have been noted. A *miotic upper respiratory syndrome* consisting of rhinorrhea, a sensation of chest constriction, cough, and conjunctival injection has also been reported (Fraunfelder, 1991).

BOTULINUM TOXIN

In the late 1970s, Dr. Alan Scott began investigating the pharmacologic treatment of strabismus. He experimented with the direct injection of various neurotoxins into the extraocular muscles, the theory being that, by causing a temporary paralysis of an extraocular muscle, a change in the alignment of the eye could be produced. This would be analogous to the acute esotropia that occurs in a sixth cranial nerve palsy. Botulinum toxin type A has proven to be useful as a substitute for, or as an adjunct to, strabismus surgery in many cases (Scott, 1981). After a ten-year investigational period under FDA (Food and Drug Administration) regulation during which time over 8000 injections were given, the drug is now available for clinical use under the trade name *Oculinum.*

Mechanism

Botulinum toxin is a large protein molecule, which following intramuscular injection is bound at the receptor sites on motor nerve terminals within 24 hours. The toxin remains at the nerve terminal for from several days to a few weeks. Here it interferes with the release of the neurotransmitter acetylcholine. When the toxin is injected in therapeutic doses, the effect remains localized to the injection region, which results in a denervation muscle paralysis with the onset three to five days after injection. The duration of total extraocular muscle paralysis can last from two to eight weeks with eventual recovery. The purpose of botulinum therapy in strabismus is to achieve lasting improvement through secondary effects of the toxin-induced paralysis. Toxin-induced paralysis lasting for several weeks can result in permanently changed ocular alignment as the injected muscle lengthens and its antagonist contracts (Figures 15.1, 15.2, 15.3, and 15.4). For this to work, the antagonist must be a functioning muscle, not restricted due to scar formation. If the patient has the potential for binocular vision the change in alignment produced by the toxin is more likely to be permanent.

Botulinum is prepared for clinical use in units. The drug is supplied in freeze-dried form and is reconstituted with unpreserved saline solution to a concentration of 5.0 units/0.1 ml. The dose can be increased or decreased to modify the effect. The estimated systemic toxic dose is 40 units/kg body weight. No systemic paralytic effect has been seen or suspected in any patient treated with the small doses used for

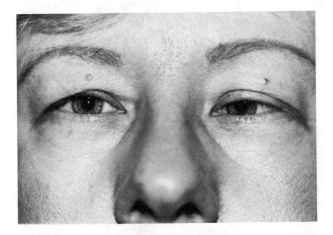

Figure 15.1 A patient with a left esotropia prior to injection of left medial rectus muscle with botulinum toxin.

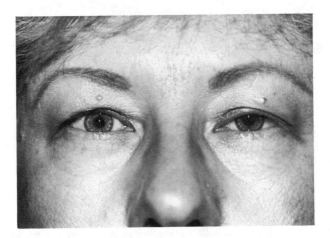

Figure 15.2 The same patient as in Figure 15.1, one week following injection, showing orthotropia in primary gaze.

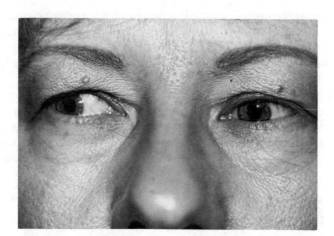

Figure 15.3 The patient has decreased adduction in the left eye secondary to toxin induced paralysis of the left medial rectus muscle.

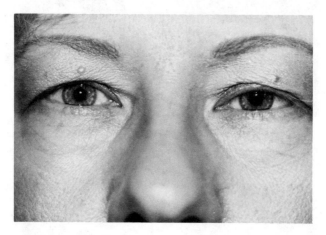

Figure 15.4 Six months postinjection, the patient remains orthophoric.

strabismus. Antibodies to the toxin have not been detected in patients given small doses for ocular use so repeat injections can be given if necessary.

Injection Technique

The injection technique involves transconjunctival injection under topical anesthesia performed in an outpatient setting. Topical vasoconstrictors are administered to help avoid bleeding at the injection site. An EMG (electromyogram) electrode

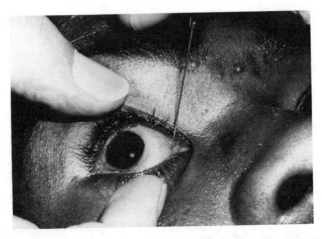

Figure 15.5 Needle is passed through the conjunctiva medially while the patient adducts the right eye.

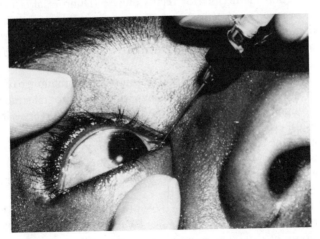

Figure 15.6 The patient is asked to adduct the right eye, and an EMG response is produced, indicating that the needle is in the muscle and that the injection is given.

needle is attached to a 1 cc syringe containing 0.1 cc of toxin. The needle is connected to an audible EMG amplifier.

The needle is passed along the surface of the globe posteriorly into the belly of the extraocular muscle. The tip is approximately 2.5 cm into the muscle from its insertion point. Once the needle is in the muscle, the patient is asked to perform a version to cause the muscle to fire. For example, when the needle is in the medial rectus muscle, the patient is told to adduct the eye.

A characteristic noise is heard as the muscle contracts and the injection is given (Figures 15.5 and 15.6). This technique involves minimal discomfort to the patient but necessitates a certain level of cooperation. There is a minimal recovery period (minutes) in most patients, and they can resume normal activities on the day of the injection.

Indications

Treatment of horizontal forms of strabismus is the area in which the greatest amount of experience exists (Scott, 1989). In patients followed six months or more after the last injection, strabismus was reduced an average of 65 percent depending on the type of strabismus. Fifty-six percent of adults injected achieved a deviation of 10 prism diopters or less. Overcorrections occurred in fewer than 1 percent of patients. Best results have been obtained with injection of the medial rectus muscle for esotropia although the lateral rectus muscle can be injected to treat exotropia. Large strabismus angles tended to return to preinjection positions and required repeat injections more frequently than smaller angles.

Vertical strabismus can be corrected in some cases, particularly hypotropia treated with injection of the inferior rectus muscle (Dunn et al, 1986). It is very difficult to inject the superior rectus muscle or the superior oblique muscle selectively. Frequently when this is attempted, a marked ptosis is produced as the toxin diffuses into the levator muscle. It is also very difficult to inject the inferior oblique muscle using present techniques.

Present indications for treatment of strabismus with botulinum toxin and for the treatment of postoperative residual strabismus include horizontal strabismus of less than 40 prism diopters. Botulinum can be used in cases where surgery is inappropriate as in prephthisical eyes or those with active thyroid disease.

Injection can be combined with strabismus surgery when there is reluctance to operate on more than two extraocular muscles in the same eye to avoid anterior segment ischemia. In some cases, the toxin is injected directly into the muscle under direct visualization in the operating room.

One of the best indications for the use of botulinum toxin is for the treatment of esotropia resulting from sixth nerve palsy (Wagner & Frohman, 1989). In these cases the antagonist medial rectus muscle is injected in the eye with the palsy. This can balance the paralysis, straighten the eye to correct primary gaze diplopia, and prevent secondary contracture of the medial rectus muscle. Future surgery may be obviated in such cases.

Relative contraindications to the use of botulinum toxin include large deviations greater than 40 diopters, restrictive strabismus as it occurs in Duane's syndrome or in some postoperative cases.

Complications that have been reported with the use of botulinum toxin include scleral perforation, retrobulbar hemorrhage, and local conjunctival inflammation. The toxin can diffuse into adjacent muscles and produce an unwanted vertical deviation. Transient ptosis, lasting for a few weeks, has been reported in as many as 16 percent of patients injected (Figures 15.7 and 15.8). No systemic illness has been produced following injection of the toxin (Scott, 1989). Many patients report having diplopia during the first few weeks following injection. This is usually short-lived as there is frequently a temporary overcorrection. This is desirable for fusion in many cases.

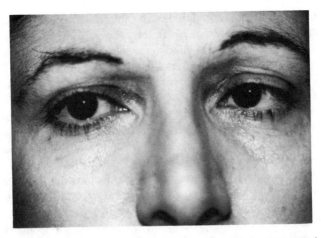

Figure 15.7 A patient with left esotropia prior to injection of the left medial rectus muscle.

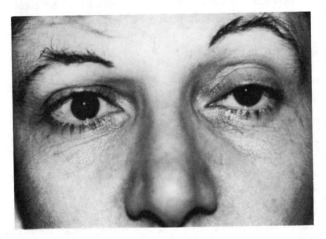

Figure 15.8 One week after injection, eyes are aligned but the patient has transient ptosis of the left upper lid.

Although the toxin is not considered a complication, patients must be warned that the effect of the toxin may not be permanent and that the strabismus may not be totally corrected. Some patients may require additional injections or strabismus surgery.

Use in Children

The treatment of strabismus in children under the age of about 12 years with botulinum toxin is still being defined. The toxin is only approved for people over 12 years of age, but many children have been treated under investigational protocols.

Some children can be nurtured through the same injection procedure as was described above for adults. Younger children and those less cooperative need to be injected in the operating room. In such cases, intravenous ketamine anesthesia is administered, which adequately sedates the child while preserving the EMG response. Some surgeons feel that if anesthesia in the operating room is required, one should correct the strabismus with the more definitive surgery.

Results in the injection of children have shown 63 percent of those injected achieved a deviation of 10 prism diopters or less. Exotropia in children was the most common undercorrected strabismus category. A recent study of 72 children injected between the ages of 4 months and 13 years reported that 85 percent had 10 prism diopters or less of deviation at the time of the last examination (Magoon, 1989). In this study, complications included transient ptosis and hyperdeviations, which always resolved in 6 months, often only several weeks following injection.

There is a great deal of interest in the treatment of congenital esotropia by injecting the medial rectus muscle in the first year of life (Magoon, 1984). These children often adopt a horizontal face turn following paralysis of the muscle with botulinum. This is evidence that they have fusional potential. Such treatment has been associated with long-term stability of alignment in some cases.

REFERENCES

Dunn WJ, Arnold AC, O'Connor PS. Botulinum toxin for the treatment of dysthyroid ocular myopathy. Ophthalmol 1986;93:470–475.

Fraunfelder FT. Ocular Toxicology. In Physicians Desk Reference for Ophthalmology. Oradell, NJ: Medical Economics Co, 1991;19.

Magoon EH. Chemodenervation of strabismic children. Ophthalmol 1989;96:931–934.

Magoon EH. Botulinum toxin chemo-denervation for strabismus in infants and children. J Pediatr Ophthalmol Strab 1984;21:110–113.

Rethy I. Stabilized accommodative factors in esotropia. In Ferrer OM ed. Ocular Motility Vol. II. Int Ophthalmol Clin 1971;27.

Ripps H, Chin NB, Siegel IM, et al. The effect of pupil size on accommodative convergence, and the AC/A ratio. Invest Ophthalmol 1962;1:127–135.

Rutstein R. Alternative treatment for amblyopia. Problems in Optometry 1991; 3:331–354.

Scott AB. Botulinum toxin treatment of strabismus. Clinical Modules for Ophthalmologists 1989;7:1–11.

Scott AB. Botulinum toxin injection of eye muscles to correct strabismus. Trans Am Ophthalmol Soc 1981;79:734–770.

Wagner RS and Frohman LP. Long-term results: Botulinum for sixth nerve palsy. J Pediatr Ophthalmol Strab 1989;26:106–108.

16

Vision Therapy for Infants, Preschoolers, and School-Aged Children

Leonard J. Press

The ability to conduct vision therapy (VT) with a pediatric patient demands considerable skill. It requires appropriate identification of the clinical concern, an individualized treatment program, and a therapist adept at interpreting the child's responses and modifying instructional sets accordingly. The therapist is rarely one individual; rather the responsibility is shared among the optometrist, an in-office assistant, and one of the child's parents.

As it was practiced from the 1930s through the 1970s, VT was primarily a treatment modality for children. Although VT has been expanded to include significant numbers of adult patients, optometrists today benefit from the wealth of techniques and activities for pediatric patients that were developed during the pioneer period. There are two contemporary aspects that have great impact on the structuring of a VT program for children. One is computerization, which allows the optometrist to present the program in an entirely different light. The demonstration of a computerized therapy activity to prospective patients shows the contemporary nature of the program and signals to the child that this will be a challenging yet enjoyable experience.

The second aspect that impacts VT is the socioeconomic forces that shape a family's experience. Who is available at home to help the child? Is the home conducive to therapy, or is the situation chaotic? Will home VT be a rewarding experience or a source of conflict between family members? In addition, the financial arrangements may be a factor and must be clearly delineated at the outset.

VISION THERAPY (VT) FROM THE CHILD'S VIEWPOINT

A common question posed by parents when they are first informed of a child's visual dysfunction is, "Why didn't Jimmy ever tell us that he was having a problem with his eyes?" The answer usually given is, "Because Jimmy presumes that everybody sees the same way he does." Sometimes the child will be afraid to verbalize a problem to a parent. At other times, as was discussed in Chapter 1, a child will have told a parent about a problem, but the parent discounts its significance until it is reinforced clinically by an optometrist.

During the initial evaluation, the examiner obtains insight into how the child utilizes vision. Some children are visually attentive; others have difficulty understanding instructional sets. From observation of the child during the evaluation and in consultation with the parents the examiner can project how well a child will do in VT. All this notwithstanding young children rarely have any conception of why they are in VT, and wonder why they are being subjected to these repetitive activities. Older children, particularly when they are asymptomatic, may perceive that nothing is wrong with their eyes or vision and see little purpose in participating. Consequently the children will be successful to the extent that they are responsive to the conditions created by the optometrist and rest of the therapy team. For younger patients this may require a lot of "show-and-tell" and promises of reward. For older children, enjoyment, discovery, and reminders of benefits to be obtained may be the key ingredients.

VISION THERAPY (VT) FROM THE PARENT'S VIEWPOINT

Most parents will extend themselves for their children to a greater degree than they would for their personal needs. When VT is explained as the treatment of choice for their child, most parents will find the time and financial resources to improve their child's performance.

Since vision is a learned process, VT is, in part, a learning experience. Parents will vary widely in their ability to be active partners in this experience. The optometrist must be sensitive to the capability of a particular parent or older sibling to be a home therapy assistant. When the parent does not have good rapport with the child at home, VT becomes one more area of potential conflict. It may be helpful to invite the parent into the therapy area during the last 5 minutes of the session to observe how the therapist interacts with the child. Whenever a new activity is prescribed for home therapy, it is advisable to have parents demonstrate their understanding of what is being asked of the child.

THEORETICAL AND APPLIED VISION THERAPY (VT)

VT can be categorized by age levels, by conditions treated, or by specific skills acquired during the therapy process. The primary emphasis in this book is on the age level of the child. The reason for this approach is twofold. First, the categorization by types of conditions treated is amply addressed in other sources. In contrast, there is a paucity of centralized information addressing techniques specifically oriented toward younger children. Second, individualizing the instructional set for children can be best done in the context of learning theory applied to various age levels. If VT is in part an education or reeducation in visual thinking, age grouping is as significant in the therapy room as it is in the classroom.

Griffin (1982) presented an in-depth discussion of learning theories applied to binocular therapy. He subdivided learning theory into two categories: stimulus-response and cognitive. The stimulus-response theory would dictate conditioning through repeated exercise, which predominates in classical orthoptic VT as well as in association of successful performance with some pleasurable experience. For younger children, this mandates that the therapy materials themselves be pleasant and that performance of the activity is directly rewarded. For older children, the reward may take the form of a sticker or of a selection from a treasure chest of miniature toys.

In contrast, the cognitive approach to learning predominates in the VT programs of the developmental optometrist. Cognitivists believe that if the appropriate conditions for learning are arranged through explanation and sequencing, patients of any age group can build intuitive thought. Piagetian cognitive theory tempers expectations of a child's performance based on the periods of cognitive development in which they exist. Griffin (1982) used convergence insufficiency therapy techniques to illustrate the extent to which a child can be expected to participate in VT in each of the four main developmental periods identified by Piaget (Table 16.1).

VISION THERAPY (VT) FOR THE INFANT

Since vision is a learned process, it would seem sensible to attribute all visual anomalies to improper learning. This, however, would be a gross assumption and oversimplification. Visual anomalies stem from a variety of sources. Some conditions are primary structural abnormalities that result secondarily in abnormal visual function. Others are primary developmental abnormalities that result in secondary structural alterations. Visual deprivation during sensitive periods in visual development results in morphologic changes at virtually every microanatomic level of the visual system.

In this section, VT for amblyopia and strabismus will be emphasized. This is not to imply that infants do not exhibit other anomalies in binocular or perceptual-motor development. Rather, these anomalies can usually be addressed by more global recommendations for an enriched visual environment such as:

> Keep a dim light on in the room at all times so that baby has something to look at during times of playful quiet.

Table 16.1 Piagetian constructs of vision therapy (VT) for convergence insufficiency

Age (years)	Period	Technique
0–2	Sensorimotor intelligence	Pencil push-ups
2–7	Preoperational representations	Physiological diplopia
7–11	Concrete operations	Chiastopic fusion
11–up	Formal operations	Aperture rule

From JR Griffin. Binocular anomalies: Procedures for vision therapy. 2d ed. Chicago: Professional Press, 1982:438–448.

Periodically change the position of the crib in the room to provide a varied binocular visual environment.

Periodically change the relative position of baby in the crib to provide a varied visual angle of commonly fixated objects.

Attach a mobile to the crib with brightly colored rotating objects so that the baby can follow the objects.

Suspend a *play-and-learn center* on the side of the crib with mirror, rotating ball, and rattle, and periodically change its position.

Give baby the opportunity to follow your eyes in different directions, moving up, down, left, right, and obliquely.

Assist baby in hand-eye coordination by giving blocks to hold, to bang, and to stack eventually.

Be a partner in baby's experimentation; when children are old enough to sit in a high chair, they will playfully knock things off their trays and watch them fall to the floor.

As baby matures, give it the opportunity to creep and develop bilateral integration; do not rush the walking stage.

Give baby wide-open spaces to explore as well as stairs to climb. Use a safety gate when not interacting with baby so that it does not fall down the stairs.

Amblyopia

Occlusion and prescriptive lenses are the centerpieces of amblyopia therapy. In strabismic amblyopia, getting the infant to accept occlusion is paramount. In refractive amblyopia, getting the infant to wear the prescription is paramount. Success in VT for strasbismic and refractive amblyopia requires individualized treatment approaches.

Strabismic Amblyopia

Strabismic amblyopia requires occlusion of the strabismic eye. The more occlusion is accomplished, the more quickly the amblyopia will resolve. It is difficult to keep an infant occluded. There are many kinds of patches. The Coverlet Eye Occlusor (see Beiersdorf, Inc., Appendix A) is preferred because it is more difficult for the infant to peel off. If its strong adhesive causes a skin rash, the Opticlude Eye Patch (see Appendix A, Personal Care Products/3M) can be used. Another alternative is the elastic band eye patch, although it is more bothersome around the head and can be removed more readily.

The ideal time to patch infants is during a nap, at which time they are unaware of the change that comes about with covering the better eye. When the infant rejects wearing the patch, a compromise must be struck. The concept of minimal occlusion, in which specific activities are done while the child is patched, is discussed in detail in the sections on preschool and school-aged VT.

Penalization is a passive approach to VT that can be considered a partial form of occlusion. It can be used in instances when conventional occlusion is unsuccessful and was discussed in detail in Chapter 15. When refractive amblyopia coexists with strabismic amblyopia, the Rx (prescription) should be used during periods of occlusion or VT. Activities that can be done during periods of occlusion or penalization are (Griffin 1982):

> Associating attention, love, and kindness with patching
> Associating reward with patching (for example, favorite foods, toys)
> Stimulating light and sound by watching television or show-and-tell
> Peek-a-boo games
> Playing with suspended toys and watching or kicking mobile
> Following or patting a rolling ball
> Motor involvement such as creeping or crawling appropriate for the
>   developmental level
> Playing with flashlight or bright objects
> Handling blocks or stacking toys, particularly if they have depth
> Catching a rolling ball with hands or capturing the ball with legs or feet

Refractive Amblyopia

Full-time wear of the appropriate Rx is the key element in refractive amblyopia. Since binocular vision is usually present, any gain in vision will be readily integrated with the contralateral eye. Consequently occlusion of the better eye may accelerate the improvement in acuity, but it is not essential unless strabismic amblyopia coexists. Some practitioners suggest that occlusion should be avoided in intermittent strabismus since it might precipitate constant strabismus. This is a concern if the patient is not being monitored on a regular basis. If the infant is being closely followed, occlusion can be discontinued or reinstituted as judged by alignment without any long-term deleterious effect on binocularity.

In anisometropia, an Rx is imperative only if there is sufficient power to account for the amblyopia, typically 3D of anisosphere or 1.5D of anisocylinder. Since meridional refractive status in infancy is highly labile, retinoscopy should be conducted monthly to confirm the astigmatic portion of the Rx. Visual acuity with the Rx should be monitored with the Teller acuity cards discussed in Chapter 3. In accommodative esotropia, which does not usually onset until after 12 months of age, the appropriate hyperopic or bifocal Rx must be worn as much as possible.

Occlusion Amblyopia

Occlusion amblyopia, an iatrogenic form of deprivation amblyopia, is of potential concern. If the patch is worn continuously, the vision of the occluded eye will decrease. This may be seen in isolated cases when the infant's arms have been immobilized and is more likely to be seen when the patient is not being monitored at frequent intervals. This has led to the suggestion that the number of consecutive days occluded should not exceed the age of the child in years. For example, a three-year-old child would have the nonamblyopic eye patched three consecutive days, then one day off, with the cycle repeating itself. If there is coexisting strabismus, the patch is transferred to the amblyopic eye on the alternate day of the cycle. For example, the three-year-old would have the nonstrabismic eye patched three consecutive days followed by one day with the patch on the strabismic eye, with the cycle repeating itself. The purpose of not allowing binocular viewing is to discourage development of anomalous correspondence.

From a practical standpoint, occlusion amblyopia is rarely encountered with older infants and young children who find a way to peek or fuss until the parent removes the patch. With infants under 12 months, docile children, or overly-aggressive parents, it is of particular concern. If a drop in acuity of the contralateral eye or a switch in fixation preference is noted, temporary discontinuation in occlusion or a brief period of reverse occlusion can usually remedy the situation.

Strabismus

In contrast to the relatively passive approach to amblyopia, strabismus requires more active intervention (Press, 1982). This discussion of strabismus centers on esotropia, as it accounts for 85 percent of all infantile strabismus (Wick, 1979). The principal goals in treatment are to optimize bilateral integration, to discourage anomalous correspondence, and to attain cosmetic alignment of the eyes. The steps to attain these goals are:

Optical compensation of refractive error
Trial period of +3.00 add for esotropia
Application of binasal tapes to spectacle frame
Fresnel prism to attain sensory fusion
Abduction calisthenics monocularly or with binasal tapes
Three-dimensional eye-hand coordination activities
Creeping and crawling with bilateral patterns
Change of crib position and direction of mobile rotation in crib
Daily exposure to gingham patterns

Binasal Occlusion

Sector occlusion, the concept of occluding only a portion of the spectacle lens, has been applied successfully as a sensory orthoptic tool in Europe for many years. Its first proponent in the United States was Louis Jaques (1950), and it has been well-recognized by now by behavioral optometrists as an effective tool in strabismus therapy (Tassinari, 1990). Binasal tapes are applied to the nasal portion of the spectacle lenses in esotropia to block the nasal visual field, and the tapes angled slightly inward to allow for convergence at near. The principles of binasal occlusion (Schapero, 1971) are:

1. To promote the alternation of fixation as objects in the right or left field of vision are fixated, since they are only visible to one or the other eye
2. Through alternation of fixation, to maintain acuity in the two eyes or to improve acuity in an amblyopic eye
3. To eliminate the use of suppression and anomalous correspondence by blocking the field of the nonfixating eye as it deviates behind the occluder

4. By using steps 2 and 3 to effect a reduction in strabismic deviation
5. To permit the possibility of binocular fixation

Translucent tape is usually used as this allows the position of the tapes to be changed when that becomes necessary. The procedure for applying binasal tapes (Figure 16.1) is:

1. Place a strip of ½-inch wide translucent tape on the front of the spectacle lens with the edge of the tape draped over the nasal bezel of the frame.
2. If the esotropia lessens, reposition the tape to keep pace with the realigned position of the eye. If the tape is moved too far toward the temporal, the eye will revert toward the original esotropic position.
3. If the esotropia does not lessen, occlude the fellow eye and leave the outer edge of the tape at the nasal pupillary border.
4. Angle the tape inward by 10 degrees to allow for convergence, and trim the edge of the tape at the frame bezel with a blade or paper clip edge.

Fresnel Prism

An infant can be kept in a state of sensory orthophoria by wearing spectacles with the amount of Fresnel prism required to neutralize the strabismic angle. Fresnel prism is available in powers up to 30 prism diopters. If the strabismus is alternating, the prism should be split evenly between both eyes. Higher-powered Fresnel prisms distort the visual image and can exert a partial occlusion effect. Consequently when there is evidence of amblyopia or a strong fixation preference, the prism should be unevenly split so that the higher prism power is placed before the fixating eye. If there is a vertical component, horizontal prism is placed on one lens and vertical prism on the other. The angle of strabismus needs to be checked at least once a week to ascertain that the amount of prism is appropriate. Fresnel prism is complementary to other means of therapy such as binasal tapes and ocular calisthenics (Greenwald, 1979).

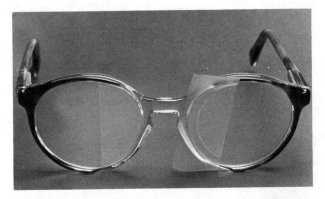

Figure 16.1 Translucent tape is placed over the frame. When the final position of the tape is determined, the edge is trimmed with a blade at the bezel of the frame.

Ocular Calisthenics

Abduction calisthenics are indicated to counteract the adduction of the esotropic eye. This consists of holding the infant's head still while moving an object of interest from the central toward the peripheral field or of moving objects inward from the periphery. It is particularly useful to do this with binasal tapes in place. The nasal tape prevents the infant from cross-fixating the opposite field with the esotropic eye. From a behavioral standpoint, this procedure also helps build peripheral awareness and decreases attention to the central field. Finger puppets and favorite foods are effective stimuli for sustaining interest during abduction. In addition, mobiles can be used with infants lying on their backs and the objects rotating in a clockwise direction for left esotropia or counterclockwise direction for right esotropia.

Spatial Localization

Research has shown that strabismic amblyopes exhibit characteristic spatial uncertainty (Bedell & Flom, 1981). Infants should therefore be engaged in tasks that require depth and spatial judgment. An activity that most infants enjoy is having a series of cups varied in size and being asked to place the smaller ones into the larger ones. A similar activity is the stacking of different sized rings on a pole (Figure 16.2). These and similar Fisher-Price items are readily available in toy stores. The procedures can be attempted on a monocular, as well as a binocular, basis.

Black Flannel Board

Anaglyphic glasses may be used to monitor suppression when suitable red and green objects are placed against a black flannel background. Place the object on the

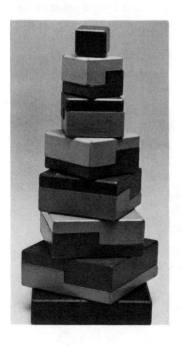

Figure 16.2   Rings, squares, or divided shapes can be stacked on a pole to aid spatial localization and depth perception.

black flannel board without the anaglyphic glasses. Note the infant's reaching behavior or reaction to the object. Compare this to the reaction obtained when the red and green glasses are in place. Try this first to confirm that the object truly cancels against the black background as opposed to being visible as a dark object.

Centration Range Extension

In therapy, take advantage of the fact that many esotropes have a proximal point in visual space where their visual axes cross and where they are therefore binocular. It is not possible to confirm this point with the preverbal child other than by performing a cover test in conjunction with critically observing the corneal light reflexes. If a centration point can be documented, the VT procedures mentioned above should be initially conducted at this distance and progressively moved outward.

Gingham Patterns

In the early 1970s, research done with cats who were rendered strabismic seemed to show that binocular neurons could be preserved by exposure to wide-field, repetitive geometric patterns (Blakemore & Van Sluyters, 1974). The basis for this observation was that, even with the eyes misaligned, corresponding retinal points were stimulated. This led to the suggestion that strabismic infants be exposed to gingham patterns as much as possible (Forrest, 1978) and an instrument designed for this purpose (Awaya, 1983). This theory has never been substantiated with infants but falls into the realm of treatment that can do no harm and may possibly be of benefit.

VISION THERAPY FOR THE PRESCHOOL CHILD

The preschooler is capable of more active VT than is the infant. VT sessions will probably need to be modified into several periods of activity interspersed with free play. Numerous activities must be programmed for the child due to the characteristically short attention spans of this age. As with infants, our emphasis here is on amblyopia and strabismus.

Amblyopia

Appropriate refractive compensation is required before amblyopia therapy is instituted. Direct occlusion should be the initial therapy approach irrespective of fixation status. Should this be unproductive, inverse occlusion can be implemented. Although constant occlusion yields the quickest result, it is difficult to obtain the child's compliance. The theory of minimal occlusion holds that brief periods of patching during intense visual activity are more efficacious than longer periods of forced patching when there is pouting or unstructured activity. Although occlusion is warranted for strabismic amblyopia, it is not essential in the treatment of refractive amblyopia.

The therapist and parent must empathize with the child who is being occluded during amblyopia therapy. Children are bright enough to know that, when the nonamblyopic eye is covered, they cannot function as well. From a child's point of view occlusion makes no sense at all, and it may be regarded as a form of punishment. It is analogous to asking them to learn how to ride a bicycle with one hand tied behind their back.

There is little solace to the child in reasoning that covering the good eye will make the weak eye stronger. A better approach is to associate patching with a time of enjoyment and reward. Rather than giving an outright bribe, if the child has favorite foods or activities, these can be indulged in while the patch is being worn. If the amblyopia is severe and the child is too disabled by total occlusion, a graded form of occlusion can be applied. This involves the successive application of filters with graduated occlusion density (see Appendix A, Franel Optical Supply).

Refractive Amblyopia

Monocular therapy activities complement the improvement that ensues by wearing the appropriate Rx. These activities can be broadly categorized as either information acquisition skills or information processing skills (Colorado Vision Consultants, 1985). Sample activities are:

Accommodative rock
Dot-to-dot drawing
Road map games and jigsaw puzzles
Groffman tracings
Figure-ground games (hidden pictures/words)
Visual discrimination games (likes/differences)
Spatial localization (stick-in-straw)
Eye-hand coordination (stringing beads; pegboard)
Saccadic activities (Hart chart; saccadic fixator)

Strabismus

In order to maintain the improvement derived from monocular activities, these skills must be integrated into the binocular behavior of the child. The concept of conducting monocular training in a binocular field was introduced to facilitate this integration (Cohen, 1981). Most of these techniques involve red-green glasses for anaglyphic cancellation. The following sections discuss the primary techniques.

Modified Brock Posture Board

Have the child "help" you draw pictures with an orange marker onto an 8″ × 10″ white sheet of paper. Place the white paper on top of an 8″ × 10″ red acetate sheet. Have the child put on anaglyphic glasses with the red filter over the amblyopic eye. Shine a white penlight from behind the red filter onto the white sheet of paper. The penlight will appear as a red light on the white sheet of paper and can only be seen by the amblyopic eye. Move the light to different locations in the picture and ask the child to identify where the light is located.

Anaglyphic Coloring Books

If the child has adequate fine eye-hand coordination, there are numerous anaglyphic coloring books that are available. These usually involve red or orange printed material that cancels with the green filter. Therefore the green filter is placed in front of the amblyopic eye while the child traces or colors the pictures.

Anaglyphic Television

When children are old enough to sustain interest in a TV show such as Sesame Street, they can view one through anaglyphic glasses. Place the red filter in the center of the TV screen with the red lens in front of the amblyopic eye. Then instruct the parents to let the child sit as close to the TV set as they please in order to make the entire picture seeable at once. The child should be questioned about any part of the screen that is black or missing. If the child is old enough to play video games, they can be used in the same manner (Press, 1981).

Lite-Brite

This is an inexpensive, commercially available toy (Hasbro) involving the placement of translucent pegs into holes that are rear-illuminated (Figure 16.3). Remove the peg screen, and place a red acetate filter beneath it (Getz, 1990). A pattern is prepunched, and clear pegs are used so that red shines through the pegs when they are placed into the holes. When the red filter of the anaglyphic glasses is placed before the strabismic eye, only that eye can see the pegs. If the contralateral eye is used, the peg looks black and is indistinguishable from the surrounding black.

Sherman Playing Cards

These are a specially designed deck of playing cards in which some are printed in red ink on a white background and others are printed in black ink on a red background. When the red filter is placed in front of the amblyopic eye, only that eye can see the black figures on the red background.

One-Half Vectogram

The Mother Goose vectogram is used with the slide corresponding to the amblyopic eye placed into the vectogram holder. The slides are polarized so that the entire slide is only seen by the eye for which it is marked. If the elements in the picture can be identified, the child is using the amblyopic eye. When the ability to memorize sets in or for variety, turn the slide upside down out of the child's view, and expose it again while asking if the king is standing on his head or on his feet.

Brock Transparencies

The Brock Transparency Set (see Appendix A, Mast Keystone Co.) is the contemporary version of the Brock Stereo Motivator. It may be used with its own

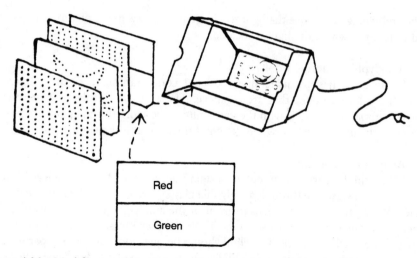

Figure 16.3 Modification of Lite-Brite to allow anaglyphic suppression control. Clear acetate sheet, horizontally divided, half red, half green, and taped together. Dimensions are the same as those of the printed picture patterns. Put the colored filter in first—before inserting either of the peg screens. (From DJ Getz. Strabismus and amblyopia, 2d ed. Santa Ana, Calif: Optometric Extension Program, 1990:26–30.)

illuminated box at nearpoint or with an overhead transparency projector at a distance to achieve anaglyphic cancellation.

Amblyoscope

The amblyoscope is useful with preschoolers who have adequate cognitive and maturational abilities (Wick, 1990). Many of the Clement-Clarke series of slides for the Synoptophore contain fusion targets with adequate suppression controls suitable to this age group (Figure 16.4). The amblyoscope provides a potent medium for encouraging fusion. The therapist can inhibit dominance of the nonstrabismic eye by varying the target illumination or by flickering the target. Success with the amblyoscope is a bridge to fusion in freespace.

VISION THERAPY (VT) FOR THE SCHOOL-AGED CHILD

Once children have attained school age, they have sufficient cognitive skills to be active participants in VT. This section discusses techniques for amblyopia and strabismus therapy that build on the principles in the preceding sections. It also introduces procedures for accommodative, vergence, ocular-motor, and developmental-perceptual therapy.

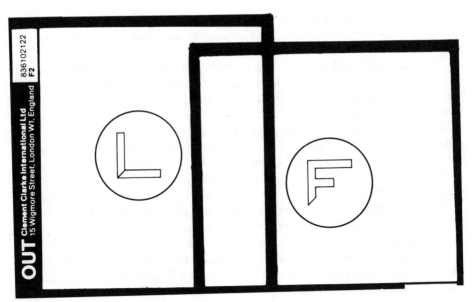

Figure 16.4 A Synoptophore slide suitable for young children. It supplies a fused percept (E) which cannot be predicted from rapid alternation of the eyes.

Amblyopia

Occlusion, the initial treatment in strabismic amblyopia, presents two significant problems for the school-aged child. First, a child will find it difficult to function in the academic environment if visual acuity is less than 20/70. Second, most children will be sensitive about their appearance and about the comments of their peers. For these reasons, occlusion should be applied initially after school hours and on weekends. It is helpful to simulate for the parent the initial level of vision that their child will have while the eye is patched. This can be done by occluding one eye and placing a fogging lens on the other eye that will reduce acuity to the same level as the child's amblyopic eye. When the child's acuity has improved to at least 20/60, the child can be sent to school with the patch on and with a request for preferential seating for the child close to the blackboard.

If the child has eccentric fixation, fovealization therapy should be instituted with Haidinger Brush/MIT, afterimage transfer, and accommodative stimulation. Pleoptic therapy is rarely used. As has been mentioned previously, direct occlusion is recommended prior to inverse occlusion. If this fails, inverse occlusion can be used to weaken the embeddedness of eccentric fixation. Improvement in accommodative amplitude and facility is an important element in normalizing the visual processing of the amblyopic child (Ciuffreda et al, 1991). Accommodative activities are similar to those used for general purposes as will be reviewed below. One specific, high-yield integrative technique uses the plexiglass letter chart slide inserted into the MIT. The therapist places minus lenses in front of the amblyopic eye while the child points to each letter. The child must keep the Haidinger Brush centered on the tip of the pointer.

Ocular-motor performance must be improved. Pursuits and fixation training can be carried out in standard fashion with the Marsden Ball, the Wayne Saccadic Fixator, and the Pegboard Rotator. The distance Hart chart is used for saccadic fixation as will be reviewed in the section on accommodation, vergence, and ocular motility later in this chapter. If the print is too small to allow fixation at a reasonable distance or when contour interaction is a problem, the chart can be cut into smaller sections and photocopied into a larger size. Ann Arbor Tracking workbooks (see Appendix A, Ann Arbor Publishers) can be used in similar fashion for nearpoint with the print enlarged or reduced on a copier to conform to the best level of resolution.

Spatial awareness and localization are two additional skills that should be developed. This can be done through use of the Wayne Saccadic Fixator, the Pegboard Rotator, and the Stick-in-Straw techniques. These procedures are elaborated in the section on visual-motor integration and organization later in this chapter. When the amblyopia is secondary to strabismus, the amblyopia will recur unless some degree of binocular cooperation is attained.

Strabismus

The older the child and the more long-standing the strabismus, the greater is the probability that anomalous correspondence (ARC) exists, particularly in constant unilateral esotropia. ARC is not a deterrent to therapy for exotropia but does lessen its prognosis as was reviewed in chapter 13. There are two basic approaches to adopt when ARC is present.

1. Break down the ARC to permit bifoveal fusion and motor alignment.
2. If the subjective angle is greater than 10 prism diopters, leave the adaptation alone and work on moving both the objective and subjective angles toward zero.

Look at strabismus from a parent's point of view. If the objective angle can be reduced to within 15 prism diopters so that it is not cosmetically noticeable and if an improvement in any aspect of binocularity can be obtained, therapy has been successful. It makes little difference to the parent or to the long-term stability of the results if fusional movements are anomalous and stereopsis is less than ideal. Therefore, it is appropriate to generalize that if the child shows the capacity for third-degree fusion in the amblyoscope or has normal correspondence under at least one test condition prior to therapy, it is worth the effort to establish normal correspondence (NRC). If not, one must question the cost-benefit ratio of the time and effort involved, particularly if the child is not motivated.

There are two broad schools of thought in doing strabismus therapy with children. One approach is to concentrate on in-instrument training to break down suppression patterns. This is predominantly an orthoptic approach. An alternative approach is to conduct primarily activities without instruments with early emphasis on equalization of monocular skills and the establishing of efficient body bilaterality. This approach is based on the theory that strabismus is not just an ocular or sensory-motor imbalance but rather a manifestation of a generalized body imbalance resulting from faulty development. There are studies that support the notion that strabismic children have abnormal body balance in gait and postural sway (Odenrick et al, 1984). A causal relationship between abnormal bilateral development and strabismus or between bilateral training and binocular abilities has yet to be firmly established (Birnbaum, 1974). Although this tempers the reliance on developmental training as an exclusive approach to eliminating strabismus, body bilaterality activities are a useful adjunct to antisuppression and fusion procedures (McGraw, 1991). Body bilaterality activities include such procedures as walk rail, balance board, angels in the snow, and bimanual chalkboard circles and are reviewed later in this chapter.

Accommodation, Vergence, and Ocular Motility

Therapy for accommodation and vergence concentrates on the range, facility, and stamina of these functions. The primary technique for remediating accommodative disorders is accommodative rock. This may be accomplished through dioptric shift in lens power or by linear change in fixation distance. Accommodative rock with lenses is typically done with loose, round plastic lens blanks or with lenses inserted into flippers. Loose lens blanks are preferable in the monocular phase and flippers in the binocular phase. Rocking with lenses bolsters the child's ability to sustain focus when reading for extended periods of time. The norms listed in Chapter 5 should be used as a guide for values to be attained through therapy. Accommodative rock through linear changes in fixation distance is done with Hart charts (Figure 16.5) (see Appendix A, Bernell Corporation). The large Hart chart consists of ten rows, each with ten letters. The letters have a visual subtense of 20/20 at a distance of 20 feet. The small Hart chart is a photo-reduced version of the large chart (Figure 16.6). Use of matched charts makes it easier for children to keep their places when switching from far to near and from near to far. Rocking in this manner bolsters children's abilities to sustain accurate focus when they are copying from the blackboard.

The general progression in therapy is to begin with monocular activities and proceed to biocular and then binocular activities. In the monocular and biocular phases, generally begin with + 0.50 and − 1.00. The minus value is always twice the plus value. In the binocular phase, the minus value is equal to the plus value. Monocular activities are done with a patch. To create the biocular phase, use the small Hart chart folded so that only two lines are exposed. A loose 8 prism diopter lens is held in one hand base up or down to dissociate the Hart chart, and the loose plus or minus lens is held in the other hand. This is the preferred technique for home therapy. An alternative technique to create dissociation is to place one half of a Spirangle vectogram in the top tier of the Polachrome Orthoptor and to place the other half in the lower tier.

Vergence posture plays a significant role in all aspects of the child's performance. Intermittent suppression can result in difficulty performing tasks such as copying from the blackboard, keeping one's place while reading, and sustaining

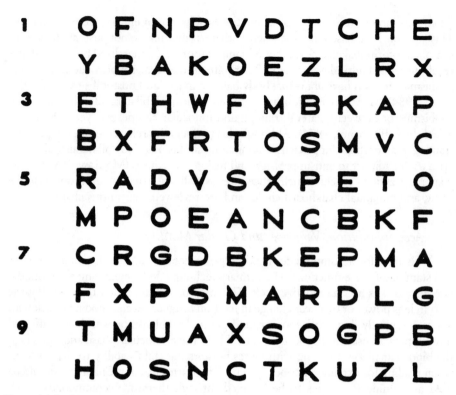

Figure 16.5 Large-sized Hart chart used for farpoint accommodative rock and saccadic fixations.

reading comfortably for extended periods of time. Vergence therapy techniques can be subdivided into slow (smooth) or dynamic (fast) vergence, spatial projection, and localization activities.

Smooth vergence is readily trained with vectograms. When working with children, accuracy of spatial localization must be monitored closely. A pointer should be used to minimize reliance on the child's language skills. Dynamic vergence can be trained easily with loose prism jumps or computerized therapy targets (Figure 16.7). The Brock String (see Appendix A, Bernell Corporation) can be used for all three phases simply by altering the instructional set. Localization is accomplished through physiological diplopia, jump vergence by jumping fixation from one bead to another, and smooth vergence by following an imaginary bug on the string moving between the beads. An additional advantage of using the Brock String with children is that the therapist can objectively monitor the relative vergence changes that the child makes

O F N P V D T C H E
Y B A K O E Z L R X

Figure 16.6 Small-sized Hart chart with two lines exposed, providing easier vertical dissociation during biocular rock.

when converging and diverging. The Correct-Eye-Scope (see Mast Keystone Co., Appendix A) is used to probe and develop the child's abilities in bilateral integration using binocular targets. Suitable targets are available for children of all ages.

Techniques for improving ocular motor performance center on pursuit and saccadic activities. Pursuit training is usually done in an oculorotary manner. Representative activities include pie pan rotations (following the circular path of a marble tilting about the inner axis of the pan), Marsden ball (following the pendular path of a ball suspended from the ceiling), and the vertical rotator (tracking a visual target on a tripod stand in clockwise or counterclockwise directions).

Saccadic activities are done at distance with the large Hart chart. The child begins with large angle saccades by calling out the first letter and last letter on each line. Smaller angle saccades are then accomplished by reading each letter aloud in sequence. Many of the techniques for training pursuits as well as saccades incorporate kinesthetic feedback through use of eye-hand coordination. Examples of eye-hand coordination activities include the Wayne Saccadic Fixator and the Pegboard Rotator, which are discussed in more detail in the following section. The numbers of activities available for training pursuits and saccades are legion and can be accessed through excellent manuals (Richman & Cron, 1988; Swartwout, 1991). Most recently, computers have been added to the optometrist's armamentarium, which add the immediacy of auditory feedback coupled with eye-hand coordination during pursuit and saccadic tasks (Figure 16.8).

To decrease motor overflow, the child may be asked to balance a book on the head. When motor overflow is manifest in postural alteration, the child can be asked to track while lying on the floor in a supine position. As training progresses, greater

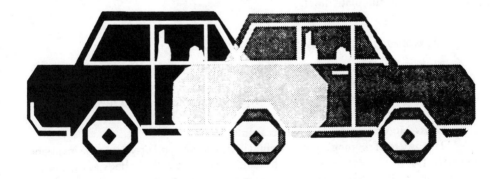

CURRENT DEMAND: 15 B.I.
HIGHEST DEMAND: B.I. 16   B.O.   0
                B.U. 0   B.O.   0

Figure 16.7 A computerized anaglyphic fusion target that is disparated through use of a joystick.

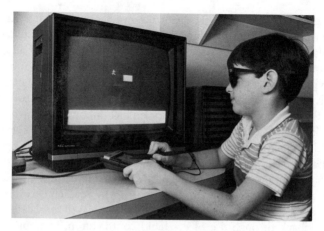

Figure 16.8   A computerized eye-hand coordination activity in which a pursuit task is accomplished through the use of a graphics tablet.

cognitive demand is added to the task. The ability to perform motor tasks while engaged in a cognitive activity such as counting to one hundred by threes has been termed cognitive stress (Barsch, 1968). The initial effect of cognitive stress or loading of the task may be a constriction of the peripheral field. It is therefore important to load the tasks in sequential and orderly fashion without rushing the child (Roberts, 1991). As noted by Richman and Cron (1988), children with attention deficit disorder (ADD) will have particular difficulty in moving performance in this area from the conscious to the automatic level.

Developmental and Perceptual-Motor Training

There are a plethora of developmental and perceptual-motor techniques that have been developed. The activities presented here match the developmental inventory of perceptual skills in the Hoffman-Richman profile discussed in Chapter 5.

Gross-Motor Control and Bilateral Integration
This aspect of training assists the child in developing and projecting the invariant (Suchoff, 1974). This process enables the child to perform with the body as the central point in space (egocentric localization). Suchoff's system for perceptual-motor therapeutics is hierarchical and summarized in Table 16.2. Progression is from more to less body involvement (egocentric to oculocentric localization) and from large to small muscle usage (gross to fine motor).

Angels in the Snow   This should first be done with the children lying on their backs to isolate the component of bilateral integration from the component of balance. The child is asked to move either the arm or the leg out to the side. The child is then asked to move both the arm and the leg outward simultaneously, first contralaterally then homolaterally.

Table 16.2 Hierarchical perceptual-motor activities

Developing the invariant (body schema)

Roll on floor over designated objects and to specific areas

Walking rail sequences (heel-to-toe, cross-walk, forward, backward)

"Slap tap" patterns (individual limbs, homolateral, contralateral)

Ball bounce patterns

Developing self-lateralization

Hammer nails into wood

Templates for chalkboard tracing

Directed jumping jacks (directional commands)

Coded ball bouncing (for example, two times right, one time left)

Marsden ball bunting with color-coded bat

Projection of self into space

Map on floor made with masking tape to follow directional commands (for example, turn left, turn right)

Map on blackboard with chalk with patient describing how to get from point A to point B

Matching directional arrows on chalkboard with hands (include verbalization)

Developing spatial coordinates

Tic-Tac-Toe configurations

Checkerboard patterns

Maps with grid coordinates (for example, find A-1)

Pegboard/parquetry block techniques

From IB Suchoff. Visual-spatial development in the child: An optometric theoretical and clinical approach. New York: State University of New York, 1974.

Slap-Tap This technique also develops bilateral integration, but involves smaller muscle movement and demands greater automaticity. The child is seated with hands on legs above the knee, palms downward. Four movements are involved beginning with the right hand tapping the leg above the knee followed by the right foot tapping with the heel, then the same is done with the left hand and the left heel. When this sequence is fluid, it is done to the beat of a metronome. The homolateral sequence is followed by the contralateral sequence of right hand, left foot, then left hand and right foot, both clockwise and counterclockwise.

Trampoline A small circular trampoline can be used to integrate visual and motor movements. Initially the patient does basic motor routines such as jumping jacks and air circles with arms. Once motor movements are fluid, intersensory integration tasks are added such as hitting a ball or catching a beanbag, while peripheral awareness is maintained. This is one example of cognitive stress, or loading, alluded to in the previous section.

Hopping This is done to develop rhythmicity in the following sequence:

1. Hop on each foot
2. Alternate hop (2 counts on each foot) with a pause
3. Alternate hop (2 counts on each foot) without a pause
4. Repeat steps 2 and 3 with a metronome
5. Hop over an object on one foot forward and backward
6. Hop over an object on both feet forward and backward

Balance Board Laterality as well as balance are involved in this activity. One can construct an 18″ × 24″ board with a central 2″ × 4″ fulcrum. There are three phases of balance (Furth & Wachs, 1975).

1. *Side balance.* The child stands near the edge of one side of the board with both feet parallel to the fulcrum and arms extended to the side. As the therapist exerts variable pressure on the other side of the board, the child must repeatedly shift weight to maintain balance.
2. *Front-back balance.* The same as phase 1 but with the child's feet perpendicular to the fulcrum.
3. *Bilateral balance.* The child straddles the center support in a seesaw manner. The child should have a visual reference point such as a cross on the chalkboard aligned symmetrically with the nose and initially be assisted in counteracting the tendency to tip to one side or the other.

Walk Rail This can be constructed using an 8-foot length of 2″ × 4″ wood that has middle and end cross supports elevating it 2″ from the floor. The child walks the rail forward in a heel-to-toe pattern, backward in a toe-to-heel pattern, and then sideways in a crossover pattern.

Bean Bag An assistant is stationed opposite the child and tosses a bean bag. The child is instructed to catch the bean bag while maintaining peripheral awareness.

Ball Bounce The child is instructed to bounce a ball in a specific sequence. This is the motor analog of the Birch-Belmont Auditory-Visual Integration Test. Once motor control is fluid with either hand, the child is asked to bounce the ball from one hand to the other and then to do the same thing to the beat of a metronome.

Visual-Motor Integration and Organization

This area generally involves smaller muscle groups as well as more direct ocular motor skill and spatial awareness. Incorporating eye-hand coordination, it is a bridge between gross motor control and visual-perceptual discrimination.

Visual-Motor Control (VMC) Bat The VMC bat can be made with a 1″ wide stick approximately 4′ long. The stick is painted with different colors arranged in a symmetrical band and is used in conjunction with a Marsden Ball that is suspended from the ceiling through an eye hook. The child is instructed to bunt the ball with "red light" or "blue left." This develops directional knowledge as well as bilateral integration.

Pegboard Rotator A variable speed rotator with holes into which pegs are inserted is used for integrating ocular motor pursuit with fine eye-hand coordination under dynamic conditions. The child is instructed to align the peg visually over the hole and follow it for one revolution before placing the peg into the hole.

Wayne Saccadic Fixator This is a multipurpose instrument with a central fixation point and a circular array of LED (light emitting diode) lights (see Appendix A, Wayne Engineering). It develops a multitude of visual skills including peripheral awareness, eye-hand coordination, and reaction time. The child is asked to touch the button adjacent to whichever light is illuminated. There are a variety of configurations for the sequences in which the lights are presented. These configurations are described in detail in the manual that accompanies the instrument.

Stick-in-Straw This technique assists in the development or enhancement of spatial localization. There are three phases of this procedure in which the patient inserts a red pointer stick into the opening of a straw. An assistant should hold the straw at the child's Harmon distance and remind the child to remain erect and well balanced.

> *Phase 1.* The child is instructed to hold the pointer stick in the dominant hand and to begin with the stick held behind the ear as if throwing a spear or javelin. The assistant holds the straw upright (*x-axis*), and the child is instructed to slowly bring the pointer in an arc downward until it is lowered into the opening of the straw. The child is instructed to keep an eye on the hole of the straw and to maintain awareness of the stick approaching the hole peripherally.
> *Phase 2.* The same as Phase 1, but the assistant holds the straw in the *straight-ahead* position (*z-axis*).
> *Phase 3.* The same as Phase 1, but the assistant holds the straw with the opening sideways (*y-axis*). The child approaches the hole on a horizontal arc.

These procedures should be performed first monocularly and then binocularly.

Chalkboard Circles These procedures provide a maximal degree of proprioception and kinesthesis. An "X" is drawn on the chalkboard opposite the patient's nose to serve as the midline reference point. A representative sequence of activities that are performed is (Kernan, 1987):

> *Harmon circles.* The child draws two circles simultaneously with one hand moving clockwise and the other counterclockwise. The circles are to be drawn as large as possible and the inner edge should be as close to the "X" as

possible. The child should keep fixation on the "X" while maintaining peripheral awareness of the hands. Both hands should move at the same relative speed.

Bimanual circles. The child draws circles in the same manner as above, but both hands move in tandem as do bicycle wheels.

Dropouts. The child does Harmon circles but synchronizes dropping one hand out of the pattern while the other continues.

Within boundaries. The therapist draws four vertical lines, two on each side of the "X." The lines indicate the diameter of the new circles to be drawn.

Groffman Visual Tracings These are a series of convoluted lines, each of which has a letter at one end and a number at the opposite end. The goal is to trace the letter at the beginning of the line visually to its corresponding number on the opposite side. There is a considerable amount of figure-ground involved in this task. If the child gets lost, a pointer can be used to trace the line. The child who gets lost easily may initially need to use a different color pen to track each letter to its corresponding number.

Pegboards These boards were originally introduced to help students understand spatial coordinates in elementary geometry. They are useful in training children about spatial relations and visualization. A representative sequence is:

1. Begin with a board that contains three rows of three nails. Use templates to show the child the pattern to be reproduced. Rubber bands are stretched across the nails to make the pattern. If there is difficulty, make the template lines different colors, and use rubber bands of corresponding colors to show the child how the lines interrelate. Advance to rows with four nails and then to rows with five nails.

2. Proceed to printed patterns of dots instead of nails, and follow the same sequence as in step 1. Use colored pens instead of colored rubber bands if necessary.

3. Proceed to the level of visualization, and ask the child to reproduce the pattern after mentally rotating it 90 degrees. If the child cannot do this, have a plastic overlay of the target to show the child the process of rotation. Repeat this for turns of 180 and 270 degrees. Have the child make the response as if sitting opposite the template and then as if viewing it from underneath.

Parquetry Blocks These activities involve the arrangement of squares, diamonds, and triangles on a page to match the shape of a template. Although there is a motor component, the primary tasks involve parts-whole analysis, figure-ground analysis, and visualization. There are two stages, each with multiple levels:

1. *Concrete to concrete.* The blocks are placed on the page directly with all internal lines of the shapes present at the first level. At the next level, the internal lines are removed, and the child must visualize the remaining space.

2. *Concrete to abstract.* The pattern is reproduced off the page with the same sequence as in concrete to concrete.

Computers The Groffman Visual Tracings and the Geoboard sequences are available in computerized format (Groffman & Press, 1989). As was previously mentioned, a computer offers a different type of visual-motor match than do pencil and paper tasks. Most children find computers interesting and challenging and are used to working at mastering the concept behind a "video game."

Visual-Perceptual Discrimination and Attention
In this aspect of training, we deal primarily with analysis and bridge the area between perceptual and cognitive processing. Motoric involvement becomes a substitute or support for verbal confirmation of the task, rather than an essential component of that task.

Spatial Coordinates The geoboard or Hart chart is used to train skills involved in tasks such as reading a map. For the 25-dot geoboard, the child is shown that the five rows across the top are labelled A, B, C, D, and E and that the five rows along the left margin are labelled 1, 2, 3, 4, and 5. The child must initially identify the coordinates at various dot locations. For example, the dot in the middle of the grid is C-3, the upper left is A-1 and the lower right is E-5. The Hart chart consists of 10 rows of 10 letters for a total grid of 100 letters. The child must determine, for example, which letter occupies position number 66 in the 100-letter grid.

Visual Coding and Grids Any grid can be constructed with a sequence of numbers, letters, or symbols and used as a template. The child is given a blank grid and asked to copy the number, letter, or symbol in the corresponding location.

Laterality and Directionality The simplest way to teach laterality and directionality is to use a Tic-Tac-Toe grid. Place an "X" in the center. The rest of the grid takes on directional coordinates—right, left, top, bottom, top right, top left, bottom right, bottom left. The child must label the correct location of each "X" or "O" before being allowed to record a response. In addition, the use of directional arrows is recommended. The child is asked to match the directions in which arrows have been drawn on the chalkboard. This should be done initially with a motoric response such as aiming one's arm in the corresponding direction. When this is fluid, the child should verbalize the direction in which the arrow is pointing.

Visual Memory Some form of tachistoscopic presentation is the usual venue for visual memory. The simplest form is the use of flash cards that work to increase the speed and span of recognition. Begin by presenting a small amount of information for a relatively long duration. The developmental progression is from digits to letters to words to sentences (Werner & Rini, 1976).

Visual Sequential Memory This area is a blend of visual memory, visualization, and speech-language development. A prominent example is children's ability to remember their telephone numbers. For speech-language integration, DLM Teaching Resources (see Appendix A) produces sets of sequential memory exercises, progressing from symbols and letters to pictures that tell a story when they are placed in proper sequence. One set of DLM cards to which children relate contains six picture cards. A child:

1. Making a selection at Coca-Cola machine
2. Pressing one panel to select a flavor
3. Reaching below to take a can from the portal
4. Opening the tab on the can
5. Drinking the soda
6. Disposing of the can

Visualization　This skill is closely aligned with visual memory, but it involves projection. For example, using the laterality and directionality activity of Tic-Tac-Toe, the child must not only picture what the configuration of the grid was when it was last seen but also what it will look like when the next move is made. The Lyons and Lyons Visualization Series (see Appendix A, Vision Extension, Inc.) is particularly useful for developing this area.

Figure-Ground　This is the ability to extract key features. This overlaps with the area of ocular-motor control as was mentioned earlier in the section describing Groffman Visual Tracings. An excellent generic activity is "hidden pictures," readily available through sources such as *Highlights* Magazine.

Visual Closure　There are numerous materials available to enhance the skill of being able to identify an object when parts of it are missing. The old TV game show "Concentration" is predicated on the extent of one's ability to make visual closure, and it can be used in its commercially available format for children. Visual closure exercises are one of a group of remedial activities available through GTVT (see Appendix A), which remediate the subcategories of visual perceptual tests contained in the TVPS (Test of Visual-Perception Skills—see Chapter 5).

Auditory-Visual Integration

There are three principal categories in this area of training. The first is intersensory integration wherein auditory rhythm is integrated with visual information. This is commonly done with a metronome. The second area is language based whereby auditory descriptors are used in the ordering of visual information. The Farnsworth D-15 test, in which colored caps are arranged sequentially, is a language mediated auditory-visual integration task. The third area is phonics.

Intersensory Integration　Have the child draw lines to the beat of a metronome. The faster the rate of the beat, the shorter the line (Wiener, 1975). Simon, a commercially available electronic game that has a circular disc with multicolored panels, is highly effective. Each of the four colored panels is linked with a different tone. The child waits to hear and see the tone and color sequence, then reproduces it by pressing the corresponding panels. The "slap-tap" procedure listed in the section on gross-motor control and bilateral integration earlier in this chapter also involves intersensory integration with rhythmicity.

Language   This area can be divided into visual integrative language and visual integrative nonlanguage (Wold et al, 1975). An example of visual integrative language is visual sequential memory as discussed in the section on visual-perceptual discrimination and attention earlier in this chapter. Some practitioners favor teaching children practical lessons in orthography, particularly when letter or word reversals or transpositions are a problem (Lane, 1988).

Phonics   In Chapter 5, the Rosner TAAS, a test designed to probe auditory analysis skills, was discussed. Vincett (1975) and Rosner (1979) designed training packages to improve deficits in phonics uncovered by these screening tests. When working in the areas of language and phonics, the optometrist should be prepared to consult with an auditory or speech-language specialist. As an analogy, one would not expect an audiologist to administer convergence exercises independently based on results of a self-devised visual screening instrument.

USE OF COMPUTERS IN VISION THERAPY

The use of computers in optometric practice has become commonplace for administrative functions, but only recently have computers developed into a basic component of VT. There have been numerous proprietary programs that have been developed for VT that have been reviewed elsewhere (Press, 1991). In the section on visual-motor integration and organization (earlier in this chapter), the Groffman cartridges that complement Cooper's Computer Orthoptics program (see Appendix A, RC Instruments) were discussed. The Computer Orthoptics program is a fast, prototypical program that serves as a good, basic work station for visual skills. Recently a liquid crystal polarization system has been developed that is particularly useful with young strabismic patients. Ludlam's Opti-Mum (see Appendix A, Learning Frontiers, Inc.) program is the other major entry in this field and has a potpourri of well-structured ocular motor and perceptual-related activities. In addition, there are numerous public domain programs that are useful in developing visual-perceptual abilities as listed by Maino (1988). Given these three major packages (Cooper, Groffman, and Ludlam) and independent visual-perceptual software, the optometrist is equipped with an excellent array of therapy techniques adapted to the video screen.

Computer programs are intended to complement rather than displace traditional therapy programs. In particular, children need observation and guidance while they are engaged in these activities. Computer programs can be used for their therapeutic value and as a reward system. The interactive nature of the computer maintains children's interest and facilitates the learning process by helping children in acquiring visual skills or in modifying visual performance.

REFERENCES

Awaya S. Management of early onset esotropia. J Ocul Ther and Surg 1983, September–October:231–235.

Barsch RH. Achieving perceptual-motor efficiency. Seattle: Special Child Publications, 1968.

Bedell HE, Flom MC. Monocular spatial distortion in strabismic amblyopia. Invest Ophthalmol Vis Sci 1981;20:263–268.

Birnbaum MH. Gross motor control and postural characteristics of strabismic patients. J Am Optom Assoc 1974;45:686–696.

Blakemore C, Van Sluyters RC. Experimental analysis of amblyopia and strabismus. Br J Ophthalmol 1974;58:176–182.

Ciuffreda KC, Levi DM, Selenow A. Amblyopia: Basic and clinical aspects. Boston: Butterworth–Heinemann, 1991.

Cohen AH. Monocular fixation in a binocular field. J Am Optom Assoc 1981;52:801–806.

Colorado Vision Consultants. Manual of esotropia therapy. Boulder: Colorado Vision Consultants, 1985.

Forrest EB. Treating infant esotropia: A case report. Am J Optom Physiol Opt 1978;55:463–465.

Furth HG, Wachs H. Thinking goes to school: Piaget's theory in practice. New York: Oxford University Press, 1975.

Getz DJ. Strabismus and amblyopia. 2d ed. Santa Ana, Calif.: Optom Ext Prog, 1990:26–30.

Greenwald I. Effective strabismus therapy. Duncan, Okla.: Optom Ext Prog, 1979.

Griffin JR. Binocular anomalies. Procedures for vision therapy. 2d ed. Chicago: Professional Press, 1982:438–448.

Groffman S, Press L. Computerized perceptual therapy programs. Optom Ext Prog 1989;61:423–430.

Jacques L. Corrective and preventive optometry. Los Angeles: Globe Print Co., 1950.

Kernan M. Developmental visual training procedures. Optom Ext Prog, Assistant's Courses, 1987;29:21–23.

Lane KA. Reversal errors: Theories and procedures. Santa Ana, Calif.: Vision Extension, 1988.

McGraw L. Guiding strabismus therapy. Santa Ana, Calif: Optom Ext Prog, 1991.

Maino DM. The process approach, microcomputers and therapy. Optom Ext Prog 1988;60:227–234.

Odenrick P, Sandsted P, Lennerstrand G. Postural sway and gait of childen with convergent strabismus. Devel Med and Child Neurol 1984;26:495–499.

Press LJ. Computers and visual training. Santa Ana, Calif.: Optom Ext Prog, 1991.

Press LJ. Electronic games and strabismic therapy. J Optom Vis Devel 1981;12(3):35–39.

Press LJ. How to manage congenital strabismus. Rev Optom 1982;August:35–40.

Richman, JE, Cron MT. Guide to vision therapy. South Bend, Ind.: Bernell Corporation, 1988.

Roberts B. The developmental sequence of visual training. Behav Optom (Australia) 1991;3(1):27–32.

Rosner J. Helping children overcome learning difficulties.. 2d ed. New York: Walker and Company, 1979.

Schapero M. Amblyopia. Philadelphia: Chilton, 1971.

Suchoff IB. Visual-spatial development in the child: An optometric theoretical and clinical approach. New York: State University of New York, 1974.

Swartwout JB. Manual of procedures and forms for in-office and out-of-office optometric vision training programs. Santa Ana, Calif.: Optom Ext Prog, 1991.

Tassinari JD. Binasal occlusion. J Behav Optom 1990;1:16–21.

Vincett WK. Optometric perceptual testing and training manual. 2d ed. Akron, Ohio: PerCon, 1975.

Werner P, Rini L. Perceptual-motor development equipment: Inexpensive ideas and equipment. New York: John Wiley and Sons, 1976.

Wick B. Vision therapy for pre-school children. In Rosenbloom AA, Morgan MW, eds. Principles and practice of pediatric optometry. Philadelphia: Lippincott, 1990:280–282.

Wick B. Prevention and care of strabismus in infants and preschool children. J Am Optom Assoc 1979;50:1161–1165.

Wiener H. Eyes OK I'm OK. San Rafael, Calif.: Academic Therapy Publications, 1975.

Wold R, Getz DJ, McGraw L. In-office vision therapy manual. Los Angeles: A-V Scientific, 1975.

17

Control of Progressive Myopia

Leonard J. Press

At first blush it may not seem warranted to devote an entire chapter to the subject of myopia control in a text on pediatric optometry, but there is strong reason for doing so. Parents are alarmed about anomalies such as strabismus or ptosis that are readily apparent. Similarly it is disconcerting for most parents to sit idly by while their child returns year after year to receive progressively thicker lenses. Cosmesis is not their sole concern. They wonder aloud when the increases in myopia will end, if blindness is a possible outcome, and if there is something that can be done to slow its progression. Although there is a school of thought that very little can be done clinically about myopia (Sivak, 1991), the majority of pediatric optometrists maintain that some components of myopia are alterable.

The differentiation of components in alterable, functional myopia from nonalterable, structural myopia has been reviewed elsewhere (Press, 1987). Strong evidence for a noninherited component of myopia comes from a study of familial trends. In a study comparing the refractive state of young myopes with their parents, Ditmars (1967) found that 63 percent had neither parent myopic. When both parents were myopic, 86 percent exceeded both parents' myopia. Myopia cannot be treated as simply an inheritable condition to be compensated for by full prescription of the refractive anomaly. Aside from the conventional wisdom of underprescribing at distance by $-0.50D$, there are three principal approaches that optometrists offer: (1) vision therapy (VT), (2) bifocals, and (3) contact lenses. Before discussing these approaches, it is necessary to differentiate from a clinical standpoint several types of myopia.

CLASSIFICATION

The myopias are a group of heterogeneous refractive anomalies sharing the common property of being compensated for by concave lenses (Curtin, 1985). Their underlying causes and management, however, are quite disparate.

Congenital/Early Onset

Myopia with onset prior to the age of six years is typically of high magnitude, usually in the range of 6–10D. High unilateral myopia invariably presents with the myopic eye in the range of 10 diopters and the contralateral eye near emmetropia. In

327

some instances, the myopia is induced by physical obstruction of the image such as with lid anomalies, craniofacial abnormalities, lenticular aberrations, or retinopathies. In other instances, there may be no apparent cause.

High myopia (above 6D) is considered pathological because it is associated with structural alterations of the posterior segment. These eyes must be monitored frequently for degenerative retinal changes. Children with high unilateral myopia should receive full optical compensation with a contact lens as early as possible. Sorsby and associates (1957) demonstrated that myopia in excess of 6D is predominantly axial. There is a pervasive theoretical notion that is based on Knapp's Law that patients with anisometropic axial ametropia should be corrected with spectacles rather than with contact lenses to minimize induced aniseikonia. Although this is true on the basis of calculated image size difference, there are no clinical studies to substantiate that children fitted with contact lenses develop a greater degree of amblyopia than do children fitted with spectacles. As was stated in Chapter 13, clinical impressions indicate that the improved image quality from a contact lens, as well as the reduction in induced prismatic imbalance, overrides the theoretical considerations of Knapp's Law. Children with unilateral myopia should be given the benefit of aggressive amblyopia therapy. High bilateral myopia is adequately managed initially with spectacle lenses.

Juvenile (Adolescent) Myopia

Myopia with onset after 6 years of age has variable expression. Girls tend to have earlier ages of onset of myopia than boys do. The earlier the onset of myopia, the greater is the probability that it will progress to the range of 6D and beyond (Goss, 1983). In contrast, myopia with onset after age 12 rarely progresses beyond 3D. Efforts to contain the progression of myopia will be more successful when the myopia has late onset and is of a low amount.

Young Adult Myopia

Practitioners are observing increases in myopia in patients who are beyond their growth years. This extends to college students as well as to persons with occupations requiring intense and extended near work. The Committee on Vision of the National Research Council (1989) concluded that doing near work places one at risk of myopia. Twenty to 40 percent of low myopes or emmetropes who enter colleges or academies involving extensive near work are likely to progress toward myopia by the age of 25.

CONVENTIONAL METHODS OF INTERVENTION

The very young child with high myopia is likely to change little in one direction or the other. Successful intervention to contain progression of myopia in the pediatric population usually begins with the school-aged child with early adaptive shifts toward increasing myopia. When parents inquire about possible intervention, the optometrists should be prepared to discuss available treatment options objectively. Too often optometrists limit themselves by not making recommendations for clinical treatment because definitive, prospective studies on treatment have not been done. Although studies of this nature are desirable, they are not what most parents are seeking. A parent ultimately wants to know what decision optometrists would make if their own children had the same clinical circumstances. Given this, what are the usual methods of treatment?

Underprescribing the Distance Prescription (Rx)

Conventional wisdom holds that the Rx given to the child with low or moderate myopia need not compensate for the full extent of distance blur. An Rx that is underminused by −0.50D thereby affording 20/30 binocular acuity is considered adequate for classroom needs. Most parents accept, and some request, a slight partial correction of this nature. Teachers are readily agreeable to preferential seating near the blackboard.

In many instances, the child with substandard distance acuity presents the optometrist with a form to be completed and returned to the school nurse. To clarify the intent of undercorrection, the optometrist should explain to the nurse as well as to the parent why the child's acuity is being corrected to less than 20/20.

Bifocal or Multifocal Lenses

If there is plus lens acceptance at near, particularly when esophoria is manifest, bifocal lenses are indicated. When myopia is one diopter or less, some practitioners simply advise the child to remove the glasses for near work. This is an impractical suggestion for younger children who do not have the maturity to know when to leave the glasses on and when to take them off. This will result in the glasses being used all the time or not being used at all. In addition, bifocals in some instances have the advantage of exerting a bases down yoked prism effect that is elaborated in the section on yoked prisms later in this chapter.

As was discussed in Chapter 12, there is latitude in the kind of bifocal that can be prescribed. The power of the add can be determined by a number of methods. The procedure favored by many pediatric optometrists is MEM (monocular estimate method) retinoscopy as was discussed in Chapter 5. The advantage of nearpoint retinoscopy is that it does not rely on the subjective responses of the child. The effectiveness of bifocals in slowing the progression of myopia has been challenged by a recent study (Grosvenor et al, 1987), which randomly assigned patients to plano, +1.00D, and +2.00D add groups. Rather than discounting the efficacy of bifocals, this study should be interpreted as underscoring the importance of selecting add powers based on the indivdiual's plus lens acceptance profile at near. Indications for plus lens application include:

High lag of accommodation (cross-cyl or near retinoscopy finding above +0.50)

High negative relative accommodation (NRA) as compared with positive relative accommodation (PRA)

Pass plus lens flippers and fail minus lens flippers

High AC/A with movement in the direction of normal near exo through plus lenses

Reduction in eso posture on Van Orden (VO) star or cheiro trace through plus lenses

Improvement in stereopsis responses through plus lenses

Vision Therapy (VT)

Three broad areas of VT are applicable to children with progressive myopia: (1) increasing the efficiency of accommodation, (2) increasing degrees of freedom between accommodation and convergence, and (3) peripheral awareness. Included are monocular and binocular accommodative rock activities, BOP/BIM (base-out through plus lenses/base-in through minus lenses) procedures, base-in therapy with vectograms, McDonald Form Fields, and the Wayne Saccadic Fixator. Some practitioners have used auditory-visual biofeedback therapy for myopia control with children as young as ten years of age. The ability to use biofeedback, visual imagery, or relaxation techniques varies more with the intellect than the age of the child. During the past decade, many psychologists have published studies indicating the importance of operant conditioning in the behavioral treatment of myopia (Leber, 1989).

Visual Hygiene

Increasing numbers of children in today's society are susceptible to various forms of stress. This may stem from tension generated in household, academic, or peer interactions. Stress can manifest itself in many forms such as skin rash, gastrointestinal disorders, headaches, or blurred vision. It is well known that the Streff Syndrome (see Chapter 10) is associated with juvenile stress, but simple low grade myopia can be stress-induced as well (Forrest, 1988). To the extent that progressive myopia is stress-induced, children can benefit from good visual hygiene. Suggestions for visual hygiene are complementary to a comprehensive vision therapy program.

1. Avoid working at near distances for extended periods of time. Look up to the distance, preferably out a window, to give the eyes an opportunity to refocus to distance viewing.
2. When you take a work break, close the eyes and take a few deep breaths to assist the mind as well as the eyes to escape overintensity to the nearpoint task.
3. Work in properly lit areas. Make sure the lighting is soft and does not create glare on the viewing surface.
4. Use a chair that affords good posture. This will reduce not only visual stress but also physical stress.

5. Avoid rotating the paper when writing. This encourages postural warps and visual maladaptation.
6. Maintain a distance from the eye to the screen or paper no closer than the distance from the elbow to the first knuckle. This is approximately 16 inches for adults and 12 inches for children. This holds true for watching television, using a computer, or doing homework.
7. Maintain good general nutrition. Most people know that vitamin A influences night vision, but there are other lesser-known associations between nutrients and focusing abilities.

Sympathetic-parasympathetic balance and its influence on myopia is related to general stress-reduction therapy as well as specific VT techniques (Birnbaum, 1984). In Japan, the use of visual hygiene activities is commonplace (Yamaji, 1981). Included are techniques for relaxation, deep winking, massaging of the temples, near to far Landolt "C" chart fixations, eye relaxation, and neck and shoulder exercises. The key to their success lies in the extent to which children make the training part of daily living.

Contact Lenses

Clinical experience has shown that rigid contact lenses slow the progression of myopia (Kerns, 1981; Polse et al, 1983; Rengstorff, 1989). Some have argued that the period during which teenagers are fitted with lenses coincides with an age when myopic progression tends to be self-limiting. The factors that might account for stabilization of myopia can be classified as optical or mechanical.

Optical Factors

An unintentional orthokeratological effect may ensue whereby flattening of the central or peripheral cornea results in arrest of myopia. Planned orthokeratology is not usually administered until the teenage years. Reviews of orthokeratology can be found elsewhere (Mandell, 1988).

Contact lenses magnify retinal image size relative to spectacle lenses. Skeffington (1966) proposed that plus lenses for nearpoint use stabilized vision due to their magnification properties. Sutton (1988) observed that any induced shape magnification relative to the habitual state should operate similarly to relative power magnification. Consequently the relative afocal magnification provided in the switch from spectacles to contact lenses might exert an effect similar to a bifocal prescription.

Mechanical Factors

A recent study by the University of Houston Contact Lens Research Institute concluded that RGP (rigid gas permeable) lenses are effective in controlling progression of myopia (Grosvenor et al, 1991). During the three-year period of lens wear, spectacle lens wearers progressed at a rate three times faster than contact lens wearers matched for age and beginning levels of myopia. Less clear is the influence of soft lenses on myopic progression. The term *myopic creep* has been used to describe the frequent requirement for increased minus power in some soft lens patients. One suggested mechanism for this induced myopia is peripheral corneal flattening due to central anterior lens dehydration (Caroline & Campbell, 1991).

ALTERNATIVE METHODS OF INTERVENTION

There are a number of approaches that have been advocated for myopia control but that are not generally practiced in pediatric optometry. These include pharmacologic and surgical intervention and dietary control.

Pharmacologic Intervention

The use of atropine to slow the progression of myopia is still practiced by a surprising number of U.S. ophthalmologists. Its efficacy is predicated on the extent to which excessive accommodation is a myopiagenic factor (Jensen & Goldschmidt, 1991). Avetisov (1990) reports that 1 percent neosynephrine administered at bedtime on alternate days is widely utilized in the countries recently part of the USSR for normalizing accommodative ability in progressive myopia. One can consider the use of these agents as a pharmacologic method of establishing a greater degree of freedom between accommodation and convergence.

Although this subject is touched upon in Chapter 15, a specific point is being emphasized here. An explanation of why some ophthalmologists treat progressive myopia with drugs can bolster one's presentation of nonpharmacologic treatment with nearpoint lenses and VT. Many parents will be receptive to bifocal or VT as an alternative to long-term drug therapy.

Surgical Intervention

Numerous procedures have been advanced for the surgical reduction of myopia. Radial keratotomy, keratomileusis, and keratophakia have been proposed to reduce low to moderate amounts of myopia. Higher amounts of degenerative myopia have been treated by scleral reinforcement (Thompson, 1985), which remains a controversial procedure. All of these procedures have potential complications as was extensively reviewed by Curtin (1985).

Dietary Control

The possible association between certain dietary deficiencies and myopia has been made by various investigators and clinicians (Lane, 1982; Kavner, 1985). These include deficiencies in trace minerals as well as vitamins. The trend toward holistic care and consumerism in health care has spurred renewed interest in the potential relationship between nutritional factors and myopia.

Yoked Prisms

Yoked prism is defined as prism used in front of both eyes simultaneously with identical base directions. Most practitioners who prescribe yoked prism for myopia control do so in the bases down direction though some advocate bases up (Press, 1990). The theory behind bases down prism is that it has a widening effect on the periphery, counteracting the constriction of peripheral space associated with progressive functional myopia. Single vision convex lenses induce a bases up yoked effect when one is reading in downgaze, whereas the same Rx in a roundtop segment preserves the bases down effect (Lagace, 1987). This is one argument for the preference of prescribing bifocals rather than single vision lenses to children.

Biofeedback

Trachtman (1987) is the principal proponent of biofeedback through the use of the Accommotrac, a device with an auditory tone through which patients can monitor accommodative output. Many children have been successful with this technique from as young an age as eight years. The procedure requires a calm, cooperative, intelligent child, which (perhaps not coincidentally) happens to be the nature of many young progressive myopes.

There is a great deal of controversy surrounding the use of this device. Two studies have strongly challenged its efficacy (Gallaway et al, 1987; Koslowe et al, 1991), whereas supportive studies have been sparse. It appears that the clinical success of some practitioners with the device is as much related to the holistic approach, involving relaxation, breathing, peripheral awareness, visual hygiene, and diet and nutrition, as it is with the device itself.

Some optometrists apply more traditional approaches to myopia containment before using the Accommtrac. If the parent makes it clear that their interest is in specifically reducing their child's myopia and if the myopia amount is in excess of one diopter, these more traditional optometrists will refer the child to a colleague who uses this device at the outset.

REFERENCES

Avetisov E. Myopia in children. In Taylor D, ed. Pediatric ophthalmology. Boston: Blackwell Scientific, 1990.

Birnbaum MH. Nearpoint visual stress: A physiological model. J Am Optom Assoc 1984;55:825–835.

Caroline P, Campbell R. Between the lines: Long term effects of hydrophilic contact lenses on myopia. Contact Lens Spectrum 1991;5(6):68.

Curtin BJ. The myopias: Basic science and clinical management. Philadelphia: Harper and Row, 1985.

Ditmars DL. A comparative study of refractive errors of young myopes and their parents. Am J Optom Arch Am Acad Optom 1967;44:448–451.

Forrest EB. Stress and vision. Santa Ana, Calif.: Optometric Extension Pro, 1988.

Gallaway M, Pearl SM, Winkelstein AM, et al. Biofeedback training of visual acuity and myopia: A pilot study. Am J Optom Physiol Opt 1987;64:62–71.

Goss DA, Winkler RL. Progression of myopia in youth: Age of cessation. Am J Optom Physiol Opt 1983;60:651–658.

Grosvenor T, Perrigin D, Perrigin J, et al. Do rigid gas permeable lenses control the progress of myopia? Contact Lens Spectrum 1991;5(7):29–36.

Grosvenor T, Perrigin DM, Perrigin J, et al. The Houston Myopia Control Study, a randomized clinical trial, Part II: Final report by the patient care team. Am J Optom Physiol Opt 1987;64:482–498.

Jensen H, Goldschmidt E. Management of myopia: Pharmacologic agents. In Grosvenor T, Flom MC, eds. Refractive anomalies: Research and clinical applications. Boston: Butterworth–Heinemann, 1991.

Kavner R. Your child's vision. New York: Simon and Schuster, 1985;201–203.

Kerns RL. Contact lens control of myopia. Am J Optom Physiol Opt 1981;58:541–545.

Koslowe KC, Spierer A, Rosner M, et al. Evaluation of Accommotrac biofeedback training for myopia control. Optom Vis Sci 1991;68:338–343.

Lagace JP. In vivo behavioral analysis. Santa Ana,Calif.: Optometric Extension Program, 1987;59.

Lane BC. Myopia prevention and reversal: New data confirms the interaction of accommodative stress and deficit-inducing nutrition. J Intl Acad Prev Med 1982;7:17–30.

Leber LL. Improving visual acuity of myopes through operant training: The evaluation of psychological and physiological mechanisms facilitating acuity enhancement. Ann Arbor, Mich.: University Microfilms International, Dissertation Information Service, 1989.

Mandell RB. Contact lens practice. 3rd ed. Springfield, Ill.: Charles C Thomas, 1988;858–860.

National Research Council. Myopia: Prevalence and progression. Committee on Vision, Committee on Behavioral and Social Sciences and Education. Washington, D.C.: National Academy Press, 1989;68.

Polse KA, Brand RJ, Schwalbe JS, et al. The Berkeley ortho-K study, Part II: Efficacy and duration. Am J Optom Physiol Opt 1983;60:187–198.

Press LJ. Topical review of the literature: Lenses and behavior. J Optom Vis Devel 1990;21(1):5–17.

Press LJ. Topical review of the literature: myopia. J Optom Vis Devel 1987;18(1):1–17.

Rengstorff RH. Refractive changes after wearing contact lenses. In Phillips AJ, Stone J, eds. Contact lenses, 3d ed. Boston: Butterworth–Heinemann, 1989;741.

Sivak JG. Clinical experience in halting myopia. Optom Vis Sci 1991;68:826–829.

Skeffington AM. Lecture I, Northwest Congress of Optometry, Portland, Ore., December 1966.

Sorsby AB, Benjamin B, Davey JB, et al. Emmetropia and its aberrations: A study in the correlation of the optical components of the eye. Medical Research Council, SRS No. 293. London: Her Majesty's Stationery Office, 1957.

Sutton A. The use of lenses to alter behavior and performance. Presented at the Annual Meeting of the College of Optometrists in Visual Development, Hilton Head, S.C., November 1988.

Thompson FB. Scleral reinforcement for high myopia. Ophthal Surg 1985;16:90–94.

Trachtman JN. Biofeedback of accommodation to reduce myopia: A review. Am J Optom Physiol Opt 1987;64:639–643.

Yamaji R. Treatment of acquired myopia. In Sato T, Yamaji R, eds. Proceedings of the second international congress on myopia. Yokohama-Shi, Japan: Sato Eye Clinic, 1981.

18

Low Vision and Multiple Impairment

Paul B. Freeman

The most recent estimate of the number of children with low vision in the United States (1991) (Table 18.1) indicated that there were approximately 110,000 children under the age of 17 who were either legally blind or visually impaired (Genensky, 1991). This number continues to increase. In the 1986–1987 school year, 27,049 visually impaired students were receiving services mandated by PL (Public Law) 94–142 (see Chapter 12) and the Education Consolidation and Improvement Act (RFR, 1990).

Children with low vision, compared with fully sighted children, often show lags in one or more areas of development (Leung & Hollins, 1989). Thirty percent of children under age five have at least one other disability (Sorsby, 1972). Surveys of visually-impaired children show the incidence of cerebral palsy in this population to be between 10 and 23 percent (Sykanda, 1984). Consequently the clinician should expect to encounter multiple impairment within a continuum of complexity. When mental retardation, hearing impairment, or physical disability accompanies visual impairment, management of the child becomes a formidable task. The assessment of the child with low vision begins with a structured interview to gain insight into the child's previous care (Hritcko, 1983).

CASE HISTORY

Taking a case history from a parent, reviewing past written reports and integrating other historical information about the visually/multiply impaired child is fraught with subtleties. In Chapter 1, the basic elements of case history were presented. Here we present the extended history required when a child has congenital or early onset impairment.

Objective Information

The majority of low-vision-inducing conditions in children are inherited or congenital (Kalloniatis & Johnston, 1990). Prior medical records will theoretically give objective findings about prenatal, perinatal, and postnatal development of the child. The optometrist should attempt to document the status of the child at birth. Specific facts should include anomalies involving length of gestation, time of labor,

335

Table 18.1 Estimates of various subsets of the visually-impaired population of the United States in 1991

(1) Age	(2) PS	(3) PS-LB	(4) LB	(5) LB&PS = LB-FB	(6) FB	(7) U.S. Population
0–4	6,200	5,000	2,000	1,200	800	18,354,440
5–19	117,200	94,000	35,400	23,200	12,200	53,067,900
20–44	390,600	313,200	106,500	77,400	29,100	99,674,690
45–64	463,600	371,700	122,200	91,900	30,300	46,371,010
65–74	394,700	316,500	101,700	78,200	23,500	18,106,560
75–84	483,300	387,500	120,900	95,800	25,100	10,055,110
85 AND UP	458,400	367,500	113,200	90,900	22,300	3,080,165
TOTAL	2,314,000	1,855,400	601,900	458,600	143,300	248,709,875

PS   = Partially sighted
PS-LB   = Partially sighted but not legally blind
LB   = Legally blind
LB&PS   = Legally blind and also partially sighted
LB-FB   = Legally blind but not functionally blind
FB   = Functionally blind

Note that the LB&PS are also LB-FB and vice versa. Therefore they are exactly the same set of people.

Also note that in each row of the table, the numbers in column 2 are the sum of the numbers in columns 3 and 5, and the numbers in column 4 are the sum of the numbers in columns 5 and 6. Thus the PS are the PS-LB added to the LB&PS and the LB are the LB&PS added to the FB.

birthweight, neonatal or perinatal anoxia, high fevers, convulsions, incubation, supplemental oxygen, jaundice, and light exposure. The Apgar score should be noted in the hospital records (Table 18.2). The score is based on a maximum point total of ten. A score of seven or higher indicates that the infant is reasonably healthy. A score of less than four means that the infant needs to be aggressively cared for to survive and is susceptible to central nervous system (CNS) damage. This information helps to determine whether the difficulties the child is experiencing are organic and whether they can be expected to be progressive or stable in nature.

Subjective Information

The child's mother should be probed about prenatal history, specifically if she was taking drugs, medications, experienced illness or nutritional deficits, smoked, drank alcohol, or was under excessive emotional or physical stress. These factors are of particular concern when they occur during the first trimester. In addition, genetic predisposition toward impairment should be determined through family history.

During this questioning it is important that the optometrist not attribute blame to anyone for the child's impairment even if causative factors are obvious. Guilt tends to create cyclic behavior and anger. Statements from either parent such as "if only I had done this" or "I should not have done that" will dilute any positive suggestions with reminders of what could have been if things had been different. Also while interacting with the child and family it is important not to patronize or minimize feelings by stating: "I know how you must feel" or "I understand." Do not project feelings or value judgements onto the patient or family.

Questions about the child's early development are best substantiated with a diary or a baby record. Absence of such documentation places questionable value on the chronological accuracy of the report though it may furnish a reliable developmental timetable of milestones in language and motor development. The further from the event the questions are posed, the more likely it might represent what the parent or caretaker would have liked to have happen or represent a compilation of other siblings (Yarrow, 1963). The perceptions of the parent or caretaker will be important, however, when subsequent recommendations are given about active vision stimulation.

During this interview, the optometrist may be able to ascertain the stage of psychological impact of the parent: denial, shock, disbelief, or acceptance. Recommendations for intervention may need to be tempered with the preparedness of the parent to rear a visually/multiply impaired child. Questions such as "How often is the child picked up?" and "Is there close body contact between the child and other family members?" should be asked. Minimal physical contact between the child and other family members may impinge on the bonding process and damage the child's self-esteem. Visual withdrawal may then be compounded by psychological or physical withdrawal.

Finally concern about child abuse needs to be delicately explored, more by observing how questions are answered than by direct questioning. Child abuse appears more commonly with unwanted children or children perceived to be defective. In New York state as an example, optometrists are included among the health care professionals who are mandated to report suspicions of child abuse. In any event, suspicion of abuse merits the suggestion of psychological consultation or referral.

Goals and Expectations

The younger or less communicative the child, the more the optometrist will need to rely on those who will help the child, specifically parents, educators, and therapists. Questions should be posed to afford an idea of both long-term and short-term goals. These will help the optometrist formulate a visual game plan based on optometric test results. Bear in mind that goals are levels for which to strive, not

Table 18.2 Apgar scores

Sign	0	1	2
Heart rate	Absent	Slow	Normal
Respiration	Absent	Hypoventilates	Normal
Muscle tone	Limp	Some flexion	Normal
Skin color	Blue	Blue-pink	Pink
Reflex irritability	None	Some motion	Cries

endpoints. Structuring realistic, intermediate levels of expectation allows goals to be attained and should create a positive and motivating environment.

EXAMINATION AND EVALUATION
Observation

When a visually-impaired child is examined, surreptitious observations are invaluable. Watching the child in the reception area will give the optometrist an idea of visual and motor function without the added burden of directed stress in responding to specific questions or commands.

Observations should be made as to whether the child is visually alert, manipulates objects, or visually interacts with the environment in any fashion. In addition, this is an excellent time to observe the parent/child interaction. Does the parent view the child as completely dependent, or does the parent allow the child some independent function? Observation of this interaction should be continued in the examination room as well. The extent of this relationship will bear on the nature of the activities that are suggested for the parent to do with the child.

Typically parents, who feel that the child is without usable sight and is dependent, will be inclined to do home visual stimulation activities for the child rather than to allow the child to manipulate and explore the environment. Conversely parents who feel their child is totally independent tend to have the child perform activities with minimal support. Extreme cases are these parents who deny the impairment and place added pressure on the child to perform as if no impairment existed. The ideal situation lies somewhere in between.

Distance Visual Acuity

When the child is in the examining room, continued observation is important. Does the child look around the room, or is the child able to connect visually with anything in the environment? While this will not give definitive information, particularly if the child has figure-ground difficulty, this can be an informal start to distance acuity assessment. Because visually-impaired children run the gamut of multiple sensory and motor impairment, the acuity procedure often needs to be customized for the child. Avoid the recording of "counts fingers" or "could not be done."

The child should be encouraged to identify Snellen or equivalent targets. These are the acuities of choice not only because they are the universal form of acuity but also because they can be used to define the child's legal vision status.

Acuities can be done either verbally or nonverbally and should be done monocularly and binocularly. A spoken response from the child when a letter or object is shown is the verbal method. Nonverbal cues can be obtained either by matching information at near with the same information on a chart at distance or by watching for behavioral changes during the testing.

A unique method of determining visual acuities of the multiply impaired, visually impaired child is through diagnostic patching. Typically this type of patching is done over time with observational notations made by either the parent, the caretaker, or support personnel. Typical observation time is ½-hour a day over the course of 1 to 2 months. The diagnostic patching regimen is

1. *A patch is placed on the child's forehead.* The reason that it is not placed directly on the eye initially is to avoid behavioral changes due to the sensation of the patch itself. The patch is to be worn until it is apparent that its placement is not creating resistance. Once a child ceases any resistance to the patch, it is safe to assume behavioral changes related to covering one eye will be due to altered vision rather than to irritation to the patch.
2. *The child's one eye should be covered.* If the child's behavior does not significantly change when that eye is occluded, it can be assumed that the unoccluded eye is used for sight. If the partner eye is then occluded at a later time and the child's behavior changes, it can be assumed that the unoccluded eye is not typically the seeing eye. If the responses are the same with either eye occluded or with both eyes open, it can be assumed that the vision is approximately the same regardless of occlusion or nonocclusion. This methodology is similar to that employed for infants or preschoolers as was detailed in Chapters 3 and 4.

Many multiply impaired children, however, will be unable to respond to these methods. Therefore other attempts at acuities should be tried. If response to objects is unattainable, the child's ability to localize light can be used as a source of information about visual status. The human postural system is basically tropotaxic, that is, it will localize a light source and orient to it. In addition, the visual system is teleotaxic, attempting to detect differences of light intensity from a single light source and to orient to that source so that light is equally distributed between the two eyes (Howard & Templeton, 1966). Using this concept, if the eyes are capable of receiving light input, the doctor can use a penlight to establish a crude form of localization acuity. This will be important for use later in helping the child appreciate doorways, windows, and other light and dark areas. This should be done monocularly as well as binocularly.

When using light as a means of determining visual response, it is sometimes helpful to modify the direction of the light in order to observe changes in postural behavior. Using monocular or yoked prisms, one can alter the location of light thereby creating postural changes to the reoriented light. Having ascertained this, prism can later be used to test as well as train postural adaptability in orienting with a prism to objects in the environment.

Although only Snellen or Landolt acuities are acceptable in defining a child's legal visual status, localization acuity and tests of light perception and projection can be used to help others understand the child's potential toward orientation and mobility. If the child is able to respond to objects, estimate of localization acuity can be made through the following formula (Carter, 1983):

$$\left(\frac{\text{the height of the object measured in feet}}{\text{the distance of the object measured in feet}} \right) \times 13760 = \frac{20}{x}$$

It is important to remember that this does not indicate discrimination acuity as was reviewed with STYCAR materials in Chapter 3.

There are several other assessments of visual acuity. Optokinetic nystagmus is often suggested as a test of visual acuity. As was noted in Chapter 3, it is at best inconclusive, testing only the visual pathway proximal to the visual cortex. Preferential looking (PL) and visually evoked potential (VEP) acuities can be obtained as was discussed in Chapter 3. VEP and PL are in good agreement in two-thirds of multiply handicapped patients tested with each technique (Orel-Bixler et al, 1990). Both, however, use grating stimuli that are known to overestimate Snellen acuity. For visual acuity less than 20/60, this difference becomes pronounced (Orel-Bixler et al, 1990).

VISUAL FIELD ASSESSMENT

The extent of the visual field is as critical for low-vision and multiply-impaired children as is the central visual acuity. Peripheral vision is survival vision for these children. It allows them to know where they are in their environment and in relation to other objects, allowing for stable spatial relationships. Incomplete or depressed visual fields can cause confusion for the child and complicate the efforts of rehabilitation professionals working with the child.

Testing Procedures

Many low-vision/multiply-impaired children are unable to use sophisticated electronic equipment in testing. In these instances, confrontation fields should be performed:

1. Sit opposite the child at approximately one meter's distance.
2. Occlude the child's eye and your own eye on the same side.
3. Bring objects inward from at least the four major quadrants.
4. Try to quantify the results with an arc perimeter. If a tangent screen or a blackboard is used, 2½ inches corresponds to 5 degrees at a 1 meter distance.
5. Repeat the procedure for the contralateral eye.
6. For lower-functioning children, use larger or brighter lights or objects to overcome figure-ground response problems.

In addition, a functional mobility field can be established by having the child navigate a specific maze path set up on the floor without bumping into any of the objects placed around the room.

COLOR VISION TESTING

Two color vision tests that are beneficial for this population are the Yarn Test and the Color Matching Block Test. In both of these tests, the instructional set given allows the child either to identify the colors being shown or to match the colors the child sees with colors the optometrist or assistant holds. Typically, the primary colors are all that are necessary for rehabilitative programs. During this testing, it is important to use only the parameter of color as the responding variable. Size or shape matching are distinct perceptual skills that can confound the results of color matching. For example, when a test with color blocks is done, use all one-inch cubes rather than mixing circles, squares, or diamonds of various colors.

ACCOMMODATION AND CONVERGENCE

It is a misconception that many children with low vision may not need near optical aids. This stems from the belief that children have adequate accommodation to shorten their viewing distance and to use linear magnification. The reduction in vision, however, limits the blur-driven component of the accommodation response. Certain children with accompanying impairment such as cerebral palsy are even more likely to have reduced accommodation because the motoric impairment limits the proximal and kinesthetic feedback loop (Duckman, 1984). Therefore when the child is tested, it is important that the child holds the reading material since kinesthetic cues maximally stimulate the proximal response component of accommodation (Sloan, 1977). Accommodative and vergence testing was discussed in depth in Chapters 4 and 5.

DEPTH PERCEPTION TESTING

Depth perception for many of these children is a more functional meaningful measure than is stereoscopic vision. Using many of the stereoscopic testing procedures will prove to be of limited value, and in fact in many monocular children or in those children with terribly unequal impaired visual acuities, stereoscopic vision will prove to be nonexistent. Testing depth perception, however, is a more appropriate way of determining where a child perceives itself to be in the environment. An easy way to test for depth is by using a penlight. The procedure for doing this is that the examiner holds a penlight in front of the child at approximately 10 to 12 inches. The child is then asked to bring a finger up to the light from below and to touch it as quickly as possible. When this is being done, the child's motor abilities must be taken into account. A reasonably accurate localization with finger to penlight, however, will suggest that the child has some awareness of spatial representation from the body. This test, as all other tests, should be done both monocularly and binocularly, and if there are noted spatial localization changes, one should attempt to relate those to the child's ability to safely ambulate through the environment.

EYE MOVEMENT EVALUATION

Considerations are similar to those reviewed in Chapter 5, particularly in comparing stimulus-generated saccades with voluntary saccades as well as in fixation and following responses. Eye movements should be done with the child in a variety of positions. This enables the optometrist to account for gravity as a factor in eye-head posture and to determine the potential for modification of eye movements based on various postures. In addition, hand-over-hand techniques can be employed to determine whether motor movement will facilitate eye movement. The technique for using hand over hand is to grasp an object in the child's hand and the examiner's hand as a unit, moving them together, and noting whether the child's eye movements improve.

RETINOSCOPY

Retinoscopy is typically performed using handheld trial lenses at conventional working distances. For the severely impaired, radical retinoscopy is performed at closer working distances. At times the optometrist must be prepared to maneuver with the child to maintain alignment on the visual axis.

OPHTHALMOSCOPY

Ophthalmoscopy should be performed under dilated conditions. Monocular indirect ophthalmoscopy is ideal for this population. The ramifications of ocular disease are discussed in detail in Chapter 4. Findings should be noted for discussion at the conclusion of the examination.

CASE PRESENTATION

Case presentation information is given to the caretaker or the individual who is present at the time that the evaluation is completed. There may be situations where a case presentation is made before an educational group in relation to the child's overall needs, for example, as in the formulation of an IEP (individual education plan) (see Chapters 12 and 20). Diagnosis and prognosis should always be presented in a positive, but not patronizing, tone. Even when the prognosis is poor, guarded optimism should be maintained to encourage caretakers to work with the child. Blindness in infants with severe ocular anomalies may not always persist (Fielder et al, 1991).

Specific tasks to enhance vision stimulation and sensory-motor control should be reviewed with those who will follow through with the activities. A limit on the child's ability should not be inferred. Short- and long-term goals should be suggested. A time table should be established to evaluate progress in the various programs with which the child may be involved. Three to 6 month optometric follow-up visits should be conducted during the first several years.

EDUCATIONAL CONSIDERATIONS

The opinion that visual needs should be a priority, while possibly correct, should not be forced on the teacher. The teacher will take this information, along with the information from professionals involved with speech and hearing, occupational therapy, physical therapy, orientation mobility, and others, and establish a hierarchy of

Table 18.3 Optical system advantages and limitations

Device	Magnification needed	Field of view needed	Work distance required	Mobility required
Microscope (MS)	Practical in +8 to +48 diopter. Special doublets preferred +32 to +80 diopters.	Full field microscope provides the largest field of view for comparable magnification. Half-eye or bifocal design will result in some loss of field of view, but will allow for mobility.	Has the shortest work distance of any system for comparable magnification.	Full-field design precludes mobility. Half-eyes or bifocals allow mobility but reduce field of view advantage.
Magnifier (MG)	2× to 5× is practical as hand magnifier. Above 5× (+20), use stand magnifier or pocket magnifier.	The magnifier is a compromise between the large field of the microscope and the small field of the telemicroscope. The patient can adjust the work distance/field of view to suit personal comfort.	Magnifiers allow a more normalized work distance and acceptable field of view for comparable magnification. This advantage dissipates at 8× magnification and above.	Magnifiers are portable and do not interfere with mobility. Acceptable for use in public.
Tele-microscope (TSMS)	Practical only up to 8× magnification (32D). Can design as a binocular with cap for greater power.	Provides the smallest field of view of all devices for comparable magnification.	Has the longest work distance for comparable magnification. Usually not a practical field of view, 6× and above, with surgicals and/or bioptic design.	Full-field precludes mobility. Surgical design allows for travel and mobility, but severely reduces field.
Telescope (TS)	Hand-held systems practical up to 10×. Bioptic design practical up to 6×. Above 10×, consider binoculars (monocular).	Not applicable; all are used for distance. A focusable telescope suffers a loss of field of view over the use of caps when used as a near telescope.	As a distance device, a telescope has a small field of view. A bioptic will have the smallest field of view of the types of telescopes typically prescribed. Hand-held systems provide a larger field of view. Consider binoculars (monocular). Fields 6 degrees and less are typically not practical. Keplerian telescopes have a larger field of view than Galilean.	Full-field precludes mobility, especially above 2×. Bioptic design, while reducing field of view, allows for travel, mobility, and even driving.
Electro-optical	System is practical from 8× to 60×.	For higher magnification, it allows a more normalized work distance. May need reading correction with CCTV.	The words moving across the screen give the patient an apparent larger field of view as it allows for faster information processing.	The system precludes mobility. Materials must be brought to the system for magnification. There are some portable systems, but to date, they are not very successful.

From PB Freeman, RT Jose. The art and practice of low vision. Boston: Butterworth–Heinemann, 1991.

the child's needs from the teacher's perspective. Allowing the teacher to arrange the conditions for learning will increase the likelihood that visual stimulation or optical suggestions will be incorporated into the child's educational program.

To recommend ergonomic, optical, and vision therapy (VT) modifications, the optometrist may need to visit the child's classroom or learning environment. Ambient and task lighting, seating arrangement, distance from objects, and size of objects to be viewed need to be considered. One might differentiate between stimulating vision by using threshold size targets and encouraging the learning of a visual concept by using suprathreshold targets.

Availability of optical devices is important as making recommendations without being able to follow through with them will frustrate the teacher and be of no value to the child. Closed-circuit televisions (CCTV), hand-held and stand lenses, and headborne systems such as telescopes and microscopes from the least complex to the most complex should be discussed. If the child is capable of independent travel, a miniature telescope mounted on a finger ring may be useful (Dowie, 1988). Formal instruction should be given with each of the devices recommended for the child as some educators are not familiar with the optical properties of low-vision devices such as field of view and fixation distance. As was reviewed by Corn (1986), the factors related to low vision and visual efficiency in the learning environment are highly individualized.

REVIEW OF OPTICAL OPTIONS

Prescribing for the low-vision child will depend on the visual needs of the child, the presenting best visual acuities and the motoric capabilities, cognitive functioning, and the other skills that the child has. Table 18.3 gives an idea of the optical systems with the limitations and advantages one must consider when recommending low-vision devices. There should be a systematic approach to prescribing low-vision devices as opposed to a random approach to magnification.

REFERENCES

Carter K. Comprehensive preliminary assessments of low vision. In R Jose, ed. Understanding low vision. New York: American Foundation for the Blind, 1983;88–89.

Corn AL. Low vision and visual efficiency. In AFB Foundations of education for blind and visually handicapped children and youth: theory and practice. New York: American Foundation for the Blind, 1986;108–111.

Dowie AT. Low visual acuity management and practice. London: Eastern Press, 1988;119.

Duckman RH. Accommodation in cerebral palsy: Function and remediation. J Am Optom Assoc 1984;55:281–283.

Fielder AR, Fulton AB, Mayer DL. Visual development of infants with severe ocular disorders. Ophthalmology 1991;98:1306–1309.

Genensky SM. Personal communication, 1991.

Howard IP, Templeton WB. Human spatial orientation. New York: Wiley, 1966;4.

Hritcko T. Assessment of children with low vision. In Jose RT, ed. Understanding low vision. New York: American Foundation for the Blind, 1983;108.

Kalloniatis M, Johnston AW. Visual characteristics of low vision children. Optom Vis Sci 1990;67:38–48.

Leung EHL, Hollins M. The blind child. In Hollins M, ed. Understanding blindness: an integrated approach. Hillsdale, N.J.: Lawrence Erlbaum Associates, 1989;141.

Orel-Bixler D, Haegerstrom-Portnoy G, Hall A. Visual assessment of the multiply handicapped patient. Optom Vis Sci 1990;66:530–536.

RFR.Vision. 3rd ed. Lexington, Ma.: Resources for Rehabilitation, 1990;67.

Sloan LL. Reading aids for the partially sighted: a systematic classification and procedure for prescribing. Baltimore: Williams and Wilkins, 1977;93–100.

Sorsby A. The incidence and causes of blindness in England and Wales, 1963–1968. DHSS Reports on Health and Medical Subjects, no. 128. London: DHSS, 1972.

Sykanda AM. The effect of motor handicap on the development of visually impaired children. Proceedings of the Fifth Canadian Interdisciplinary Conference of the Visually Impaired Child. Vancouver, 1984;191–199.

Yarrow LJ. Research in dimensions of early maternal care. Merril-Palmer Quarterly 1963;9:101–114.

19

Pediatric Ocular Pharmacology

Bruce D. Moore

This chapter discusses some of the significant differences in the use of diagnostic and therapeutic pharmacologic agents between children and adults. Particular care must be exercised in the use of pharmacologic agents in young children because of the increased risk of potentially catastrophic adverse reactions due to their small size and their immature mechanisms for drug excretion and biotransformation.

GENERAL
Drug Excretion and Biotransformation

Drug excretion and biotransformation are quite different in young children than they are in adults, especially in neonates. It is very important to keep these differences in mind when drugs are used and prescribed in the pediatric population to reduce the risk of adverse drug affects.

The kidneys are the major site of drug excretion from the body. The renal glomerular filtration rate usually does not reach adult levels until approximately one year of age, but there is variability in this function with some normal infants having adult function as early as three months of age while others do not reach adult function until they are 2 years of age. Similarly, renal tubular secretion is very reduced in the neonatal period but is usually well developed by six months of age. Young children with various medical problems may have impairment of drug excretion through the kidneys. This is especially so in children that are dehydrated. This decreased rate of excretion increases the period of bioavailability of the drug in the system, possibly exaggerating the effects of the drug and increasing the risk of toxicity. Drugs that are excreted primarily through the kidneys must be given in lower dosages and less frequently to neonates than they are to adults to reduce the risk of toxicity.

The primary organ responsible for drug metabolism (especially of lipid soluble drugs) is the liver, through its microsomal enzyme system. The activity of the microsomal enzyme system is much reduced in normal neonates and even more reduced in premature infants and those with medical problems affecting the liver. The microsomal enzyme system reaches adult levels of function by about one year of age. The nonmicrosomal enzyme system, although involved in the biotransformation of fewer drugs than the microsomal enzyme system, is important for some drugs (particularly for aspirin and sulfa drugs). This system is also immature in young children.

347

Plasma protein binding of drugs within the serum is important both in the distribution of the drugs throughout the body and in their bioavailability. Infants have significantly reduced plasma protein binding in comparison to that of adults thus affecting the distribution and activity of certain drugs, in particular aspirin, Dilantin, and phenobarbital. The fluid composition of young children is usually much greater proportionately than it is in adults, necessitating somewhat higher dosages for certain drugs than would be estimated using a ratio of child to adult body weight. An additional factor that is important in arriving at the proper dosage of certain drugs is the decreased effectiveness of the blood-brain barrier in young children. This may lead to increased drug effect on the central nervous system (CNS).

Determining Pediatric Drug Dosage

Several formulae have been developed to derive the proper pediatric dosage of pharmaceutical agents from those used for adults. All have inherent inaccuracies and should be used cautiously. Young's rule is based on the child's age. Since there are such wide differences in children's sizes at any given age, this rule is clinically worthless. Clark's rule is based on the child's weight but may be inaccurate because it does not take into account a child's proportionally higher fluid weight as compared to adults, which is of great importance in determining the actual clinical effectiveness of a drug. Augsberger's rule is similar but has been modified to be more accurate for infants. Neither is particularly useful clinically. Somewhat more accurate is a determination of pediatric dosage based on a child's surface area. This is arrived at by looking up in a table the approximate relationship between the child's weight and the child's surface area as a percentage of adult values. This may be the most clinically useful method arrived at for determining the correct pediatric dosage by formula, but it still may have clinical limitations that could be problematic for some patients.

By far the safest approach to pediatric drug dosage is to follow the recommendations that the manufacturers have arrived at as part of the FDA (Food and Drug Agency) clinical evaluations for each individual drug. These recommended dosages are always conservative and minimize the potential for adverse drug effects. Many drugs, however, have not been evaluated specifically for pediatric use, and consequently there will not be any recommendations for pediatric dosages. Optometrists should not use or prescribe any pharmaceutical agent that has not been specifically FDA-approved for pediatric use on any of their young patients unless there are very specific reasons to do so—for example, the pediatric use of beta-blockers for the treatment of glaucoma. None of this class of agents is currently approved for pediatric use although they are very widely used for this purpose.

Administration

The two main routes of drug administration by optometrists are topical and oral. Topical vehicles are divided into ointments and liquids, which include drops, suspensions, and solutions. There are advantages and disadvantages to use of each vehicle. Drops (including the other liquid vehicles) are perhaps easier to instill than are ointments (at least in cooperative children); they are less messy; and they have only a minimal and transitory affect on vision after instillation.

Drops probably have a somewhat greater potential of systemic absorption via the nasolacrimal duct if the punctum is not completely blocked and if, therefore, there is an increased risk of systemic toxicity. There is also a minimal contact time with the cornea before the drug is effectively diluted and then removed by tearing. This is obviously hastened by the child crying. The effect of this minimal contact time is to reduce the absorption into and through the cornea. Less of the drug actually gets to the intended location. There may also be some uncertainty about whether a drop of medication actually even gets into the eye of a struggling, hysterical child.

Ointments may have less potential of systemic toxicity because they pass through the nasolacrimal duct more slowly than do drops. Most importantly, they have a much longer contact time on the cornea, thus ensuring that more of the drug gets to the desired location. Ointments, therefore, often have improved pharmacologic effect over drops, particularly in the case of antibiotics and steroids that need to penetrate the cornea and reach the anterior chamber. It is also more obvious that an ointment has gotten onto the eye than is the case with a drop. In general, ointments for therapeutic purposes are best when that option is available.

There are two categories of oral pharmacologic agents, liquid in the form of suspensions and solutions, and solid in pill, capsule, or tablet form. Solids are usually more difficult for children to swallow than are liquids, and hence they are not the first choice when liquids are available. Commonly used oral agents that are prescribed by optometrists include antihistamines, decongestants and antibiotics.

DIAGNOSTIC AGENTS

By far the ocular pharmacologic agents most commonly used by optometrists are the diagnostic drugs that are used for dilation, cycloplegia, and tonometry. They have been used on a majority of patients seen by optometrists since the advent of diagnostic drug legislation throughout the United States. Most optometrists have completed didactic and clinical education on their use, but the specific pediatric indications have not always been emphasized in these courses. An overview of their clinical use is therefore presented here.

Anesthetics

There are several indications for the use of anesthetic agents in children. The most common is for applanation tonometry. Although routine applanation tonometry measurements are not as necessary for children as they are for adults, they are advisable whenever possible. The technique of applanation tonometry in older children is identical to that for adults. The technique is different in younger or less cooperative children, however, and is not considered necessary in these patients unless there is a suspicion of glaucoma or unless the child has been using steroids for over a period of several weeks. In these younger patients, a hand-held applanation or air-puff tonometer is used instead of the slit-lamp mounted applanation tonometer. A drop of a combination anesthetic and fluorescein agent is instilled in the eye prior to applanation. The anesthetic is almost always .4 percent benoxinate or .5 percent proparacaine. There is an increased risk of causing a corneal abrasion in these younger patients because it is less likely that the child will maintain a steady gaze and will sit still during the procedure. It is wise to check for abrasions with a cobalt blue filter on the slit lamp or with a hand-held ultraviolet light after completing the technique. If there is a deep abrasion, patching and prophylactic antibiotics may be indicated.

The second main indication for the use of an ocular anesthetic is to reduce ocular irritation prior to instillation of other diagnostic agents such as mydriatics and cycloplegics. The discomfort from the second and later drops is reduced after anesthetic instillation, but the initial discomfort from the anesthetic itself remains a problem for many children. This discomfort from the initial anesthetic drop may cause behavioral difficulty with instillation of the mydriatic or cycloplegic agents themselves. An important effect of anesthetic use is to disrupt the corneal surface, increasing absorption of any subsequent drops and potentiating their effects. In addition if the child rubs an anesthetized eye, there is a risk of abrading the already "softened-up" cornea.

In general, the routine use of an anesthetic agent prior to instillation of other diagnostic agents is not recommended. Its use significantly does not lessen the physical or emotional trauma of eyedrop instillation, and there is increased potential for adverse affects. Children that get upset at the use of eyedrops will get upset even if an anesthetic is used. If the child does get upset from use of the drops, they invariably get over it within minutes. There is no apparent reason to accept the notion that some practitioners have that the use of drops damages the relationship with the patient or in some way prevents a continuation of the examination.

Dilating Agents

This category of pharmaceutical agents is used to provide pupillary dilation for the purpose of examination of the anterior and posterior segments of the eye. This is particularly important in young children because they will not sit as still for as long during ophthalmoscopic or slit-lamp examination as most adults will. The examiner must be able to get as good a view as possible as quickly as possible and can't depend on a slower, more methodical examination technique. Dilation is particularly essential to rule out serious pathology in patients with strabismus and amblyopia.

There are two clinically useful dilating agents in addition to the various cycloplegic agents that will be discussed shortly. Phenylephrine hydrochloride is the only useful direct-acting adrenergic agonist (also sometimes categorized as a sympathomimetic agent). Hydroxyamphetamine is an indirect-acting adrenergic agonist that was occasionally used in the past as a dilating agent but that has fallen into disuse recently. There is little reason for the optometrist to consider its use today.

Phenylephrine is a very widely used drug, particularly in adults. Phenylephrine provides rapid dilation without any cycloplegic effect. It has a relatively short period of action except in patients with light irides. Use of this drug in children, especially young children, must be with caution because of the potential for cardiovascular side effects. There have been documented cases of rapid and dangerous increases in heart rate and blood pressure in premature infants and even in adults—although with higher dosages. Pediatric use should be restricted to no more than two drops of the 2½ percent concentration spaced five minutes apart. Never use the 10 percent concentration; do not use it in children under three years of age and not in any child with a history of cardiovascular problems.

Use instead a cycloplegic agent in lieu of phenylephrine when possible, reserving it for concurrent use with a cycloplegic agent when both cycloplegia and maximum dilation is required. If the patient is to be dilated, consider performing a cycloplegic refraction as well. There is a somewhat greater risk of potentially catastrophic adverse reaction with phenylephrine than there is with the cycloplegic agents.

Although tropicamide is technically a cycloplegic agent (a cholinergic antagonist), its cycloplegic effect is weak and unpredictable and best thought of as a useful dilating agent. It performs well as a short-acting and short-duration mydriatic agent in patients with light irides and is a very effective dilating agent for binocular indirect ophthalmoscopy in patients with darker irides when it is used in conjunction with phenylephrine. It is the safest dilating agent available. The dosage is one drop of .5 percent or 1 percent tropicamide repeated after five minutes.

Cycloplegic Agents

Cycloplegic refraction is extremely important in any child with strabismus, amblyopia, or significant refractive error. Although noncycloplegic refraction techniques are useful and acceptable in older patients, a cycloplegic refraction and binocular indirect ophthalmoscopy is absolutely essential in ruling out the presence of potentially serious ocular abnormalities in younger patients. The information obtained by cycloplegic refraction is then used to determine the proper prescription, and should be considered only another important piece of information that is used in making the correct diagnosis, along with noncycloplegic data. Attempting a diagnosis on a child with strabismus or amblyopia without a cycloplegic refraction and dilated fundus examination borders on malpractice and should never be contemplated or tolerated by the optometrist.

There are two cycloplegic agents (cholinergic antagonists) that should be of historical interest only for the purpose of cycloplegic refraction (Moore, 1988). Scopolamine has properties that are similar to atropine but is somewhat less predictable and less effective in action. It is still used in the treatment of uveitis but is not generally used or recommended for cycloplegic refraction since it has no advantage over atropine when a strong agent is required. Similarly homatropine resembles cyclopentalate but is less predictable and has a greater risk of adverse affects. It is still used by some for cycloplegic refraction, but its use is based more on habit than on reason. Both scopolamine and homatropine have nothing to recommend their use of in lieu of atropine and cyclopentalate respectively.

As was just mentioned in the section on dilating agents, tropicamide is technically a cycloplegic agent but is best used primarily as a dilating agent. It is the weakest and least predictable cycloplegic agent and is clinically useless for cycloplegia in all patients but those with very light irides where its use may be acceptable.

Atropine is the most effective cycloplegic agent and has the longest and most predictable action. It is not the agent to be used on a routine basis because its active duration is much longer than is clinically required, lasting up to two weeks in some patients. It is better to restrict its use to patients that are inadequately cyclopleged with cyclopentalate due to darkly pigmented irides, patients with high hyperopia or accommodative esotropia, and patients in whom the use of an in-office drop will preclude by their behavior an adequate examination after instillation. Generally only a small percentage of patients require cycloplegia. When it is used, the ointment form is the preferred medium to minimize the amount of systemic absorption through the nasolacrimal duct and to reduce the risk of adverse reactions. Prescribe 1 percent atropine ointment used once or twice a day for the three days before the examination—to be instilled by the parents at home. No medication is used on the day of the examination to prevent the ointment from affecting the clarity of the retinoscopic reflex. Parents are both clearly warned and given a written instruction sheet describing the potential adverse reactions from atropine. Clinically this is usually restricted to mild fever and irritability, but potentially it could be more significant. If such reactions do occur, the parents are instructed to call immediately. These more serious problems are certainly of concern but actually happen only rarely.

Our cycloplegic drug of choice for in-office use is cyclopentolate. This is a rapidly acting agent with a usual duration of action of 6 to 12 hours but occasionally longer in patients with light irides. Although theoretically somewhat less complete in action than atropine, it is clinically effective enough for most patients. There may be slightly more residual accommodation remaining than with atropine. Use one drop of the 1 percent solution, repeated after about 5 minutes by a second drop. Often a third drop at least 45 minutes later is considered with older patients that are not adequately cyclopleged, but never do this with younger children. The 2 percent drop has a much higher incidence of adverse effects and should never be used. It is important to note that the degree of mydriasis does not necessarily correlate with the degree of cycloplegia. The eyes may therefore be well dilated but poorly cyclopleged or vice versa. The degree of cycloplegia is best checked by assessing the consistency of appearance of the retinoscopic reflex and not by the degree of pupillary dilation.

The most common adverse effect is what is often described as a *transient psychotic episode* where the child exhibits bizarre behavior and hyperactivity for a short time. This is always self-limited and not a cause for great concern as it leaves no significant long-term effects, but it is certainly quite dramatic for the parents and the optometrist. Antidotes are not required. Some patients may alternatively exhibit fever and irritability, particularly younger and smaller children. The best way to minimize any of these adverse effects is to block the punctum carefully when instilling the drops to minimize systemic absorption through the nasolacrimal duct and to never use more than two drops of 1 percent solution.

One point about adverse reactions to cycloplegic agents worth mentioning concerns their use in patients with Down syndrome (trisomy 21). There have been anecdotal concerns about particular hypersensitivity to cholinergic antagonists in these patients along with warnings about their use. Apparently, the same anecdotal concerns exist in the anesthesia literature as well. There are, however, no published studies that document these concerns, and those optometrists, ophthalmologists, and anesthesiologists with extensive experience with Down syndrome patients cannot relate any greater incidence of this hypersensitivity than in normal patients. Nonetheless, optometrists should be particularly careful to prevent overdosage of these agents in this population.

Cyclopentolate used by itself provides both effective cycloplegia and mydriasis for the vast majority of patients. It can be used concurrently with phenylephrine when maximum dilation in patients with very dark irides is required for binocular indirect ophthalmoscopy of slit lamp examination. The effect of cycloplegia that is so disturbing to adult patients is generally not much of an issue with children. It is worth mentioning to the parents that the child's vision will be somewhat blurred for the rest of the day at near and that reading and homework may be impossible.

Therapeutic Agents

This section will address only those areas where there are significant differences in use between adults and children. For the most part, there is little difference in the use of antimicrobials and anti-inflammatory agents in children and adults. The only real difference is in the vehicle to be selected, which was stated earlier in this chapter in the section on administration. Ointments allow for a longer contact time on the cornea, thus guaranteeing a greater concentration of the drug actually getting to the desired area. Since not all of the anti-inflammatory agents are available in ointment form, the specific choice of agents is somewhat restricted. This leaves dexamethasone as the best steroid agent for children. The choices are wider with antibiotics. Both bacitracin and erythromycin are only available in ointment form, although other agents, in particular the new quinolone agent Ciloxan, is currently available only in drop form. If culture and sensitivity reports indicate the choice of an agent that is not available in ointment form, the use of that drop is clearly warranted. The recommendation to use ointments is certainly not a rigid one, and some may prefer to use drops as a first choice. As always, the practitioner should always be guided by what is best for the patient.

The pharmacologic treatment of glaucoma is considerably different in children than it is in adults. Almost without exception, the treatment of congenital and early onset glaucoma requires surgical intervention, usually at a very early stage (DeLuise & Anderson, 1983). Open angle glaucoma in adults is almost always initially treated medically. The reason for these different treatment modalities lies in the difference in etiology of the glaucomas. Early childhood glaucoma is generally caused by anatomical abnormalities in the structure of the angle that are not treatable by medication. Various filtering procedures or cryotherapy are often used along with Diamox to decrease aqueous production. Diamox is the most useful and most widely prescribed antiglaucoma agent in young children. Some of these children may be kept on the drug for years. An important side effect of Diamox involves gastrointestinal upset, which in young children may lead to failure to thrive. This possibility must be monitored carefully.

Miotic agents such as pilocarpine and adrenergic agonists such as epinephrine and dipivefrin, which are widely used in adults, are not used much in young children. The beta-blockers, in spite of the fact that they are not currently FDA-approved for use in children, are widely used (Boger & Walton, 1981). Although there has been concern about the beta 2 effect in children with asthma, both timolol (both beta 1 and 2) and betaxolol (beta 1 only) are used in many children with glaucoma, particularly in older children where the concerns are not as great. It must be stated again that the more definitive treatment for many pediatric patients with glaucoma is surgical and not medical.

REFERENCES

Boger WP and Walton DS. Timolol in uncontrolled childhood glaucoma surgery. Ophthalmology 1981; 88:253–258.

DeLuise VP and Anderson DR. Primary infantile glaucoma (congenital glaucoma). Survey Ophthalmol 1983; 28:1–9.

Moore BD. Cycloplegic refraction of young children. NE J Optometry 1988; 41: 10–15.

20

Vision Screening
and School Consulting

Leonard J. Press

Vision screening is the principal function provided by optometrists who render school-related services (AOA, 1973). It addresses an important public health need, is an indispensable practice building tool, and tops the list of services provided by school vision consultants:

Provides or advises on school vision screenings
Provides in-service staff workshops on vision and learning
Interprets eye or vision reports from other professionals
Addresses parent-teacher organizations
Serves as a resource for information on vision and eye health and safety.

There have been suggestions that school vision screening should not be conducted since it gives a false sense of security about the adequacy of visual skills involved in classroom performance (OEP, 1968).

School vision screening is pervasive. Yet there are no nationally accepted standards for vision screening (Trief & Morse, 1987). Thirty-three states and the District of Columbia have statutes mandating vision screening for school-aged children. Six of these states mandate screening for preschool children. Even in states where screening is mandated, the functions to be screened are rarely mandated. Table 20.1 summarizes the status of vision screening as regulated by state law in each of the 50 states.

The optometrist is therefore in a position to exert professional influence on the scope of local vision screenings. Information on the historical development of vision screenings is helpful and is well-covered elsewhere (Schmidt, 1990). This discussion is adapted from the guidelines of the American Optometric Association (AOA, 1979), which delineates minimum versus expanded levels of vision screening.

PRESCHOOL/SPECIAL CHILD
VISION SCREENING

Preschool vision screenings are rarely mandated by local authorities. Optometrists will therefore find relatively few programs of ongoing screening conducted in local preschool programs and are usually free to recommend whatever level of

Table 20.1 Summary of state requirements for school vision screening in the United States

State	Mandate/Law	Procedures Listed
Alabama	Yes	Unlisted
Alaska	Yes	Snellen test
Arizona	No	
Arkansas	No	
California	Yes	Snellen test, plus lens test, color perception, muscle balance
Colorado	Yes	Snellen test (all grades), cover test (preschool, K, 1); other optional procedures
Connecticut	Yes	Snellen test
Delaware	No	
District of Columbia	Yes	Snellen test, color vision, muscle balance
Florida	Yes	Unlisted
Georgia	Yes	Snellen test, plus lens test, color perception
Hawaii	Yes	Snellen distance acuity
Idaho	No	(Most do Snellen and color vision)
Illinois	Yes	Snellen distance acuity, plus lens tests, muscle balance; other optional procedures
Indiana	Yes	Unlisted
Iowa	Yes	Unlisted; only for students evaluated for special education
Kansas	Yes	Snellen test
Kentucky	No	
Louisiana	Yes	Unlisted
Maine	Yes	Unlisted
Maryland	Yes	Unlisted
Massachusetts	Yes	Unlisted (Massachusetts Visual Test Guidelines—Titmus)
Michigan	Yes	Acuity monocular and binocular, eye muscle function, color vision
Minnesota	No	(Most do Snellen test, cover test, color)
Mississippi	No	(Most do Snellen test)
Missouri	No	(Most do voluntary screening)
Montana	No	
Nebraska	Yes	Snellen test
Nevada	Yes	Unlisted
New Hampshire	Yes	Snellen acuity, muscle balance or motility; Hirschberg corneal reflex done by school nurse

Table 20.1 *(continued)*

State	Mandate/Law	Procedures Listed
New Jersey	No	
New Mexico	No	(Most do Snellen test, plus lens test, muscle balance, color perception)
New York	Yes	Snellen test, plus lens test, color perception
North Carolina	Yes	Snellen test
North Dakota	No	
Ohio	Yes	Distance acuity, ocular motor balance, color perception (males only)
Oklahoma	Yes	Tracking, red reflex, Hirschberg
Oregon	Yes	Snellen test
Pennsylvania	Yes	Snellen test, plus lens test, color perception
Rhode Island	Yes	Snellen test
South Carolina	No	(Most do Snellen test)
South Dakota	No	(Most do Snellen test)
Tennessee	No	
Texas	Yes	Snellen test or other acuity chart
Utah	Yes	"Test for amblyopia and other visual defects"
Vermont	Yes	Unlisted (most use Titmus)
Virginia	Yes	Unlisted
West Virginia	Yes	Snellen test, stereoscope screener (muscle balance, depth perception, color perception)
Wisconsin	No	(Most do screening; procedures unlisted)
Wyoming	Yes	Snellen acuity; color perception

Source: AOA. State health care committee bulletin. September 19, 1990; 49(23).

screening they are prepared to implement. Because the cognitive abilities of special children parallel the abilities of preschoolers, it is appropriate to include them within this category. A suggested program for children ages three to five and special children is:

I. *Minimum preschool screening*
   A. *Visual acuity (distance).* Usually a preliterate chart picture of a Stycar chart (see Chapter 4) at 10 feet. Criterion for referral is 20/50 or poorer (misses three out of five symbols on the 20/40 Snellen equivalent line.)
   B. *Binocular alignment.* Cover test, Hirschberg corneal light reflex, or equivalent. Criterion for referral is any strabismus.
   C. *Stereopsis.* Usually the Random Dot E (RDE) plates administered in a

forced-choice paradigm. Criterion for referral is less than a 50 percent correct response level (incorrect choice on two out of three trials or three out of five trials).

II. *Expanded preschool screening:* Modified clinical technique (MCT)
    A. *Visual acuity.* Same as item IA.
    B. *Ametropia.* Retinoscopy. Criteria for referral are
       1. Myopia: $-0.75D$ with visual acuity loss
       2. hyperopia: $+2.00D$
       3. astigmatism: 1.00D
       4. anisometropia: 1.00D
    C. *Binocular alignment.* Same as item I:B with the addition of referral criteria for phoria:
       1. Esophoria: eight prism diopters distance and near
       2. Exophoria: ten prism diopters distance and twelve prism diopters at near
       3. Hyperphoria: two prism diopters distance and near
       4. Convergence: CNP (convergence nearpoint) more remote than three inches
    D. *Accommodative facility.* Inability to clear 20/30 through $+/-$ 2.00D flippers within seven seconds
    E. *Visual acuity (near).* 20/50 or poorer (misses at least three of five symbols on 20/40 Snellen equivalent line)
    F. *Eye movements.* Frequent loss of fixation or gross over/undershooting
    G. *Color vision.* Standard pseudoisochromatic plates and criteria
    H. *Eye health.* External observation and ophthalmoscopy

III. *Expanded Preschool Screening:* Stereoscope cards. There are several companies that produce preschool screening cards for Brewster-type stereoscopes. Bernell (see Appendix A) distributes a pre-K set of cards, and Mast Keystone manufactures the Peek-A-Boo Series (Figure 20.1, also see Appendix A). This series screens functions similar to the regular Keystone Visual Skills set including heterophoria and fusion at distance and near but with animated figures. It is difficult to elicit responses from preschoolers in a stereoscope because of the verbal skills involved as well as the spatial mismatch.

SCHOOL VISION SCREENING

Unlike preschool screening, school vision screening is mandated in the majority of states. Implementation varies widely across the United States. Many private schools have no vision screening, and these present a fertile opportunity for optometric input. Public school screening is usually done with either the Snellen chart of the Titmus or with Keystone Stereoscope screeners. A suggested program for school-aged children is:

I. *Minimum school screening*
    A. *Visual acuity (distance).* Usually a Snellen chart at 15 or 20 feet. Criterion for referral is 20/40 or poorer.

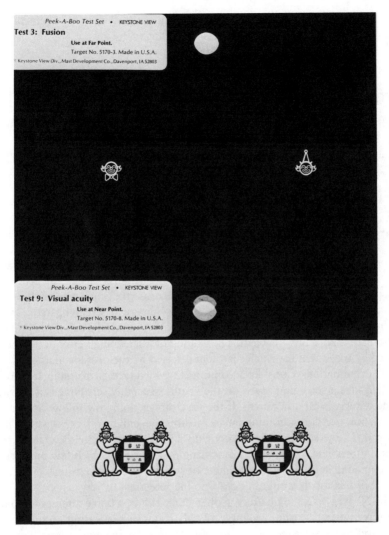

Figure 20.1 Keystone Peek-A-Boo stereoscope cards used for vision screening of preschool children.

B. *Adverse hyperopia.* Plus lens test. Criterion for referral is being able to read the 20/30 line through + 2.00D.

C. *Binocular alignment*
    1. Strabismus: any manifest strabismus
    2. Esophoria: eight prism diopters distance and near
    3. Exophoria: ten prism diopters distance and twelve prism diopters at near
    4. Hyperphoria: two prism diopters distance and near

D. *Stereopsis.* Same as minimum preschool screening

II. *Expanded school screening.* Same as expanded preschool screening, except for visual acuity being more stringent
A. *Visual acuity (near).* 20/40 or poorer.

FREQUENCY OF SCREENING

The AOA (1979) recommends that children should be screened on entry or transfer into a school system, and then at least every three years thereafter. Peters (1963) suggested that the MCT be administered once at the first grade level, followed by the Snellen chart every two years thereafter. The recommendation of the AOA appears to be the standard in the field.

PRACTICAL CONSIDERATIONS OF SCREENING

For a screening battery to be accepted, its items must have reliability and validity. Furthermore, the validity should be high in terms of its sensitivity to correct referrals and its specificity in minimizing false positives. Because the Snellen test is universally administered and interpreted, it has the greatest validity of all screening items. In other words, if the child fails the screening based on Snellen acuity, the examiner is likely to find that there is an acuity problem. The validity of a screening item can therefore be influenced by the extent to which that item is tested by the professionals conducting follow-up examinations. Consider accommodative facility as an example. It is possible that a child fails a screening based on the results of facility screening but passes the screening criteria in all other areas. If the practitioner doing the follow-up examination does not test for accommodative facility, the child will be classified as an overreferral. The screening item was not truly a false positive since the child in reality has a facility problem. But if one is practicing in a locale in which few professionals test accommodative facility, a high number of false positives will ensue. Consequently most local professionals would not endorse the screening battery.

The NYSOA screening battery (Cohen et al, 1983), a noble attempt at comprehensive screening, is a prime example of this issue. Incorporating accommodative facility as well as saccadic and visual-motor integration testing, the battery required 15 minutes to administer to each child. The screening itself proved to be more sensitive than the examination administered by most ophthalmic professionals in the state. Based on the low degree of professional acceptance the ensuing resistance was predictable, and thwarted adoption of the NYSOA screening battery by the State Education Department. In making recommendations, the individual optometrist must therefore strike a balance between the ideal vision screening and one that has a probability of being adopted.

IMPLEMENTING A VISION SCREENING

When a vision screening does not exist in an area or when the existing screening is inadequate, the optometrist should offer recommendations. The approach must be politically sensible and pragmatic. It is most effective and appears less self-serving when the recommendations are made by a group or society rather than an individual optometrist.

In California, where it originated, the MCT (Blum et al 1959) is a widely adopted screening tool. Although it has good reliability, validity, and professional acceptance, it requires a doctor's assistance. If the resources of the local school system are limited, this may be prohibitively expensive unless the doctor volunteers the necessary time. Ophthalmologists and volunteer organizations such as the National Society to Prevent Blindness (NSPB) have traditionally opposed screenings that require a doctor's participation.

In metropolitan areas where school budgets are usually constrained, screenings that can be administered by volunteers are welcomed. In smaller towns, the likelihood is that school nurses will administer stereoscope screenings. To successfully implement a screening or to effect a change, one must be aware of what had previously transpired as well as of who makes the final decision on these matters. Smaller towns have a medical officer, usually a pediatrician who dictates policy to the school nurses. In larger cities, there is usually a division of school health services within the board of education that establishes vision screening policy.

Implementation of preschool screening is comparatively much simpler. Preschools and day care centers basically set their own policies and are receptive to an optometrist's input. It may be necessary, however, to secure parental consent prior to screening the children.

CONDUCTING A VISION SCREENING

The nature of the screening will influence the amount of staff and the space required. The optometrist must visit the site prior to the screening and plan a layout for the flow of students. When large numbers of students are involved, each function screened should have a station with its attendant equipment readied.

Visual acuity is usually the first station. For school aged children, a wall chart is taped at a distance of 20 feet. A piece of tape is placed on the floor to mark the spot where the child is to stand. To avoid backlog, two acuity lanes should be readied. When the screening battery is extensive, two functions can be combined in one station, such as NPC (near point of convergence) and cover testing. The MCT requires a physical setup where lighting can be controlled due to the need for retinoscopy.

Forms must be used to communicate the results of the screening. Information must be conveyed to the parent, who serves as a conduit between the screener and the examiner. The reason for failure of a screening should be clearly indicated. The form must emphasize that the screening is not intended to serve as an eye or vision examination. Discussion is not usually held during the screening. The form that is sent home with the results should invite parents to contact a specific person should they have questions about the results of the screening. It is unethical to refer failures to a specific source for examination. The school must follow-up to ascertain that the parent has taken the child for care.

PHOTOREFRACTION

Photorefraction should be considered as a distinct entity in screening because of its potential for mass screening of infants. In Chapter 3, a self-styled apparatus that required interpretation of photographic crescents to determine refractive status was discussed. To date there is no device commercially available in the United States for this purpose. In England, Clement-Clarke markets the Cambridge Paediatric Video-refractor (VPR-1). This device is quite expensive; it takes three flash snapshots of the child. With the manipulation of a cursor, this information is fed into the unit's computer and the child's refractive status is displayed and printed out. The concept behind mass photoscreening of infants is to enable a lay person with a computerized device to substitute for an experienced retinoscopist. These devices will probably soon become more prominent in the United States.

IN-SERVICE WORKSHOPS

Shapiro (1973) offers an excellent presentation on how to become a school consultant and what consultancy involves. A pivotal element is the opportunity to speak with staff or parent-teacher groups. There are a number of prepackaged audio-visual programs available through the American Optometric Association (AOA) or the Optometric Extension Program (OEP) from which to draw ideas for in-service workshops for educators, school nurses, other professional personnel, and parents (see Appendix A). A workshop is most successful when it incorporates direct involvement through a show-and-tell approach. Two levels of workshop presentation that include demonstration and invite listener participation can be given, a basic workshop that includes

> Defining and illustrating Snellen acuity
> Differentiating Snellen acuity (eyesight) from vision
> Explaining and demonstrating nearsightedness, farsightedness, and astigmatism using members of the audience to represent these conditions (eyeball their Rxs [prescriptions])
> Explaining and demonstrating accommodation by showing how the projector should autofocus and what happens when children don't focus accurately
> Presenting the concept of why bifocals are necessary for some children. If an overhead projector is available, it would be helpful to place someone's multifocal Rx on the platform to demonstrate what it is and what it does
> Demonstrating binocular vision using the concept of physiological diplopia with the listener's finger as the near fixation target and the optometrist's head as the far target
> Showing how vision affects balance by having everyone in the audience do Standing Balance: Eyes open (SBO) vs. Standing Balance: Eyes Closed (SBC) (see Chapter 5) simultaneously as a group. The induced sway when the eyes are closed is dramatic.

and an advanced workshop that includes

Differentiating learning to read from reading to learn

Elaborating on the hierarchy of perceptual-motor development with a demonstration of figure-ground, visual closure, visualization, and sequencing abilities

Discussing and demonstrating intersensory integration with emphasis on auditory-visual and implications in language development

Explaining the interrelationship between optometry and the child study team for the child with special education needs.

Discussing and demonstrating select VT (vision therapy) techniques. Keep it simple at the outset. A simple demonstration is the stick-in-straw technique in the x, y, and z axes to show spatial localization.

Presenting information about sports vision including protective eyewear, emergency care, contact lenses, and performance enhancement through VT.

SCHOOL VISION REPORTS

Teachers do not expect to be told how to teach by the optometrist, nor do they anticipate that intervention by the optometrist will solve all of the child's problems (Freidus, 1973). They do expect the optometrist to offer interpretations of the child's visual problems, to analyze the strengths and weaknesses, and to make recommendations in understandable, nontechnical language.

Reports sent to schools by practitioners should be concise and explicit (Bintz, 1991) and should elaborate on practical matters such as intentionally undercorrecting a child's distance acuity and the need to sit closer to the blackboard or the suggestion to seat a child with amblyopia of the left eye on the right side of the classroom. There are specific instances where the child has a purposeful head turn to dampen nystagmus or compensate for a muscle weakness, and the teacher needs to be advised to encourage rather than discourage this behavior. In other instances, the report will have to elaborate on specific visual-perceptual skills and suggestions for work in a resource room that will be implemented in an IEP (individual education plan). The school vision consultant may assist in interpretation or implementation of suggestions for visual guidance contained in outside reports.

SPECIAL EDUCATION SERVICES

Special education services are provided under various titles such as Committee on the Handicapped or Child Study Team. The team usually consists of a learning disability teacher or consultant (LDT/C), a psychologist, and a social worker. Speech and language pathologists are often included, and there may also be a health service specialist. Increasingly, occupational therapists are being consulted and are providing perceptual and motor training.

Under due process accorded by PL 92-142, every child is entitled to special education services. Even students attending private and parochial schools are eligible for special education services from the jurisdiction in which they reside. Depending on

Table 20.2 Items included in IEP

Objectives	Evaluation	Related Services
Reading	Reporting (teacher, parent, standardized tests)	Supplemental instruction
Language		Reading instruction
Math	Monitor (teacher, administrator, team)	Speech/language instruction
Social studies/science		Vocational assessment
Study skills	Time line (annual, biannual, quarterly, monthly)	Occupational therapy
Social/emotional		Adaptive physical education

the number of children to be serviced and the resources within a particular system, there may be a considerable time delay between the point at which a child is identified as needing services and the point at which evaluations can be conducted by a team. In this instance, the parent may go outside the team and obtain an evaluation through independent professionals. After the child is referred to a special education team, a conference is held with the parent and team members present. All relevant evaluation reports are gathered, and a classification conference is held. Based on the results of this conference, the child is classified, and a basic plan is generated. During the conference, an IEP is generated. This includes objectives; goals; evaluation procedures including timely review, recommended program, and related services placement; and implementation. The parent must sign a statement indicating approval of the recommendations for programming and placement. The items addressed in an IEP are listed in Table 20.2.

The optometrist may enter this picture as an internal consultant or as a related service professional. A report from the optometrist or the presence of the optometrist during the IEP conference may be influential in classifying the child as perceptually impaired (PI). It is this classification that is most pertinent to optometric evaluation and treatment recommendations. VT, if it is indicated, might be included in the IEP as a related service (Lemer, 1990). The optometrist can be helpful in identifying what activities can be done in a resource room environment and what activities must be rendered in-office with direct optometric guidance. As was discussed in Chapter 6, the role of the optometrist in this process is shaped by the individual nature of local special education service policies.

REFERENCES

AOA (American Optometric Association). State health care legislation committee bulletin. 1990;49(23.)

AOA. Guidelines for school vision screening. St. Louis: AOA, 1979.

AOA. Vision consultant to educational programs. St. Louis: AOA, 1973.

Bintz DG. Form letters. Optom Economics 1991;1(7):41–43.

Blum HL, Peters HB, Bettman JW. Vision screening for the schools: The Orinda study. Berkeley: University of California Press, 1959.

Cohen AH, Lieberman S, Stolzberg M, et al. The NYSOA vision screening battery—a total approach. J Am Optom Assoc 1983, 54:979–984.

Freidus E. What the classroom teacher needs to know from the optometrist. In Vision Consultant to Educational Programs. St. Louis: AOA, 1973;45.

Lemer PS. Education for all handicapped children act, public law 94-142. J Behav Optom 1990;1:150–153,

Trief E, Morse AR. An overview of pre-school vision screening. J Vis Impair Blind May 1987;197–200.

OEP. Manual for optometric school consultants. Duncan, Okla.: Optometric Extension Program, 1968.

Peters HB. Vision screening. In Hirsch MJ, Wick RE, eds. Vision of children: An optometric symposium. Philadelphia: Chilton, 1963;333–359.

Schmidt PP. Vision screening. In Rosenbloom AA, Morgan MW, eds. Philadelphia: Lippincott, 1990;467–485.

Shapiro IL. On being an optometric sched consultant—accomplishments and pitfalls. Optometric Extension Program, 1973;45:33–37.

21

Office and Practice Management

Leonard J. Press

Many practitioners are adept at communicating with and examining children, but relatively few present themselves as pediatric optometrists. The economics of the professional marketplace usually preclude the limiting of one's practice to infants and children. The more common scenario is the family practice in which the practitioner develops a niche for pediatric optometry or the group practice in which one practitioner sees the majority of the children. For example Dr. Alva Pack markets the pediatric segment of his practice as The Children's Vision Clinic, A Division Of Drs. Ezell & Pack. P.A., through a vivid pictorial brochure.

This chapter limits itself to practice management issues unique to pediatric optometry, and forgoes discussion of general business principles found in standard texts on the subject.

MARKETING

Professionals in marketing speak of the concept of positioning one's practice. This is the manner in which the public conceptualizes the practice. This occurs through the impact of either internal or external marketing.

Internal Marketing

To cultivate children in a family eyecare practice, the office must make it known that it specializes in the care of children. There are eight categories of opportunities to cater to children listed below:

1. *Reception area.* Since this is the first patients see of your office, they must be convinced that this is an okay place for children to be. This is less important to the older child. Table 21.1 lists the basic ingredients in a children's reception area. If the reception area is effectively designed to cater to children, parents may presume that adult patients are not accepted. To counteract this perception, a sign in the reception area that says something like: "Our adult patients receive the same care and attention as our children" is helpful.

367

Table 21.1 Suggested checklist for a children's reception area

Posters	Dog or cat wearing glasses
Paintings	Depicting children having fun
Books	Read-aloud or informational
Magazines	*Highlights, Sports Illustrated for Kids,* and so on
Playthings	Blocks, educational toys, dolls (avoid small objects that can clutter or can be swallowed); use a milk crate for storage.
Kids corner	Isolated from adults by table/chairs or counter space; washable wall paper and/or plexiglass splash recommended
Pamphlets	Educational material for parents from AOA/OEP/COVD* addressing issues in children's vision care
Bulletin board	Pictures of children in the practice; thank you letters from schools or organizations; timely information about the doctors or vision care, particularly from local newspaper clippings
Plaques	Certification or recognition of practitioner as specialist in children's vision

*COVD = College of Optometrists in Vision Development

2. *Patient education videos.* Tapes on children's vision, as available through American Optometric Association (AOA) and the OEP Foundation (see Appendix A), should be available and played when appropriate in the reception area. When there are children in the reception area who have behavioral difficulties, a well-timed cartoon is captivating for the children and appreciated by the adults.

3. *Pretesting.* Dedicate a separate space in the office to pretesting children between the ages of 3 and 12. A mural painted onto the wall might greet the children as they enter the room. An example of such a poster is shown in Figure 21.1. Some children's games such as those shown in Figure 21.2 might also be used as part of the pretesting room. The stations that comprise the pretesting are listed in Table 21.2. The primary purpose of pretesting is to ensure that children are not apprehensive when they are escorted into the examination room. Secondarily it alerts the optometrist to the possibility of problems in the respective areas tested. In addition, it is a conversation piece for new families.

4. *Examination room.* It is also a good idea to devote some space in the pretesting room to testing infants, for example a horizontal surface with a small crib pad onto which infants are placed for examination. The Preferential Looking unit and the pediatric OKN drum are kept there because they generate discussion whenever patients or visitors view the area. The room has no windows so that it can be darkened easily for Mohindra retinoscopy. In the main examination room, finger puppets of Sesame Street characters might greet young children so that their first

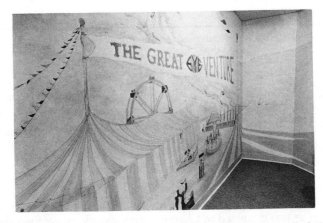

Figure 21.1 Mural on the wall of a pretesting room. The mural is called "The Great Eye Venture."

identification with the optometrist is through familiar faces. Younger children might be placed into a booster seat in the main examination chair and a TV set might be placed in the room and used for retinoscopy and ophthalmoscopy as was reviewed in Chapter 4.

5. *Frame selection area.* The optical area of the office is an opportunity to showcase pediatric care. A number of colorful, wall mounted frame displays that read "Just For Kids" (by Clear Vision) might be used. In addition, several frame manufacturers have display units which feature their product line, complete with point-of-purchase props. Some are timeless such as Disney characters; others are fleetingly popular because

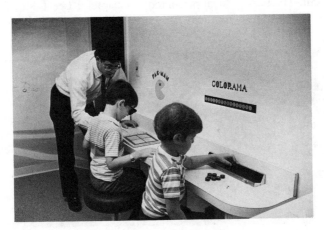

Figure 21.2 Two components of pretesting: Pac-Man (TNO anaglyphic stereopsis) and Colorama (Farnsworth D-15 test).

Table 21.2 Test components of the Great Eye Venture

1. Pac Man	TNO anaglyphic random dot stereopsis test (one series of targets resembles Pac Man)
2. Colorama	Farnsworth D-15 color cap test
3. Fun house	Telebinocular cards for vertical phoria, lateral phoria distance and near, and fusion at distance and near
4. Video game	Diagnostic phoria of Computer Orthoptics* program

*See Appendix A

they are linked with current movies. Yet others are associated with trendy clothes as was discussed in Chapter 12. A specific area within the optical section should be devoted to children with furniture and displays scaled to size. Frame design features and accessories are reviewed in Chapter 12.

6. *Postexamination.* Some token should be given to the children so that they will remember the office visit as a pleasant experience—stickers (Figure 21.3), miniature rulers, key chains, a "prescription pad" that entitles the child to a free kiddie-sized yogurt as is offered by TCBY stores across the country.

7. *Office stationery.* The practice's stationery should make it evident that the office caters to children, for example, Figure 21.4 was designed with the child pictured in between two adults; this positioning shows that the child is the central figure in the practice.

8. *Professional correspondence.* Every opportunity should be taken to communicate about the children to their teachers and pediatricians. This is a bridge for developing and maintaining a relationship with school and medical personnel. The parent's permission must be sought before reports are sent. The history form presented in Chapter 1 (see Table 1.1) has a space asking: "To whom may we send a report of our findings?" Parents

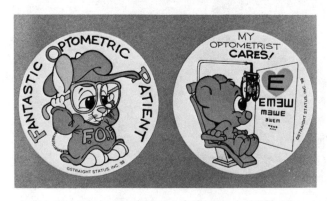

Figure 21.3 Stickers used as a good patient reward incentives.

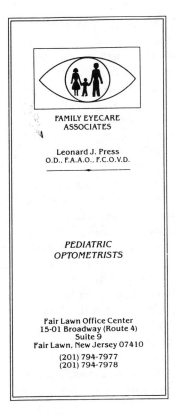

Figure 21.4 A custom-designed practice logo that positions the child as the central figure in the practice. This logo is used on all stationery, brochures, and business cards for the practice.

tend to check the treatment plan proposed by other health care practitioners with the child's pediatrician. A well-written report to the pediatrician explaining your treatment plan can be influential.

External Marketing

This area is defined as things done outside of the office to cultivate potential pediatric patients. Traditionally pediatric optometrists have relied on referrals through current patients, educators, and other health professionals. Recently, some practitioners have become more aggressive at marketing directly to the public. This is done in a manner that plants the idea with the parent that the child may have signs or symptoms that are amenable to lenses or vision therapy (VT). The theory is that the parent makes the final decision about where to take the child.

A practice that caters to children should have a strong pediatric identity in its advertising. Here are eight areas of development for external marketing:

1. *Practice brochure.* A brochure describing one's practice is a crossover item that can serve as both an internal and an external marketing vehicle. Committee work, postgraduate certification, and organizational affiliations

associated with children's care should be included as well as pictures or descriptions of how the office caters to children.

2. *Newsletter.* If the practice produces a newsletter, at least one piece on children's vision should be included in each issue. There are numerous sources of preprinted material on children's vision available in newsletter format through OEP and AOA.

3. *Yellow pages.* A perusal of the local phone book will reveal many practitioners who have an interest in children's vision. An advertisement might indicate that the practice has special facilities for infants and children (see Figure 21.5).

4. *Direct mail.* The most common pieces focus on back-to-school promotions. These are structured around either the introduction of a new line of eyewear, discounted eyewear, savings on the examination fee, or donation of a portion of the fee to an organization that fights illiteracy.

5. *Media exposure.* Talks given to local parent-teacher groups will assist in identifying the optometrist as a local authority on children's eye care. Programs such as "Save Your Vision Week" by the AOA always tie in to children's vision. Poster contests sponsored by the practice are well-received by local schools. A wealth of ideas can be found in the *AOA News Backgrounder on Optometric Care and Advice for Infants and Children,* or in the AOA's Practice Enhancement Program (PEP) monograph on *Patient Communications in Your Community* (#MN18).

6. *School affiliation.* School consulting was discussed in detail in Chapter 16 and is a natural calling card for a pediatric optometrist.

DR. LEONARD J. PRESS
OPTOMETRIST
Fellow, American Academy of Optometry

FAMILY EYECARE
ASSOCIATES

Eye Health Care, Contact Lenses,
Children's Vision and Eyewear

15-01 Broadway
Suite 9
Fair Lawn, N.J. 07410   (201) 794-7977

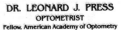

DR. LEONARD J. PRESS
OPTOMETRIST
Fellow, American Academy of Optometry

FAMILY EYECARE
ASSOCIATES

*Vision care of infants,
children and adults.*

15-01 Broadway   315 Park Avenue So.
Suite 9   New York, N.Y. 10010
Fair Lawn, N.J. 07410   (212) 982-5850
(201) 794-7977   (212) 420-4959

DR. LEONARD J. PRESS
OPTOMETRIST
Fellow, American Academy of Optometry
Diplomate, Binocular Vision Perception

FAMILY EYECARE
ASSOCIATES

Pediatric & Adult Vision Therapy

15-01 Broadway
Suite 9
Fair Lawn, N.J. 07410   (201) 794-7977

DR. LEONARD J. PRESS
Fellow, American Academy of Optometry
Diplomate, Binocular Vision/Perception

FAMILY EYECARE
ASSOCIATES

*Specializing in the vision care
of infants and children*

15-01 Broadway
Suite 9
Fair Lawn, N.J. 07410   (201) 794-7977

Figure 21.5 Different versions of a business card targeted to specific potential referral sources.

7. *Office field trip.* A field trip to the office is ideal for a local school class or cub scout pack (Canterman, 1982). A sufficient number of adults should accompany the children to maintain decorum. The children can all participate in a vision screening. An office assistant can demonstrate contact lenses as well as different types of ophthalmic lenses. Demonstration can be done with ultraviolet (UV) light and photogray lenses as well as the interaction of fluorescein and UV. Children perceive these as magic acts. The advantage of a field trip, as compared with the practitioner going to the school, is exposure of the children and accompanying adults directly to the practice. The disadvantages are that fewer children can be accessed at once and that considerable staff time and coordination is involved in presenting a good program.

8. *Public relations.* There are many opportunities to sponsor events and organizations within the community, for example, sponsoring a baseball team from a local school. In this example, the team's uniforms might bear the practice name. Another venture such as sponsoring a young patient in a preteen beauty pageant might bring attention to the practice especially if the patient becomes a finalist. Affiliations with local Lions Clubs and other special interest groups dealing with children will definitely assist the practitioner in networking with others who are occupied with child care.

REFERRAL SOURCES

Direct referrals from parents of current patients and other professionals are the backbone of a pediatric practice. Parents speak with one another during activities in which their children are mutually involved, and casual conversation often leads to referrals. The balance of this section addresses referrals from professional sources.

Levels of Referral

There are three levels of referral through which patients come to the office:

1. *Unconditional referral.* This implies that you will implement whatever treatment or management is necessary. This is the usual route when a nonoptometrist refers a patient. This relationship may also exist with an optometrist, particularly if the patient is an infant or a toddler.

2. *Consultation.* This implies that the results will be conveyed to the referral source who will then guide the patient accordingly. This may be the route from an optometrist who has a difficult time refracting the patient or who needs assistance in constructing a home VT program for a hyperactive child.

3. *Co-Management.* This implies that you will be rendering ongoing care to the patient in conjunction with the referral source. This is the common avenue of referral from a primary care practitioner. It is understood that

patients will return to the referral source for all services, such as eyewear and contact lenses, that source provides, unless other arrangements were stipulated in advance.

Cultivating Referral Sources
Optometric Referral Sources

Co-management between the pediatric and primary care optometrists should model the symbiotic relationship between the primary care optometrist and the cataract surgeon. The optometrist in a busy corporate practice generally prefers a relationship in which the optometrist manages the case to completion. Conversely the privately practicing optometrist expects the patient back for all dispensing, contact lens, and eye health services. In the latter case, it is important to explain to the family that the optometrist will render only the services for which the child has been referred. Even if patients are aware that the optometrist dispenses eyewear and insist that they would rather not return to the referral source for eyewear, they must be directed back to the referral source in a positive manner. It is important to compliment the referring practitioner to the family for insight in detecting the cause for concern and sending the child to you.

Co-management is a professional marriage, and as with marriage, the most important element in the relationship is communication. It is a good idea to send local optometrists pamphlets designed to answer the questions of parents who wonder why they are being referred to a specialty practice (Figure 21.6). Timely reports on the initial assessment as well as progress reports on any change in status are vital. As with all areas of specialty practice, referral sources should be acknowledged thoughtfully.

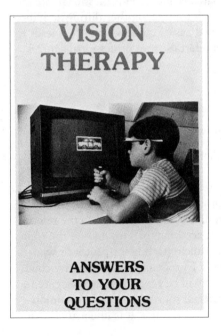

VISION THERAPY

ANSWERS TO YOUR QUESTIONS

Figure 21.6 Cover of a customized brochure given to primary care optometrists that stresses the co-management concept. It also addresses office policies and procedures for VT.

Nonoptometric Referral Sources

1. *Pediatricians.* Since they are the central figures in children's health care, local pediatricians must be made conversant with optometric services. It is a strong endorsement of a practice when a child is referred to it directly by the pediatrician. An in-office seminar to give to pediatricians is helpful and might include a laminated Snoopy eye chart (available through Avante-Garde eyewear) and a demonstration of preferential looking acuity (see Chapter 3).
2. *Psychologists and educators.* As was reviewed in chapter 20, interaction with these professionals is usually through some need related to special education services. The AOA/OEP (American Optometric Association/ Optometric Extension Program checklist for teachers is a proven vehicle for communication about potential vision problems. Psychologists should be particularly interested in the connection between vision and stress in children as manifested in relation to the Streff syndrome (see Chapter 13).
3. *Allied health care professionals.* Occupational therapists are principal among those with whom pediatric optometrists overlap. Areas of shared interest include developmental disabilities and perceptual-motor training. Some chiropractic physicians are beginning to experiment with applied kinesiology and neuro-organization techniques that overlap the ocular motor aspects of learning disabilities. Although there are radical aspects to this approach that warrant healthy skepticism (Worral, 1990), there are practitioners with whom a more conservative approach can be mutually beneficial.
4. *Agencies for the handicapped.* Referrals from agencies such as State Commissions for the Blind and local Cerebral Palsy or Developmental Centers are discussed in Chapter 18.

PERSONNEL

Practices caring for large numbers of children require assistants and technicians who truly love working with children. Children in the reception area can be trying at times, climbing the chairs, strewing objects about, and raising the noise level. Office staff must display a higher-than-average tolerance for this behavior. Employees who exhibit warmth when a child enters the office, who come out from behind the reception desk with a big smile and sincere greeting, and who talk to, not at, the child, are well worth retaining.

PARENT CONFERENCES

After the examination of the child has been completed, it is important to conduct a conference with the parents to explain the results. It is preferable to have both parents present, particularly if a VT program is being recommended. Conclude the conference by restating the options and the primary recommendation. The following is an example of a case summation for pseudomyopia:

> Joey's eyes are very healthy. What we are finding, though, is that he has a focusing problem that gives him the appearance of being nearsighted. This means that things are easy to see close up, but blurred far away. Some children have this condition simply because an eyeball is too long. Others, like Joey, are blurred for a different reason. There's a little lens in your eye that does the fine tuning or focusing and is controlled by a muscle. When we're young we have a lot of focusing power—so much that children sometimes get sloppy with it. A child should be able to focus his eyes automatically, just like a slide projector. Joey's problem is that he doesn't autofocus—he has to focus manually every time he changes where he's looking. There are three choices we have in dealing with this:
>
> 1. Do nothing, and his blur will probably get worse.
> 2. Prescribe glasses to make things clear at distance. This is like taking aspirin for a headache. The glasses do nothing for the cause of the focusing problem; they just put things back into focus for a period of time.
> 3. Undertake vision therapy, which would enable Joey to learn how to focus his eyes properly. If Joey were my child, I would choose vision therapy at this point since he hasn't gotten used to glasses yet.

SELLING PEDIATRIC OPTOMETRY

Not long ago the use of the word *selling* in professional circles met with disdain. Today there is no need to substitute the euphemism of patient education when patients must be sold on the benefits of a particular service. Rowley (1990) addressed the need for selling behavioral optometry to patients because of the lack of recognition of its benefits by optometrists as well as the general public.

Too many parents harbor the misconception that the pediatrician will detect any vision defect necessitating referral. An equal number persist in the belief that the school nurse's screening is tantamount to examination. It is therefore incumbent upon the optometrist to educate parents about the consequences of ignoring children's eye and visual care. Parents should have a firm understanding of when the child should be examined. Children should be seen by an optometrist by six months of age if there is any family history of eye or vision disorders. If the child is not at risk by family history and has no demonstrable signs of difficulty, the first examination should be no later than the third birthday. Examinations thereafter should be yearly.

There are many economic and time-consuming forces bearing on today's family with both parents usually working and with challenging psychodynamics in the household. All professionals who deal with children tend to consider themselves essential ingredients in the welfare of the children. Remember that you are only one source among many who ask the parent to make an investment in their child's future. You must ask convincingly and well.

THE PERSONAL TOUCH

The pediatric optometrist is limited only by imagination when considering the ways in which a practice can reflect a caring attitude for the child. These suggestions should stimulate further possibilities:

1. Arrange office hours so that they coincide with times conducive to seeing children. During the school year, children have time off from school during teacher conference days and vacation periods. Obtain these dates at the start of the school year, and let it be known that your office will be open extra days and hours for the convenience of children and their parents.
2. When you learn of a pediatric patient in your practice who is ill or has surgery, send balloons to the child. Children of all ages are cheered by this gesture. Do this also for any child who has been referred for strabismus surgery. Having balloons waiting at home shows concern. A note accompanying the balloons lets the child *and* the parents know that you hope the child is doing well and look forward to seeing you all in the office soon. This reinforces your identity as the case manager—the primary eyecare practitioner.
3. When parents bring young siblings to the office, it can be difficult to have the parent in the examination room. Have one staff person with flexible clerical duties who can assist in the care of the sibling in the reception area while the parent is with the patient being examined. Although siblings accompanying the child for the appointment is discouraged, it seems an inevitable fact of life. The appreciation of the parent for providing an informal babysitting service will pay dividends.
4. Have facilities for changing infants' diapers, as well as some extra diapers. This not only shows compassion, but it also makes a statement that the practice is prepared to deal with infants.

REFERENCES

Canterman, DD. A field trip to your office? Optom Management 1982;18(8):59–63.

Rowley E. Selling behavioral optometry. Optometric Extension Program, Assistant's Courses, Nov 1990.

Worral RS. Neural organization technique: Treatment or torture. Skeptical Inquirer 1990;15(1):40–50.

Afterword

Leonard J. Press

If we have done our job well, this book has read almost like a novel. We have, among other things, intended to give you a chairside insight or an over-the-shoulder look at our clinical thinking. Caring for children is an art as well as a labor of love. Among the many pleasures in this sort of caring is the opportunity to conduct show-and-tell. Six years ago, when my daughter was in fourth grade, I did a presentation on the eye for her class. To spice up the standard presentation, I did three special things:

1. Poured some clear gel (from a Gefilte Fish jar) into a model eye to simulate the vitreous
2. Demonstrated a variety of contact lenses and children's eyewear
3. Had each child view through vertical prism to experience abnormal diplopia, then contrasted that with the type of physiological diplopia they might see when they are daydreaming.

I leave you with three precious notes that I received in the mail following the presentation.

> Feb. 13, 1986
> Dear Dr. Press,
>
> Thanks a lot for the ring and your time. Now I now how discusting and usefull the eye can be.
>
> From,
> L

Feb. 13, 1986

Dear Dr. Press,
    Thank you for showing us parts of the eye. I enjoyed it very much. Question: If someone gets glasses can they get sort of blind can they get contac lenses? A nother question: Wich are better glasses (not the kind you drink out of) or contac lenses? Pleas answer me. Thank for the rings. I like it alot. Did you know this bef ore you was a doctor?
            Sincerly,

February 13, 1986

Dear Dr. Press,

Thank you very much for taking your time and showing us how the eye works. Though you have told us many things I still have one question. Here it is: Why do I see double sometimes?

A baffled student.

P.S. Please answer my question.

Thank You
for the ring!

Appendix A

Resource Guide to Pediatric Materials/Equipment

Academic Therapy Publications
20 Commercial Boulevard
Novato, CA 94947
MVPT, Jordan L-R, Wold Sentence Copy Test

Allbee Optometric Printers
224 West Park Avenue
Waterloo, IA 50704
Amblyopia tracing book, Root rings

American Optometric Association
243 N. Lindbergh Boulevard
St. Louis, MO 63141
Patient education pamphlets (Bifocals For Children, Signs of a Child's Vision Problems, Educators Guide to Classroom Vision Problems, Toys For Your Children), Student Vision Report Form

American Psychological Association
1200 17th Street NW
Washington, DC 20036
Psych/SCAN: LD/MR—quarterly issue of summaries of latest research in LD

Anadem Publishing
P.O. Box 14385
Columbus, OH 43214
Newsletter on pediatric optometry & vision therapy (VT)

Ann Arbor Publishers
P.O. Box 7249
Naples, FL 33940
Michigan Tracking Series

(Note: This listing is adapted from Curtis R. Baxtrom, O.D.)

Baby Optics
P.O. Box 1162
St. George, UT 84771
Ophthalmic sunlenses Ultraviolet (UV) sized for children from birth to age 8

Beiersdorf, Inc.
South Norwalk, CT 06854
1-800-233-2340
Coverlet Eye Occlusor heavy adhesive, junior and adult sizes

Bernell Corporation
750 Lincolnway East
South Bend, IN 46634
Broken Wheel Test, NYSOA K-D Test, assorted VT equipment, major distributor of VT-related tests and books

Billy Ludlam VT
P.O. Box 145
Forest Grove, OR 97116
Prism and accommodative flippers

Biofeedtrac Inc.
56 Schermerhorn
Brooklyn, NY 11201
Accommotrac for myopia control

Bubbles
2120 St. Peters Lane
Charleston, SC 29407
Picture story introduction to VT

Butterworth–Heinemann
80 Montvale Avenue
Stoneham, MA 02180
Textbooks on pediatric optometry and binocular vision

B.W. Laboratory
201 Worthington Avenue
Cincinnati, OH 45215
Wolff Wands

Cheldaro Enterprises
515 North Third
Stayton, OR 97383
Patient education pamphlets (perceptual skills dysfunction, accommodative dysfunction, esophoria, exophoria, strabismus/amblyopia)

Childcare Company
1122 E. 3rd Street
Loveland, CO 80537
Form boards, circus puzzle, assorted perceptual materials

Childcraft Education Corporation
20 Kilmer Road
Edison, NJ 08818
Developmental materials

Circle International Group
4019 Gravois Road
House Springs, MO 63051
Variety of cheiroscopic tracing forms

College of Optometrists in Vision Development (COVD)
P.O. Box 285
Chula Vista, CA 92012
Patient education pamphlets, journal, annual meeting

Concepts
P.O. Box 400
Tehachapi, CA 93561
Learning systems devised by Ben Stoebner, O.D.

Creative Ideas Company
Tooties Division
5328 West 142nd Place
Hawthorne, CA 90250
Tootie materials

C & R Croisant
17401 SE 39th St., No. 102
Camas, WA 98607
Regional OEP conference transcripts

Cuisenaire Company of America
12 Church Street, Box D
New Rochelle, NY 10805
Geoboard and assorted developmental materials

DLM Teaching Resources
P.O. Box 4000
One DLM Park
Allen, TX 75002
Developmental materials including computer software

Efficient Seeing Publications
7510 Soquel Drive
Box 28
Aptos, CA 95003
Alphabet pencils, fusion targets, assorted VT material

Franel Optical Supply
P.O. Box 96
Maitland, FL 32751
Ryser graded occlusion filters for amblyopia

Frontier Technologies, Inc.
2444 Solomons Island Road
Suite 205
Annapolis, MD 21401
Opti-mum computer assisted VT

Goffe Torgeson Vision Technology (GTVT)
17907 25th Drive, SE
Bothell, WA 98012
Custom Brock String with letters, anaglyphic letter charts, assorted VT and developmental materials

Good-Lite Company
1540 Hannah Avenue
Forest Park, IL 60130
Dot visual acuity test, HOTV test, illuminated test cabinet

Harper and Row
2350 Virginia Avenue
Hagerstown, MD 21740
Illinois Test of Pyscholinguistic Abilities (ITPA)

Hoyle Products
302 Orange Grove
P.O. Box 606
Fillmore, CA 93015
Pencil grips, 20-degree angulated lapdesks/bookstands

Ideal School Supply
11000 S. Lavergne Avenue
Oaklawn, IL 60453
Harmon walking rail, balance disc, assorted perceptual/developmental material

Interagency Committee on Learning Disabilities
P.O. Box 2911
Washington, DC 20040

Ladoca Publishing Foundation
5100 Lincoln Street
Denver, CO 80216
Denver Developmental Screening Test

Lafayette Instrument Company
P.O. Box 5729
Sagamore Parkway
Lafayette, IN 47903
Tachistoscopes and assorted electronic devices related to perception/development

Learning Frontiers, Inc.
190 Admiral Cochran Drive
Suite 180
Annapolis, MD 21401
Opti-Mum Computer Vision Therapy (Ludlam)

Lighthouse Low Vision Services
New York Association for the Blind
111 E. 59th Street
New York, NY 10022
Preschool acuity cards (apple, house, umbrella)

LVI Elekrton Optikk A/S
Ullevalsveien 117
N-0359
Oslo 3, Norway
Hyvarinen acuity and fixation targets for infants and young children

Mafex Learning Materials
90 Cherry Street
Box 519
Johnstown, PA 15907
VT manual oriented toward teachers and therapists

Mast Keystone Co.
4673 Air Center Circle
Reno, NV 89502
Stereoscope testing and training, Correct-Eye-Scope, assorted VT materials

Mentor, Inc.
3000 Longwater Drive
Norwell, MA 02061-1610
B-VAT acuity monitor.

MKM Materials
809 Kansas City Street
Rapid City, SD 57701
Materials to test and train visual memory related to learning

Modern Curriculum Press
13900 Prospect Road
Cleveland, OH 44136
Beery-Buktenica VMI Test, Frostig Test

Morrison Gardner
Children's Hospital
Publications Dept., OPR-110
P.O. Box 3805
San Francisco, CA 94119
TVPS and other testing/training material on visual perception

Mosier Materials
63128 Yakwahtin Court
Lend, OR 97702
Assorted perceptual training materials

NFER-Nelson
Darville House
2 Oxford R. East
Windsor, Berkshire SL41DF, England
STYCAR materials for infant and retardate acuity and developmental testing

OEP Foundation
2912 S. Daimler Street
Santa Ana, CA 92705
Journal of Behavioral Optometry (see also Vision Extension, Inc.)

Pacific Prisms
P.O. Box 554
Forest Grove, OR 97116
Prisms, lens flippers, fixation targets for near retinoscopy

Percon, Inc.
3575 Looker Avenue
Akron, OH 44319
G.O. Board, Groffman tracings, parquetry workbooks and blocks

Personal Care Products/3M
St. Paul, MN 55144
Opticlude adhesive eye patches

Psychological Corp.
7500 Old Oak Blvd.
Cleveland, OH 44130
Goodenough-Harris Draw-A-Man Tests and related materials

RC Instruments
99 W. Jackson Street
Cicero, IN 46034
Computer Orthoptics (Cooper) and Perception (Groffman)

Solomon K. Slobbins, O.D.
1200 Robeson Street
Fall River, MA 02720
Acetate bull's eye rock, McDonald Form Field Card

SOI Systems
P.O. Box D
Vida, OR 97488
Mary Meeker test materials, VMC bat, advanced balance board

Special Child Publications
P.O. Box 33548
Seattle, WA 98133
Books on visual perception and development

Sports Vision Enhancement Institute
P.O. Box 506
Huntington, NY 11746
Sports vision testing and training

Stereo Optical Co.
3539 N. Kenton Avenue
Chicago, IL 60641
Vectograms and stereoscope materials

Straight Status, Inc.
P.O. Box 445
New Castle, IN 47362
Wide array of stickers with eye care themes

Stoelting Company
1350 S. Kostner Avenue
Chicago, IL 60623
Equipment in electrophysiology and experimental psychology

Sunburst Communications
101 Castleton Street
Pleasantville, NY 10570-3498
Computerized perceptual software

Titmus Corp.
P.O. Box 191
Petersburg, VA 23804
Vision screening devices

Vision Extension, Inc.
2912 S. Daimler Street, Suite 100
Santa Ana, CA 92705-5811
Wide range of VT materials, publications, tests including Birch-Belmont AVIT

VisTech Consultants, Inc.
1372 N. Fairfield Road
Dayton, OH 45432
Teller infant acuity cards and contrast sensitivity tests

Walker Educational Book Corp.
720 Fifth Avenue
New York, NY 10019
Perceptual skills curriculum and textbooks on learning by Jerome Rosner, O.D

Wayne Engineering
1825 Willow Road
Northfield, IL 60093
Saccadic Fixator, Vis-Flex, variety of electronic devices

Western Optical
1200 Mercer Street
Seattle, WA 98109
Hand-held slit lamps, pediatric goniolenses, and condensing lenses

Western Psychological Services, Inc.
12031 Wilshire Boulevard
Los Angeles, CA 90025
Ayres Southern California perceptual testing and training materials

Wimmer-Ferguson, Inc.
P.O. Box 100427
Denver, CO 80250
Developmental vision and vision stimulation products for use with infants

Appendix B

Pediatric Lens Manufacturers

Company	BCs	Powers	Phone
Stock Soft Lenses			
Streiter	7.6–9.2 mm	−20 to +20D	(800) 851-4557
Aquaflex (W.J.) V4	7.8–9.0 mm	−20 to +10D	(800) 348-9595
Ciba STD	8.3–8.9 mm	−10 to +6D	(800) 241-5999
Wesley-Jessen D2T3	8.2–8.5 mm	−20 to +20D	(800) 348-9595
Allergan-Hydron	8.1–8.9 mm	−20 to +20D	(800) 347-4500
Softcon (Ciba)	7.8–8.7 mm	−8 to +18D	(800) 241-5999
Permalens	7.7–8.6 mm	−20 to +20D	(800) 538-7824
Lombart	7.5–8.7 mm	+8 to +35D	(800) 446-8301
Silicone Elastomer Lenses			
B&L Silsoft	7.5–8.3 mm	+12 to +32D	(800) 828-9030
Custom Soft Lenses			
Coastvision	Spheres, torics		(800) 341-2020
Kontur	Spheres, torics		(800) 227-1320
Salvatori	Spheres, torics		(800) 237-2280
Sunsoft	Spheres, torics		(800) 526-2020
Strieter	Spheres, torics		(800) 851-4557
Optech	Spheres, torics		(800) 525-7465
Ocu-Ease	Spheres, torics		(800) 521-8984
Flexlens	Spheres		(800) 223-3539
White Ophthalmic	Spheres, torics		(800) 661-9175
White Ophthalmic	Occluders, masking		(800) 661-9175
Narcissus Foundation	Masking		(800) 992-9224
Wesley-Jessen	Masking		(800) 348-9595

Index

393